HIV Infection in Women

For Churchill Livingstone

Publisher   Peter Richardson
Project Editor   Lowri Daniels
Production Controller   Mark Sanderson
Sales Promotion Executive   Kathy Crawford

HIV Infection in Women

Edited by

Margaret A. Johnson MD MRCP

Consultant Physician in HIV/AIDS, Thoracic Unit,
Royal Free Hospital, London, UK

Frank D. Johnstone MD FRCOG

Senior Lecturer, Department of Obstetrics
and Gynaecology, Edinburgh University;
Consultant Obstetrician and Gynaecologist,
Simpson Memorial Maternity Pavilion, Edinburgh, UK

CHURCHILL LIVINGSTONE
EDINBURGH LONDON MADRID MELBOURNE NEW YORK AND TOKYO 1993

CHURCHILL LIVINGSTONE
Medical Division of Longman Group UK Limited

Distributed in the United States of America by Churchill
Livingstone Inc., 650 Avenue of the Americas, New York,
N.Y. 10011, and by associated companies, branches and
representatives throughout the world.

First published 1993
  Reprinted 1994

ISBN 0 443 04885 1

British Library Cataloguing in Publication Data
A catalogue record for this book is available from the British
Library.

Library of Congress Cataloging in Publication Data
A catalog record for this book is available from the Library of
Congress.

The
publisher's
policy is to use
**paper manufactured
from sustainable forests**

Printed and bound in Great Britain by
Butler & Tanner Ltd, Frome and London

Contents

Preface

HIV infection is clearly a major calamity for world health, with features unique to the disease casting a shadow over the world's population. Women occupy a central place in the development of the epidemic, in its consequences for population health, and in strategies to limit the disease and its effects.

This book aims to explore issues about HIV infection which have particular implications for women, and to define current medical knowledge as it relates to women. These areas have previously not attracted sufficient attention.

The authors are all established leaders in their field and, despite heavy workloads, have con-

tributed within a tight time schedule. Churchill Livingstone has produced the book rapidly, with the result that the content will remain up to date at publication.

We thank all involved in the writing and production of this book. We also hope that it focuses attention on the place of women in this pandemic, and helps direct more research, prevention, treatment and resources on their behalf.

London and Edinburgh 1993

M.A.J.
F.D.J.

Contributors

Rosemary Ancelle-Park MD
Deputy Director, European Centre for the
Epidemiological Monitoring of Aids, St Maurice,
France

Jane Anderson PhD MRCP
Senior Lecturer in HIV Medicine, Medical
College of St Bartholomew's Hospital, London,
UK

Patricia Antoniello PhD
Medical Anthropologist; Assistant Professor,
Department of Health and Nutrition Sciences,
Brooklyn College, City University of New York,
USA

Chris Carne MA MD MRCP
Consultant in Genitourinary Medicine,
Addenbrooke's Hospital, Cambridge, UK

Anne Cockroft MB ChB MD DIH FRCP FFOM
Consultant and Senior Lecturer in Occupational
Medicine, Royal Free Hampstead NHS Trust
and Royal Free Hospital, London, UK

Susan F. Crane BA
Executive Director, International Family Health,
California, USA

Katherine Davenny MPH(Epidemiology)
Clinical Medicine Branch, Division of Clinical
Research, National Institute on Drug Abuse,
National Institutes of Health, Rockville,
Maryland, USA

Isabelle De Vincenzi MD MPh
Epidemiologist, European Centre for the
Epidemiological Monitoring of AIDS, St
Maurice, France

Loretta P. Finnegan MD
Senior Advisor on Women's Issues, Office of the
Director, National Institute on Drug Abuse,
National Institutes of Health, Rockville,
Maryland, USA

Eleanor Goldman MB BCh
Associate Specialist, Royal Free Hospital
Haemophilia Centre, London, UK

Diana Hartel MPH DrPH(Epidemiology)
Women's AIDS Studies Coordinator, Community
Research Branch, National Institute on Drug
Abuse, National Institutes of Health, Rockville,
Maryland, USA

Roger Henrion MD
Professor of Obstetrics and Gynecology,
Maternité Port-Royal, Paris, France

Guro Huby MA
Research Associate, Department of General
Practice, University of Edinburgh, UK

Margaret A. Johnson MD MRCP
Consultant Physician in HIV/AIDS, Thoracic
Unit, Royal Free Hospital, London, UK

Frank D. Johnstone MD FRCOG
Senior Lecturer, Department of Obstetrics and
Gynaecology, Edinburgh University; Consultant
Obstetrician and Gynaecologist, Lothian Health
Board, UK

Frederick Mambwe Kaoma MBBS
Medical Officer, Department of
Dermatovenerology, University Teaching
Hospital, RW1 Lusaka, Zambia; Fogarty
International Fellow, Division of Pediatric
Immunology, Department of Pediatrics,
University of Miami, USA

Katherine Duer LaGuardia MD MP
Associate Professor of Obstetrics and Gynecology;
Director, Division of Women's Health,
Department of Obstetrics and Gynecology, The
New York Hospital–Cornel Medical Center, New
York, USA

Marc C. I. Lipman MRCP
Clinical Research Fellow, Departments of
Thoracic Medicine and Immunology, Royal Free
Hospital, London, UK

Kathryn H. McCarthy MBBS
Research Registrar, Royal Free Hospital and
School of Medicine and King's College Hospital
and School of Medicine, London, UK

Laurent Mandelbrot MD
Chef de Clinique-Assistant, Obstetrics and
Gynecology, Hôpital Robert Debré, Paris, France

Danielle Mercey MB ChB MRCP
Consultant Genito-Urinary Physician, Middlesex
Hospital, London, UK

Riva Miller BA Soc. Sc.
AIDS Counselling Coordinator, Royal Free
Hampstead NHS Trust; Honorary Senior
Lecturer, Royal Free Hospital School of
Medicine, London, UK

Jacqueline Mok MD FRCP(Edin) DCH MBChB
Consultant Paediatrician, Regional Infectious
Diseases Unit, City Hospital; Department of
Community Child Health, Lothian Health Board,
Edinburgh, UK

Veronica A. Moss MBBS DTMDCH DObst RCOG
Medical Director, Mildmay Mission Hospital,
London, UK

Stephen Norman MRCOG
Senior Registrar, King's College Hospital,
London, UK

Mike Porter BA MPhil
Senior Lecturer, Department of General Practice,
University of Edinburgh, UK

Malcolm D. Potts MB BChir PhD
President, International Family Health; Professor
of Population Studies and International Health
(in Department of Social and Administrative
Health Sciences), University of California, USA

Anton L. Pozniak MRCP
Senior Lecturer and Honorary Consultant,
Departments of Medicine and Genitourinary
Medicine, King's College School of Medicine and
Dentistry, London, UK

J. Roy Robertson MB ChB FRCGP
General Practitioner, Edinburgh, UK

Gwendolyn B. Scott BS MS MD
Professor of Pediatrics; Director, Division of
Pediatric and Infectious Diseases, University of
Miami School of Medicine, USA

Peter Selwyn MD MPH
Associate Director, AIDS Program; Associate
Professor of Medicine, Epidemiology and Public
Health, Yale University School of Medicine, Yale–
New Haven Hospital, New Haven, Connecticut,
USA

Lorraine Sherr BA (Hons) Dip Clin Psych (BPS) PhD
Churchill Fellow; Principal Clinical Psychologist,
St Mary's Hospital, London, UK

Jason B. Smith NPH
Research Associate, Family Health International,
North Carolina, USA

Rhoda S. Sperling MD
Associate Professor, Department of Obstetrics,
Gynecology and Reproductive Science, Mount
Sinai School of Medicine, New York, USA

Edwin R. van Teijlingen MA (Hons) Sociology
Research Associate, Department of General
Practice, University of Edinburgh, UK

I. G. Williams BSc MRCP
Senior Lecturer, Academic Department of
Genito-Urinary Medicine, University College
London Medical School, London, UK

1. Epidemiology and natural history of HIV/AIDS in women

R. Ancelle-Park and I. De Vincenzi

INTRODUCTION

The first cases of the disease which was to be called AIDS were diagnosed in 1980 among homosexual men in the United States. Although in the early years of the epidemic a majority of cases were diagnosed among this population group, it was soon realized that the disease was also striking injecting drug users (IDU), haemophiliacs, transfusion recipients, heterosexual males and females and children born to infected mothers. Since, the epidemic has spread by waves through populations and continents and today approximately 500 000 cases of AIDS have been reported throughout the world. It has been estimated that more than 10 million subjects have been infected by the HIV (WHO 1992b) and among these 50% are females (Fig 1.1). This chapter will focus on the epidemiology and the natural history of the disease among women.

Availability of information varies from one area to another. In the industrialized countries where the virus was introduced at an early stage and the logistical availabilities for surveillance are adequate, the quality of the AIDS surveillance is excellent and surveillance of HIV through national sentinel surveys is only just producing results. In non-industrialized countries like Thailand and those of Africa, the setting up of sentinel surveillance of HIV infection was undertaken in different population groups at an earlier stage and information coming from these surveys gives a more up-to-date picture of the present situation.

The terms 'high risk' and 'low risk' populations will be used throughout this chapter. The populations at high risk: prostitutes, bar girls and females attending sexually transmitted disease (STD) clinics. The populations at low risk: pregnant women. These populations are used for sentinel surveillance as indicator groups of the spread of the infection.

SURVEILLANCE

The geographical spread of the epidemic among women follows different patterns of place and time according to the area. Nevertheless it is noted that in areas where the virus was introduced at an early stage among homosexuals and IDU the sex ratio of male-to-female AIDS cases is decreasing regularly, 'picturing' the progression of the spread among the female population. Similarly, in northern America the rates decreased from 10.7 : 1 in 1987 to 6.5 : 1 in 1991, from 9.7 : 1 in 1987 to 5.5 : 1 in 1991 in Brazil and from 7.5 : 1 in 1987 to 5.2 : 1 in 1991 in Europe (Pan American Health Organization 1992, European Centre 1991a). In Australia the sex ratio has remained very high at 24 : 1 in 1987 and 31 : 1 in 1991 (National Centre on HIV and Clinical Research 1992). In other areas where the virus was introduced first in the heterosexual population and therefore where the sex ratio was already close to 1 : 1, no notable changes have been observed over time. Rates in the Caribbean Islands reached 2.5 : 1 in 1987 and 2 : 1 in 1991 (Pan American Health Organization 1992). In Africa where the virus was introduced in the heterosexual population and is still spreading in this population, overall trends are not available. Nevertheless, the sex ratio of AIDS cases is available for some countries and it is thought to be slightly lower than one (0.8 : 1 in Kinshasa and 0.9 : 1 in Uganda in 1989), whereas in the Ivory Coast and Senegal men outnumbered female patients by 2 : 1 and 4 : 1, respectively (Piot et al 1990). In Asia, and in par-

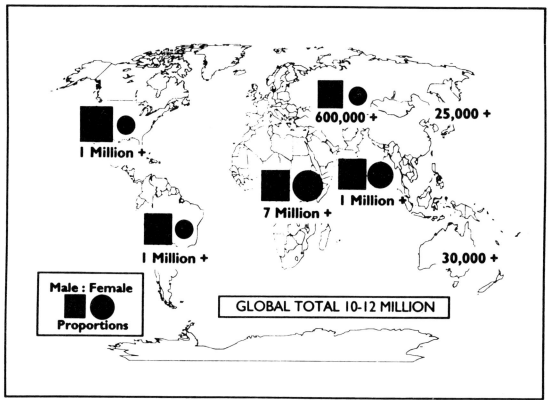

Figure 1.1   Estimated global distribution of cumulative adult HIV infections mid-1992 (WHO global programme on AIDS, July 1992)

ticular in Thailand, where the virus was introduced at a later stage, the number of AIDS cases are yet small and among these cases male cases predominate but no trends are available.

Industrialized countries

AIDS surveillance

Although the number of persons with AIDS in industrialized countries is large – 242 146 cumulative cases in the USA and 81 849 in Europe by October 1992 (Centers for Disease Control 1992b, European Centre 1992c) – it is apparent that the majority of cases remain yet to develop. Overall the rates of infected women among AIDS cases have increased from 6.6 to 14% in the USA (Ellerbrock et al 1991, Centers for Disease Control 1992b) and from 9.4 to 15% in Europe (European Centre 1991a, 1992c). Among the heterosexual cases of AIDS, females represent approximately

34% in the USA and 28% in Europe. In both these areas the majority of these cases have been infected by use of injecting drugs (55 and 59%, respectively), whereas transmission by heterosexual contact accounts for 37 and 32%, respectively (Table 1.1).

Although changes in trends among homosexual men and IDU have been noted in the USA due to the decline in the underlying infection rate and to the development of effective therapies that may delay AIDS diagnosis (Brookmeyer 1991), the incidence in persons reported to have been infected by heterosexual contact shows no indication of slowing down. In each of the last 5 years the percentage increase in annual AIDS incidence in this group has been higher than that of any other transmission group (Green et al 1992). An increase of 40% was noted between 1989 and 1990. In 1990 a study of women with AIDS showed that most women with AIDS were Black or Hispanic (72%), residents of large metropolitan areas

Table 1.1 Distribution of percentages of female adult AIDS cases by transmission group in selected geographic areas – August 1992

Transmission group	USA (n = 23 301) %	South America (n = 4921) %	Caribbean Islands (n = 3419) %	Europe (n = 10 337) %	Australia (n = 91) %	Africa (n = 75 169) %	Thailand (n = 271)** %
Injecting drug users	55	35	>1*	59	31	—	5*
Heterosexual contact	37	51	98	32	27	94*	92
Transfusion recipient	8	14	1	9	42	6*	3*

* Estimates: detailed data not always available; ** includes AIDS-related complex

(73%), especially in cities along the Atlantic coast, and that 85% were of reproductive age (15–44 years) (Ellerbrock et al 1990).

In Europe changes in trends have also been noted (Downs et al 1991). Modelling of data reported by December 1989 and adjusted for reporting delays, shows that trends among the homosexual transmission group are closer to the linear fit whereas the trends among IDU are still closer to the exponential model with nevertheless an approaching peak predicted by the Box Cox model. In the heterosexual transmission group, incidence between 1986 and 1989 appears to have a closer fit to the exponential model than to the linear model and it was estimated that the incidence of transfusion-associated AIDS cases could peak between 1992 and 1994 (Downs et al 1991).

The largest numbers of women reported with AIDS by October 1992 have been reported in France (3144 cases), Italy (2729) and Spain (2546) (European Centre 1992c). Among adults, the percentage of women infected varies from 0% to 45% according to the country. In the two countries with proportions higher than 40% (Romania and USSR), more than half the female cases belong to the 'transfusion recipient' or 'unknown' transmission group. Apart from these two countries, percentages are highest in countries with a high proportion of cases infected through heterosexual contact (Belgium 22%), or a high proportion of IDU (Italy 19%, Spain 17%).

Nearly all the women with AIDS (90.7%) were of reproductive age (15–49 years) at diagnosis. In order to compare the age distribution of women with that of men, the cases in the homo/bisexual, haemophiliac and other/unknown transmission groups were excluded. The proportions of women and men aged 13–24 years at diagnosis are 18.4%

and 11.8% respectively. Between 1986 and the first 9 months of 1991, the proportion of cases diagnosed in the 13–24-year age-group has decreased from 27.8% to 13.2% in women, and from 22.7% to 4.6% in men, while the proportion aged 25–34 years has increased from 49.7% to 63.1% in women, and from 50.8% to 67.9% in men. The trend is similar in both sexes. This change in age distribution is mainly observed in the IDU group (European Centre 1991a).

HIV surveillance

Estimates of the numbers of adults infected reach over 1 000 000 cases in the USA (World Health Organization 1992a) and 500 000 in Europe (European Centre 1991b).

In the USA large-scale serologic surveys have been under way since 1986 undertaken on populations ranging from high risk patients attending drug treatment centres and STD clinics to average risk among women in reproductive age, sentinel hospital patients and child-bearing women (Dondero & Gill 1991). Overall the results of these surveys show that HIV is widely spread across the country but with a highly varied distribution in populations similar to the distribution of the AIDS cases.

Results among surveys involving child-bearing women using the anonymous unlinked method show that nation-wide in 1989–1990 rates were 1.5 per 1000 with a range by state from 0 to 5.8 per 1000 (Gwinn et al 1991). At women's reproductive health clinics in the USA prevalence ranged from 0 to as high as 26 per 1000 (Dondero & Gill 1991). Although HIV infection has been found in individuals from almost all studied areas, the rates are nevertheless much

Table 1.2 European HIV prevalence data base: HIV infection among neonates (rates per thousand)

	1988 (/1000)	1989 (/1000)	1990 (/1000)	1991 (/1000)
United Kingdom				
Inner London	0.22	0.69	1.28	2.0
Three Thames regions	0.22	0.32	0.48	0.59
Scotland	—	—	0.29	0.29
Edinburgh	—	—	2.46	1.64
Italy				
Lazio	2.14	2.70	3.29	—
Rome	—	—	4.05	—
Lombardia	3.00	—	2.17	—

higher in individuals from urban than rural areas (Dondero & Gill 1991). In Europe, anonymous unlinked HIV prevalence monitoring programmes have been under development (European Centre 1991c) in the UK since 1988 (Gill et al 1989, Peckham et al 1990) and in Scotland a little later (Tappin et al 1991). In Italy cross-sectional surveys using all Guthrie cards collected over a 4 month period were set up in nine regions in 1988, repeated in eight regions in 1989 and extended to all 20 Italian regions in 1990 (Ippolito et al 1991).

Results show the prevalence of antibodies among neonates in the UK to be greatest in London and in Edinburgh (Table 1.2), and a four fold increase is noted between three Thames regions and inner London in 1991. Moreover, there was a ten fold increase in inner London between 1988 and 1991 (PHLS AIDS Centre 1991; Ades et al 1991).

Among the regions surveyed in Italy, the highest seroprevalence rates were observed in Lazio, the region including the city of Rome (2.14 per 1000 in 1988; 3.29 per 1000 in 1990), and in Lombardia, the region including the city of Milan (3.00 per 1000 in 1988). These two regions have also reported the highest number of AIDS cases in Italy. The HIV seroprevalence rates in Lazio and Lombardia were much higher than those observed in the Thames regions in England which include the city of London (0.22 per 1000 in 1988; 1.28 per 1000 in 1990) (European Centre 1991b).

In France, an anonymous unlinked cross-sectional survey on pregnant women (Couturier et al 1992) was undertaken in 1990 in the Paris area (inner Paris plus the three peripheral districts) over a 4-month period in all medical settings dealing

with outcome of pregnancy. All women, regardless of pregnancy outcome (delivery; ectopic pregnancy; spontaneous, elective or therapeutic abortion) were included. Blood samples were collected from any available maternal or neonate sources (maternal blood, placenta, cord). This cross-sectional survey will be repeated in each region every 2 years.

Overall rates among pregnant women in the Paris area reached 4.14 per 1000. As in this study pregnant women were tested at the end of pregnancy independently of outcome, all women having an abortion were included, and these women had a higher HIV prevalence rate (7.00 per 1000) than women who delivered (2.75 per 1000).

Voluntary screening of pregnant women has been developed in Norway and Sweden and the Amsterdam area in the Netherlands (Jenum 1988, Lindgren et al 1991, Bindels 1991); results show that rates are much lower and range from 0.07 and 0.04 in 1988 in Norway and Sweden, respectively, to 0.06 to 0.09 in the same countries in 1990 (refusal rates reached 7–8%). In Amsterdam, rates of infection for HIV1 and HIV2 in 1990 were higher among women undergoing abortion than among women delivering (5.6 vs 1.0 per 1000), and it is to be noted that the refusal rate reached 23%; therefore, if the women refusing are at higher risk the infection rate could be even higher.

Although data resulting from specific studies undertaken on high risk groups are not representative of these populations, they may be used as indications. Rates among high risk populations, in particular female patients of STD clinics, are high and ranged from 7.5% in Madrid, Spain to

0.0% in the UK (England and Wales) (European Centre 1992a). Results of a European (nine European countries) concerted action on HIV infection among prostitutes shows that overall rates of infection are higher among IDU prostitutes (35/110, 31%), especially in southern European countries, than in non-IDU prostitutes (11/756, 1.5%) (European Centre 1992b).

Non-industrialized countries

In non-industrialized countries the majority of the adult cases were infected by heterosexual contact. In South America, 51% of female cases were infected by heterosexual contact compared to 35% by use of injecting drugs. In Africa and the Caribbean Islands, 50% of the heterosexual cases are females and more than 94% of these cases have been infected by heterosexual transmission. In Australia and Thailand the number of AIDS cases is still low and does not reflect the present situation (Table 1.1)

Only the situation in Thailand and Africa will be described in this article.

Thailand

Because of the situation in industrialized countries and the fact that a few AIDS cases had already been reported, sentinel surveillance, the systematic collection of data on HIV infections in selected populations, was set up in Thailand in 1989. At that time 14 cities were selected for participation in the sentinel surveillance programme (Division of Epidemiology 1989) and others were progressively included until the entire country was under surveillance. The results of the programme showed that the virus has spread progressively throughout the country following several population waves. Antibodies to HIV were first detected in 1985 among male prostitutes in Bangkok (Wangroongsarb et al 1985). Surveys among IDU showed very low infection rates of 0–1% between 1985 and 1987 but prevalence rates in 1987 increased at a dramatic speed (Vanichseni et al 1989, 1990). These increases were also noted, but to a lesser extent, for prostitutes (Ungchusak et al 1990). The first national survey detected HIV infection in 44% of low-charge brothel-based pros-

titutes in Chang Mai (Northern region). This was confirmed by follow-up studies in August 1989 in which 37% were HIV-positive, presenting monthly seroconversion rates of 10% (Siraprapasiri et al 1991). Incidence rates given by a cohort study 7 and 11 months later showed monthly rates of 4.8% and 3.4%, respectively (Sawanpanyalert et al 1991). National median provincial (13 provinces) prevalence rates for low-charge brothel-based prostitutes increased steadily from 3.5% (range 0–44%) in 1989 to 15% (range 2–63%) in 1991 (69 provinces). The same sentinel surveys were also undertaken among high-paying prostitutes and rates rose steadily from 0% (range 0–5%) in 1989 to 5% (range 0–29%) in 1991 (Weniger et al 1991). Rates for low-paying prostitutes have been consistently higher in the Northern part of the country where the provinces border with Burma and Laos (Fig. 1.2). The annual census of prostitution undertaken by the Department of Communicable Disease Control recorded 86 494 female prostitutes working in 6160 establishments nationwide in 1990. These census data yield a rate of 157 prostitutes per 100 000 population or 1 prostitute for 146 men of age 15–44 years (Weniger et al 1991).

High rates of turnover and migration are common among female prostitutes. Changes in worksite were studied and it was estimated that changes occurred within the same town or to other provinces every 3–4 months (Weniger et al 1991).

Men who have sex with prostitutes also put their regular sexual partners (wives, girlfriends and acquaintances), and also indirectly their newborn children, at risk. The anticipated new wave of infection was detected in 1991. Prevalence rates produced by national sentinel survey among women attending antenatal clinics reached 0.7% (range 0–12%). The proportion of HIV-positive pregnant women infected by their husbands (33%) exceeded that of prostitutes (20%) and IDU (6%) (Weniger et al 1991).

Estimates of the total number of infected people in Thailand have been revised periodically in accordance with the results of seroprevalence data and estimates of the population subgroups. Based on the WHO extrapolation method (Chin & Lwanda 1991), the burden of infection and disease by the year 2000 in Thailand was estimated to

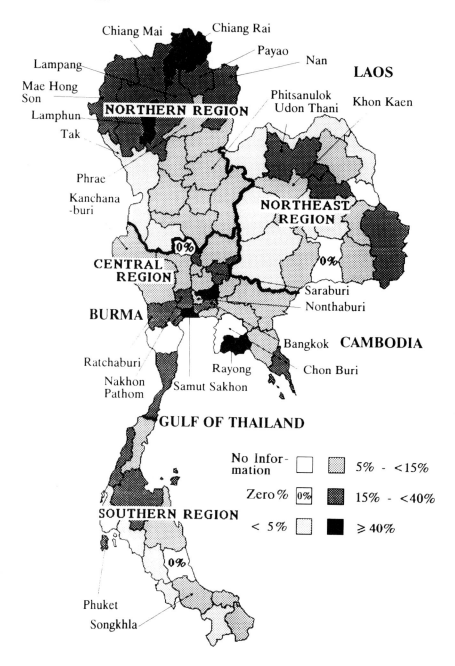

Figure 1.2 HIV seroprevalence rates from December 1990 national sentinel survey among brothel-based (lower-class) female prostitutes, by province. Rates not available for Chon Buri (in June 1991: 33%, 31 out of 93) and for the northeast province of Mukdahan (in June 1991: 5%, 1 out of 20). Mapping by Population Division, United Nations Economic and Social Commission for Asia and the Pacific, Bangkok (data source: Division of Epidemiology, Ministry of Public Health). (From Weniger B G et al 1991 The epidemiology of HIV infection and AIDS in Thailand. AIDS 5 (suppl 2))

Table 1.3 Trends in seroprevalence of HIV among four population groups in Nairobi 1989 to 1991. (From Kitabu MZ et al 1992 VIII International Conference on AIDS, Amsterdam, July)

Nairobi	1989			1990			1991		
	n	HIV+	%	n	HIV+	%	n	HIV+	%
Prostitutes	656	441	67	981	724	74	525	395	75
Pregnant women	1396	228	16	2251	388	17	1422	235	17
STD patients	2507	777	31	2738	970	35	3631	1604	44
Truck drivers	299	86	29	429	132	31	411	124	30

STD, sexually transmitted disease

reach 1–3.4 million cumulative HIV infections. These figures, however, depend on how well future transmission can be slowed and more precisely on the impact of information and education on behaviour change of the population.

Africa

The HIV2 is predominantly found in West Africa; nevertheless Angola and Mozambique, which have historical connections with Portugal (Saimot et al 1987) and therefore the other Portuguese-speaking African countries like the Cape Verdian Islands or Guinea Bissau, where the HIV2 virus predominates, have high prevalence rates. This type of virus seems to spread at a much lower rate than HIV1 (De Cock & Brun-Vézinet 1989). In addition, whereas HIV2 infections are high (8.9%) among adults in a community-based survey in Guinea Bissau, HIV2 antibody was absent among infants and young children (Poulsen et al 1992). This suggests that HIV2 is transmitted less efficiently from mother to child than HIV1 (Ancelle et al 1987), though such transmission certainly occurs (De Cock et al 1991).

The HIV1 has spread over most of the African countries and has rapidly become the predominant human immunodeficiency virus – however, with higher rates in Central and Eastern countries. (It is to be noted that the distinction HIV1, HIV2 will not be made in this chapter.)

As in all areas in the world, there exist variations between countries but also variations within each country. In Africa there is a disproportionate distribution of HIV infection in local urban areas even though the viruses may have existed in rural areas for longer periods of time (Boyle Torrey & Way 1990).

Several factors determining the spread of the virus are probably acting simultaneously. These factors include demographic, behavioural, biological and probably also political and economic factors. Because of difficulties in rural areas many people, especially men, have been attracted to large cities where jobs appear to be plentiful. Population movements towards these large urbanized areas to secure jobs (Lwanga 1992) as well as trading results in concentrations in large cities of communicable agents and also young sexually active people. These people are far from their homes, families and usual sexual partners and in many cities, but also on the roadside leading from one city to another, core groups of prostitutes provide sexual services. There also prostitution provides attractive easy money (Non-governmental co-ordinating committee Zambia 1992). Truck drivers driving from one area to another are at high risk of infection and dissemination, although it seems that for some of them use of condoms may have become habitual (Laukamm-Josten et al 1992).

In these areas accessibility of existing health services is often insufficient for women, and self-medication and inadequate antimicrobial treatment all contribute to the problem (Laga et al 1991).

General sexual behaviour that involves contacts with a small but highly infected core group are associated with the most rapid spread of HIV. Studies among prostitutes have been developed in the frame of research programmes or programmes for sentinel surveillance. Prostitutes and patients attending STD clinics have consistently higher seroprevalence rates than sample groups taken from the general population, such as pregnant women (Nkowane 1991). In the Cameroon in 1990 rates among prostitutes reached 8.6% (Kaptue et al

1990), 2.9% among STD patients (male and female) and 0.2% among pregnant women (Ndumbe et al 1990). In Nigeria during the same year rates among prostitutes were 2.9 and 2.3% among STD patients (male and female) and 0.3% among pregnant women (Harry et al 1990). In Kinshasa rates reached 35% among prostitutes in 1990 (Kivuvu et al 1990) and were close to 5% among pregnant women in 1989 (Piot et al 1990).

Trends in these high risk populations show a continuous high increase (Kitabu et al 1992), whereas increases in rates among pregnant women are very much lower (Table 1.3) (Temmerman et al 1992). The prevalence of HIV1 is alarmingly high in women who do not report risky behaviour, which suggests that the epidemic has spread well beyond the core group and that a substantial proportion of women of child-bearing age are now infected. While the adverse role that HIV infection plays on pregnant women has still to be clarified, the detrimental impact of HIV infection on children born to HIV-infected mothers is now clear. In a prospective study in children born in Kinshasa, during the 1st year of life there were 100 (21%) deaths among the 468 children of HIV-seropositive mothers compared with 23 (3.8%) deaths among children born to seronegative mothers (Nsa et al 1989).

The rate of sexual partner change, the type of sexual intercourse and the nature of partners with whom one mixes are all critical in determining the spread of a sexually transmitted infection. It appears that HIV infection has become one of the leading causes of morbidity but also of potential life lost per capita in urban populations in sub-Saharan Africa (Over 1989).

NATURAL HISTORY AND RISK OF HIV INFECTION IN WOMEN

Much of what is currently known about the natural history of HIV disease has been learned through the prospective study of large cohorts of gay men. In contrast, the description of HIV disease in women consists of case reports, cross-sectional and retrospective studies published primarily in conference proceedings with no detailed descriptions of research methodology. The overwhelming predominance of men with clinically evident HIV disease in the developed world explains, at least in part, the lack of data concerning women. Since the development of the HIV epidemic in women is still recent, numbers of women infected with HIV in a single setting were often inadequate for the performance of epidemiological studies investigating factors potentially associated with progression of the disease. On the other hand, there has been a disproportionate focus on pregnancy in the study of HIV disease and women, a perspective that tended to conceptualize women as vectors of HIV transmission.

In non-industrialized countries, the sex ratio among AIDS cases is nearly 1, but little information is available concerning AIDS-defining diseases among women. Furthermore, since the date of infection is difficult to assess in countries where the HIV infection is endemic in the general population, no data are available on cohorts of patients with known dates of infection, followed prospectively.

With regard to HIV infection and women, studies on heterosexual transmission give data on the risk of infection of uninfected women as well as data on the risk of transmission of HIV to their sexual partners.

Incubation period and cofactors of progression

An incident cohort including men and women is the most reliable study design to estimate and compare incubation time. However, few data are available to date from ongoing cohort studies, either because few women are included or because the follow-up is still too short for the progression to AIDS to have occurred in women included. A total of 234 women and 422 men have been enrolled in an Italian cohort (Dorrucci et al 1992); 7 women and 31 men developed AIDS and no differences in rates of progression to AIDS have been observed between men and women. The risk of developing AIDS was only associated with older age at seroconversion. The dynamic of CD4 decrease was similar whatever the gender.

Analyses of prevalent cohorts (Sacks et al 1992, Creagh et al 1992), which controlled for CD4 counts at entry, did not show any difference in progression rates between men and women.

The modelling of the incubation time using data from AIDS patients having acquired HIV infection through transfusion has also been used to estimate incubation time according to age, sex and year of transfusion. The modelling of European data on transfusion-associated AIDS cases reported before 1990 (Downs et al 1991), based on the Weibull distribution, gave estimates of 9.4 and 10.5 years for men and women, respectively. The difference was not statistically significant ($p < 0.08$). An earlier study (Medley et al 1987) suggested a trend towards a better evolution in women (median incubation time of 8.4 years for women and 5.5 years for men), although the introduction of a sex difference in the model was not statistically significant ($p < 0.20$).

Cofactors of progression have been studied mainly in men. To date, the only cofactor which has been clearly shown to be associated with more rapid progression is an older age at seroconversion (Medley et al, 1987, Downs et al 1991, Dorrucci et al 1992). Results concerning other potential cofactors of progression such as infection with other viruses (e.g. cytomegalovirus), continued use of intravenous drugs, or human leukocyte antigen (HLA) type are conflicting.

One potential cofactor specific to women is pregnancy. Several studies have been performed to study the influence of pregnancy on the course of HIV infection. Most of these studies, often based on small sample sizes, found no influence (MacCallum et al 1989, Bledsoe et al 1990, Berrebi et al 1991, Mazzarello et al 1991), but two studies do appear to support an association between pregnancy and the clinical progression of HIV disease (Deschamps et al 1989, Delfraissy et al 1989). Some studies have suggested an impairment of cell-mediated immunity during pregnancy, especially for women who were in advanced stages of HIV infection before pregnancy (Lapointe et al 1991, Weedon et al 1992). Further studies are clearly needed before any conclusion can be drawn, and a potential differential influence of pregnancy in asymptomatic and symptomatic women may be analysed.

Survival following AIDS diagnosis

The AIDS case definition used until now has been defined on clinical manifestations related to HIV infection described among patients before 1987. At that time, women were under-represented among patients with symptoms, and it is possible that the definition does not include illnesses that affect specifically women. Thus, women who received an AIDS diagnosis according to Centers for Disease Control criteria may be at a later stage of clinical deterioration and immunodeficiency than men with a similar diagnosis, and may thus appear to have shorter survival following an AIDS diagnosis.

Early reports suggested that women have a markedly shorter survival after AIDS diagnosis than do men (Rothenberg et al 1987, Kloser et al 1989). Since then, several studies have examined comparative survival among men and women who have AIDS while controlling for important variables such as access to health care and to antiviral treatment before AIDS. In some US studies (Lemp et al 1990, Moore et al 1991, Friedland et al 1991, Araneta et al 1991, Horsburgh et al 1991), a differential survival was observed in univariate analysis. However, in all but one (Friedland et al 1991), no gender effect was found after adjustments. The poorer prognosis earlier described for women might be due to a late diagnosis of HIV-associated illnesses among women, such that specific treatments were delayed. In some countries like the USA, many HIV-infected women have poor access to health care services and do not always receive adequate case management in time because of low socio-economic status (Moore et al 1991, Turner et al 1991). Data from two European studies (Pedersen et al 1990, Patris et al 1991), did not show any difference in survival, either in univariate or in multivariate analyses.

After controlling for the AIDS-defining disease, factors reported to be associated with poor survival, whatever the gender, are older age at diagnosis and lack of access to antiviral treatments before diagnosis of AIDS. Patients diagnosed in more recent years show a better prognosis than those diagnosed earlier.

AIDS-defining diseases in women

Without regard to gender, the more frequent diseases indicative of AIDS in industrialized countries are opportunistic infections including *Pneumocystis carinii* pneumonia, *Candida* esophagitis, cryptococcal meningitis, herpes simplex virus disease, cytomegalovirus disease, tuberculosis and toxoplasmosis. Other frequent AIDS-defining conditions are wasting syndrome, lymphoma and Kaposi's sarcoma (Centers for Disease Control 1992b, European Centre 1992c).

Women with AIDS rarely develop Kaposi's sarcoma. However, the occurrence of Kaposi's sarcoma seems to be associated with the mode of infection rather than the gender. Homo- and bisexual men are more likely to develop Kaposi's sarcoma than male intravenous drug users (Beral et al 1990, Couturier et al 1990), and sexual contact with a bisexual man has been reported more frequently as the source of infection among women with Kaposi's sarcoma compared with women with other AIDS-defining conditions (Couturier et al 1990). Such associations are consistent with the hypothesis that Kaposi's sarcoma is related to a sexually transmitted agent that is highly correlated with HIV exposure in homo/bisexual men. While Kaposi's sarcoma in HIV-infected men often occurs early in the course of HIV infection and shows a better prognosis than most other AIDS-defining conditions (Patris et al 1991), Kaposi's sarcoma in HIV-infected women has been reported to be diffuse and progressive and may be associated with severe immune depression (Lassoued et al 1991, Benedetti et al, 1991).

In several studies, esophageal candidiasis has been reported more frequently among female than male AIDS cases (Fleming et al 1991, Castro et al 1992). A few authors reported that women more often show wasting syndrome and herpes simplex disease, but such differences were not observed in other studies. Again, the frequency of each opportunistic infection seems to be closely related to the transmission group and the geographical origin of the patient, and these parameters have to be taken into account before any conclusion can be drawn with regard to gender-specific susceptibilities to AIDS-defining illnesses. For example, the frequency of wasting syndrome and *Pneumocystis*

carinii pneumonia among AIDS cases reported during the first semester of 1992 in the USA are respectively 10% (Centers for Disease Control 1992a) and 50%, while in Europe (European Centre 1992c) these conditions are less frequent (respectively 6% and 30%). On the other hand, toxoplasmosis is less common in the USA than in Europe, since the frequency of latent toxoplasmosis infection in the general US population is lower.

Most of these comparisons have been performed on surveillance data, using only the first AIDS-defining disease and rarely all events occurring during the course of AIDS. One possible field of research would be to examine a potential differential timing of these events.

Non-AIDS-defining diseases in women

Studies examining the clinical features of HIV-related disease in women have frequently identified fungal and viral infections, in particular of the genital tract, as the most prevalent disease manifestations preceding the diagnosis of AIDS. Some studies have reported an association between decreased immune function and *Candida* infection of the vagina, human papillomavirus disease, and genital herpes. Whether women with HIV infection are disproportionately affected by various gynaecological conditions is not always clear since data drawn from comparative populations of women who are not infected with HIV are rarely presented. Such comparative data are imperatively needed since the risk factors are similar for HIV infection and for other genital infections (e.g. rate of partner change).

For example, one study (Iman et al 1990) examined the severity and location of *Candida* infections in women in relation to the degree of immunosuppression measured by CD4 counts. Both oral and esophageal candidiasis were associated with marked immunosuppression, but recurrent and often severe vaginal candidiasis was observed in the absence of immunosuppression. In another study (Anderson et al 1990), vaginal candidiasis and herpes simplex virus infection were observed at all stages of HIV disease. These data suggest that the high prevalence of vaginal *Candida* infections observed in HIV-infected women may not be related to HIV-induced immunodepression.

An association between HIV infection and cervical intraepithelial neoplasia has been reported (Centers for Disease Control 1990, Klein et al 1992, Regevik et al 1992, Anastos et al 1992). In most studies, the lack of a comparison group of women not infected with HIV and/or small sample sizes tend to limit analysis. The human papillomavirus has an established role in the aetiology of cervical diseases. Since most clinic-based studies include women likely to have human papillomavirus infection or risk factors associated with cervical disease, a potentially independent role of HIV in the aetiology of cervical disease remains to be determined. In several studies, comparisons of results from cervical screening with those from biopsies indicate that the Papanicolaou test alone may not reliably detect abnormalities in women with HIV infection (Maiman et al 1991). If these results are confirmed, other strategies for cervical screening among HIV-infected women should be defined.

In conclusion, it is not clear whether these gynaecological disorders are related to the degree of immunodeficiency or not. However, these disorders seem frequent among women infected with HIV, and the medical care of these women should include genital examination. More information is needed to define with precision the extent and frequency of check-ups to be recommended. However, the Centers for Disease Control recommend the performance of a Pap test every year for HIV-infected women (Centers for Disease Control 1990), and has recently decided to include cervical neoplasia as a new AIDS-defining illness.

Risk of HIV infection among women

In countries where blood donors are systematically screened, where haemophiliacs use heated blood products, and where medical instruments are not used for several patients without sterilization, the risk of nosocomial HIV infection is nearly zero. Two, and only two, modes of infection are responsible for the diffusion of HIV infection among women: using injecting equipment of infected intravenous drug users, and having unprotected sexual intercourse with infected men.

The primary source of infection world-wide is

clearly heterosexual contact, although there is considerable geographical variation in the extent to which intravenous drug use contributes to exposure to HIV. In Europe and North America, about 55% of women with AIDS reported intravenous drug use (Beral et al 1990, European Centre 1992c). However, since a lot of female drug users have sexual partners who are themselves drug users (and thus at risk of HIV infection), and because drug use can lead to exchange of sex for money or drugs, there might be a lot of unrecognized cases of infection through sexual contact.

Heterosexual transmission of HIV

Several studies have examined the risk of sexual transmission of HIV from infected men to their female partners (European Study Group 1992; Haverkos & Battjes 1992). HIV prevalence ranges from 15 to 30% in most studies from Europe and the USA. In addition to unprotected sexual intercourse, anal sex and advanced clinical or immunological stage of HIV infection in men have been shown to significantly increase the risk of transmission. Other factors have been reported as potentially increasing the susceptibility of women to HIV infection, such as perimenopausal status, defloration, pain during sexual contacts, cervical ectopy, use of oral contraceptives, and use of an intrauterine device (European Study Group 1992, Haverkos & Battjes 1992).

The role of previous genital lesions is difficult to interpret. Because all sexually transmitted diseases (STD), including HIV infection, have the same mode of transmission, and because the prevalence of genital infections might be increased in people infected with HIV due to immunodeficiency, it is difficult to design studies to examine the independent effects of other genital infections as cofactors for HIV transmission. Nevertheless, several studies in Africa and in developed countries have presented strong arguments to support the hypothesis that genital infections, especially ulcerative infections, are cofactors for transmission.

Since many more men are infected with HIV than women in most developed countries, transmission from infected women to their male sexual partners has been poorly studied. Even in regions where HIV is predominantly acquired through heterosexual contact, few data are available. Factors which may enhance the infectivity of female-to-male transmission are an advanced clinical or immunological stage of HIV infection and the presence of blood in the vagina at the time of sexual contacts (e.g. sex during menses), STD, and circumcision of the male (European Study Group 1992 Haverkos & Battjes 1992).

The role of most of the factors reported in different studies as potential cofactors of transmission remains to be confirmed. However, all these reports add weight to the argument that, besides the immunological status of the infected partner, all factors (traumatic, infectious, hormonal) able to impair the genital mucosa might be considered as factors which increase the risk of sexual transmission.

In a review of 16 partner studies (Haverkos & Battjes 1992), male-to-female and female-to-male transmission rates were compared. Transmission rates varied widely among the studies, with higher rates generally observed in couples recruited in Africa or Haiti (female-to-male transmission, 58% (83/143); male-to-female transmission 53% (171/324)) than couples recruited in Europe or the USA (female-to-male transmission, 15% (67/461); male-to-female transmission 28% (411/1485)). Transmission rates were statistically greater for couples in whom the male was the index case among US and European couples (relative risk = 1.9), but not among couples from Africa and Haiti. However, in regions such as Africa and Haiti where HIV infection is endemic in the heterosexual population, and when both partners of a couple are HIV-infected, it is often difficult to know whether the man or the woman was the first infected, and thus difficult to assess the direction of transmission. Furthermore, heterosexual patients in these regions may have been infected earlier than in industrialized countries, and it has been reported (European Study Group 1992) that the difference in efficiency of transmission may be reduced when the infectious partner is in an advanced stage of the disease.

Although estimations of the magnitude of the relative risk of male-to-female vs female-to-male transmission of HIV are still imprecise, it might not be much greater than that observed for other sexually transmitted diseases such as gonorrhoea

(approximately 3.0). Thus, controversies about the exact rate of female-to-male transmission rate should not lead men (some with multiple heterosexual partners) and HIV-infected women, to consider safer sex practices (e.g. use of condoms) as useless.

The risk of transmission through oral sex during homosexual (between men as well as between women) and heterosexual contacts is another controversial field. Several case reports suggest that transmission can occur through this route. However, the magnitude of risk is difficult to estimate. During the follow-up (Detels et al 1989) of initially seronegative homosexual men in a US highly infected population (HIV prevalence of 40% at the beginning of the study), two seroconversions occurred among men practising fellatio but not anal sex, leading to a seroconversion rate of 0.6 per 1000 persons followed for 1 year. For comparison, the rates of seroconversion were 3.5 and 15.5 per 1000 persons, respectively, among men having anal sex protected with condoms for each sexual contact, and among those not using condoms systematically. These results suggest that, compared to the risk of transmission through protected anal sex, the risk of HIV transmission through unprotected fellatio might be less or similar. These results may be explained by the risk of condom failure during sex, which has been estimated at 1% during vaginal intercourse and nearly 5% during anal intercourse (Anonymous 1991).

However, if sex with condoms should not be considered as 'safe sex', it is truly considered as 'safer sex'. During the follow-up of heterosexual couples in which one partner was HIV-negative (De Vincenzi et al 1991), no seroconversion occurred among 100 partners using condoms for each episode of vaginal or anal intercourse, while 10 seroconversions occurred among 104 partners not systematically using condoms. As for condom use, oral sex might be considered as a safer, but not safe, sexual practice.

CONCLUSION

It is increasingly clear that the epidemiology of the HIV is becoming more heterogenous, is affecting more and more women and is changing rapidly in some areas, especially in areas where the virus has been introduced very recently.

The epidemic has not yet reached a stable situation in many populations and several factors determining the spread of the virus are probably acting simultaneously. These factors include demographic, behavioural, biological and probably also political and economic factors.

The identification of behavioural and biological risk factors for HIV is important for the control of this disease, and a better knowledge of the natural history of HIV infection and of the interaction with other diseases is important for patient management and resource allocation.

Most of the biomedical aspects of HIV/AIDS in women are still under debate. Incubation time and survival after AIDS diagnosis do not seem different between men and women infected with HIV, but few cohort studies have enrolled enough women to have observed any statistical differences or gender-specific cofactors of progression. Other important outcomes of interest for future studies include timing of onset of gynaecological disease in relation to the level of immunodeficiency due to HIV infection. Much remains to be learned regarding the impact of pregnancy on clinical progression.

The recruitment and prospective study of women with HIV infection in both industrialized and non-industrialized countries are critical for the elaboration of effective prophylactic and therapeutic regimens. It can no longer be assumed that simple extrapolation of results from studies of men is adequate for the development of clinically appropriate therapy approaches for women.

REFERENCES

Ades A E, Parker S, Berry T et al 1991 Prevalence of maternal HIV-1 infection in Thames regions: results from anonymous unlinked neonatal testing. Lancet 337: 1562–1565
Anastos K, Denenberg R, Solomon L et al 1992 Relationship of CD4 cell counts to cervical cytologic abnormalities and gynecologic infections in 150 HIV-infected women. VIII International Conference on AIDS, Amsterdam, Abstr TuB 0532
Ancelle R, Bletry O, Baglin A C et al 1987 Long incubation time for HIV-2 infection. Lancet 1: 688–689
Anderson J, Horn J, Atkinson J et al 1990 Gynecologic infections in women with HIV infection. VI International Conference on AIDS, San Francisco, Abstr 2052
Anonymous 1991 12000 preservatifs jugés par leurs utilisateurs. 50 millions de consommateurs. 212: 42–47
Araneta M R, Lemp G J, Cohen J B et al 1991 Survival trends among women with AIDS in San Francisco. VII International Conference on AIDS, Florence, Abstr MC 3122
Benedetti P, Greco D, Figoli F et al 1991 Epidemic Kaposi's sarcoma in female AIDS patients. AIDS 5: 466–467
Beral V, Peterman T, Berkelman R et al 1990 Kaposi's sarcoma among persons with AIDS: a sexually transmitted infection? Lancet 335: 123–128
Berrebi A, Chraibi J, Kobuch W E et al 1991 Influence of pregnancy on HIV disease. VII International Conference on AIDS, Florence, Abstr WB 2046
Bindels P J E 1991 Resultaten van de screening op HIV-antistoffen bij zwangere vroumen, bezoeksters van infertiliteitspoliklinieken in de regio Amsterdam in 1990. Ned Tijdschr Geneeskd 135 (45): 2123–2128
Bledsoe K, Olopoenia L, Barnes S et al 1990 Effect of pregnancy on progression of HIV infection. VI International Conference on AIDS, San Francisco, Abstr ThC 652
Boyle Torrey B, Way P O 1990 Seroprevalence of HIV in Africa: Winter 1990. CIR Staff Paper no55, Center for International Research, Washington
Brookmeyer R 1991 Reconstruction and future trends of the AIDS epidemic in the United States. Science 253: 37–42
Castro K G, Valdiseri R O, Curran J W 1992 Perspectives on HIV/AIDS epidemiology and prevention from the eighth international conference on AIDS. Am J Publ Health 82: 1465–1470
Centers for Disease Control 1990 Risk for cervical disease in HIV. infected women – New York City. MMWR 39: 846–849
Centers for Disease Control 1992a AIDS cases reported through June 1992. HIV/AIDS Surveillance
Centers for Disease Control 1992b AIDS cases reported through September 1992. HIV/AIDS Surveillance
Chin J, Lwanda S K 1991 Estimation and projection of adult AIDS cases: a simple epidemiological model. Bull WHO 69: 399–406
Couturier E, Ancelle-Park R, De Vincenzi I et al 1990 Kaposi's sarcoma as a sexually transmitted disease. Lancet 335: 1105
Couturier E, Brossard Y, Larsen C et al 1992 HIV infection at outcome of pregnancy in the Paris area, France. Lancet 340: 707–709
Creagh T, Thompson M, Morris A et al 1992 Gender differences in the spectrum of HIV disease. VIII International Conference on AIDS, Amsterdam, Abstr MoC0032
De Cock K M, Brun-Vézinet F 1989 Epidemiology of HIV-2 infection. AIDS 3:589–595
De Cock K M, Brun-Vézinet F, Soro B 1991 HIV-1 and HIV-2 infections and AIDS in West Africa. AIDS 5: S21–28
De Vincenzi I, Ancelle-Park R et al 1991 Heterosexual transmission of HIV: Follow-up of a European cohort of couples. VII International Conference on AIDS, Florence, Abstr MC 3028
Delfraissy J F, Pons J C, Sereni D et al 1989 Does pregnancy influence disease progression in HIV positive women? V International Conference on AIDS, Montreal, Abstr MBP 34
Deschamps M M, Pape J W, Madhaven S et al 1989 Pregnancy and acceleration of HIV-related illness. V International Conference on AIDS, Montreal, Abstr MBP 6
Detels R, English P, Visscher B et al 1989 Seroconversion, sexual activity, and condom use among 2915 HIV seronegative men followed for up to 2 years. The Multicenter AIDS Cohort Study. J Acq Immune Dis Synd 2: 77–83

Division of Epidemiology 1989 First sentinel surveillance June 1989. Wkly Epidemiol Surv Rep (Thailand) 20: 376–389

Dondero T J, Gill O N 1991 Large-scale serologic surveys: what has been learned? AIDS 5: S63–69

Dorrucci M, Rezza G, Pezzotti P et al 1992 Age accelerates the progression from HIV-seroconversion to AIDS in women. VIII International Conference on AIDS, Amsterdam, Abstr MoC0033

Downs A M, Ancelle-Park R A, Brunet J B 1990 Surveillance of AIDS in the European Community: recent trends and predictions to 1991. AIDS 4: 1117–1124

Downs A M, Ancelle-Park R A, Costagliola D et al 1991 Transfusion associated AIDS cases in Europe: estimation of the incubation period, distribution and prediction of future cases. J Acq Immune Defic Synd 4: 805–813

Ellerbrock T V, Bush T J, Chamberland M E et al 1991 Epidemiology of women with AIDS in the United States, 1981 through 1990. JAMA 265: 2971–2975

European Centre for the Epidemiological Monitoring of AIDS 1991a AIDS cases in women: European non-aggregate AIDS data set (ENAADS). AIDS surveillance in Europe quarterly report no31

European Centre for the Epidemiological Monitoring of AIDS, 1991b Prevalence: estimates of the total number of HIV seropositive subjects in Europe. AIDS surveillance in Europe quarterly report no32

European Centre for the Epidemiological Monitoring of AIDS 1991c Unlinked anonymous testing among pregnant women and neonates in Europe: data from the European HIV prevalence database. AIDS surveillance in Europe quarterly report no32

European Centre for the Epidemiological Monitoring of AIDS, 1992a European Community concerted action on monitoring HIV seroprevalence in a sentinel population of STD patients (June 1990–December 1991). AIDS surveillance in Europe quarterly report no33

European Centre for the Epidemiological Monitoring of AIDS, 1992b European Community concerted action on HIV infection among female prostitutes (September 1990–November 1991). AIDS surveillance in Europe quarterly report no34

European Centre for the Epidemiological Monitoring of AIDS 1992c Update at 30th September 1992. AIDS surveillance in Europe quarterly report no35

European Study Group on Heterosexual Transmission of HIV 1992 Comparison of female-to-male and male-to-female transmission of HIV in 563 stable couples. Br Med J 304: 809–813

Fleming P L, Clesielski C A, Berkelman R et al 1991 Sex-specific differences in the prevalence of reported AIDS-indicative diagnoses. VII International Conference on AIDS, Florence, Abstra MC 3210

Friedland G H, Saltzman B, Vileno J et al 1991 Survival differences in patients with AIDS. J Acq Immune Defic Synd 4: 144–153

Gill O N, Adler M W, Day N E 1989 Monitoring the prevalence of HIV. Br Med J 299: 1295–1298

Green T A, Karon J M, Nwanyanwu O C 1992 Changes in AIDS incidence trends in the United States. J Acq Immune Defic Synd 5: 547–555

Gwinn M, Pappaioanou M, George J R et al 1991 Prevalence of HIV infection in child-bearing women in the United States. JAMA 265: 1704–1708

Hankins C A, Handley M A 1992 HIV disease and AIDS in

women: current knowledge and a research agenda. J Acq Immune Defic Synd 5: 957–971

Harry T O, Gashau W, Ekenna O et al 1990 Growing threat of HIV infection in a low prevalence area. V International Conference on AIDS in Africa, Kinshasa, Abstra TOB6

Haverkos H W, Battjes R 1992 Female-to-male transmission of HIV. JAMA 268: 1855

Horsburgh C R, Hanson D F, Fann S A et al 1991 Predictors of survival in HIV infection include CD4 + cell counts, AIDS-defining condition and therapy but not sex, age, race, or risk activity. VII International Conference on AIDS, Florence, Abstr MC 3175

Iman N, Carpenter C C J, Mayer K H et al 1990 Hierarchical pattern of mucosal candida infections in HIV-seropositive women. Am J Med 89: 142–146

Ippolito G, Costa F, Stegano M et al 1991 Blind serosurvey of HIV antibodies in newborns in 92 Italian hospitals: a method for monitoring the infection rate in women at time of delivery. J Acq Immune Defic Synd 4: 402–407

Jenum P 1988 Anti-HIV screening of pregnant women in south-eastern Norway. NIPH Annals 11: 53–58

Kaptue L, Zekeng L, Feldblum P et al 1990 HIV-2 infection among high-risk groups in Yaounde, Cameroon. V International Conference on AIDS in Africa, Kinshasa, Abstr WPB3

Kitabu M Z, Maitha G M, Mugai J N et al 1992 Trends in seroprevalence of HIV among four population groups in Nairobi, 1989 to 1991. VIII International Conference on AIDS, Amsterdam, Abstr PoC 4018

Kivuvu M, Malele B, Nzila N et al 1990 Syphilis among HIV + and HIV − prostitutes in Kinshasa: prevalence and serologic response to treatment. V International Conference on AIDS in Africa, Kinshasa, Abstr TPC7

Klein R S, Adachi A, Fleming I et al 1992 A prospective study of genital neoplasia and HPV in HIV infected women. VIII International Conference on AIDS, Amsterdam, Abstr TuB 0527

Kloser P, Bais P, Lynch A et al 1989 Women with AIDS: a continuing study 1988. V International Conference on AIDS, Montreal, Abstr A 563

Laga M, Nzila N, Goeman J 1991 The interrelationship of sexually transmitted diseases and HIV infection: implications for the control of both epidemics in Africa. AIDS 5: S55–63

Lapointe N, Boucher M, Samsom J et al 1991 Significant markers in the modulation of immunity during pregnancy and post-partum in a paired HIV positive and HIV negative population. VII International Conference on AIDS, Florence, Abstr WB 2054

Lassoued K, Clauvel J P, Fegueux S et al 1991 AIDS-associated Kaposi's sarcoma in female patients. AIDS 5: 877–880

Laukamm-Josten U, Ocheng D, Mwizarubi B K et al 1992 HIV and syphilis seroprevalence and risk factors in truckstops and nearby communities in Tanzania. VIII International Conference on AIDS, Amsterdam, Abstr PcC 4162

Lemp G F, Payne S F, Neal D et al 1990 Survival trends for patients with AIDS. JAMA 263: 402–406

Lindgren S, Bohlin A B, Ottenblad C et al 1991 Swedish national antenatal screening program for HIV-1. Three years' experience. VII International Conference on AIDS, Florence, Abstr WC3278

Lwanga J S 1992 Factors which put adolescents at risk of HIV/STD in Uganda. VIII International Conference on AIDS, Amsterdam, Abstr PoC 4198

MacCallum L R, Cowan F M, Whitelaw J et al 1989 Disease progression following pregnancy in HIV seropositive women. V International Conference on AIDS, Montreal, Abstr MBP 3

Maiman M, Tarricone N, Vieira J et al 1991 Colposcopic evaluation of HIV-seropositive women. Obstet Gynecol 78: 84–88

Mazzarello G, Canessa A, Melica F et al 1991 Influence of pregnancy on HIV disease progression. VII International Conference on AIDS, Florence, Abstr WC 3235

Medley G, Anderson R, Cox D et al 1987 Incubation period of AIDS in patients infected via blood transfusion. Nature (London) 328: 719–721

Moore R D, Hidalgo J, Sugland B W et al 1991 Zidovudine and the natural history of AIDS. N Engl J Med 324: 1412–1416

National Centre on HIV Epidemiology and Clinical Research 1992 Australian HIV surveillance report 8, suppl 3

Ndumbe P M, Andela A, Ndoumou A et al 1990 HIV infection in selected populations in Cameroon. V International Conference on AIDS in Africa, Kinshasa, Abstr WPA14

Nkowane B M 1991 Prevalence and incidence of HIV infection in Africa: a review of data published in 1990. AIDS 5: S7–15

Non governmental coordinating committee Zambia 1992 HIV and prostitution in Zambia. VIII International Conference on AIDS, Amsterdam, Abstr PoD 5643

Nsa W, Manzila T, Mvula M et al 1989 Cause-specific morbidity in the first 18 months of life in 477 infants born to seropositive mothers in Zaire. V International Conference on AIDS, Montreal, Abstr WGO4

Over M 1989 A production function approach to estimating the aggregate macroeconomic impact of AIDS on Central African economics. V International Conference on AIDS, Montreal, Abstr THO15

Pan American Health Organization 1992 AIDS surveillance in the Americas: update 10 September 1992. PAHO/WHO Global Program on AIDS/Americas

Patris C, Delmas M C, Pillonel J et al 1991 Survival after diagnosis among Paris AIDS cases. VII International Conference on AIDS, Florence, Abstr MC 3178

Peckham C S, Tedder R S Briggs M et al 1990 Prevalence of maternal HIV infection based on unlinked anonymous testing of newborn babies. Lancet 335: 516–519

Pedersen C, Gerstoft J, Tauris P et al 1990 Trends in survival of Danish AIDS patients from 1981 to 1989. AIDS 4: 1111–1116

Piot P, Laga M, Ryder R et al 1990 The global epidemiology of HIV infection: continuity, heterogeneity, and change. J Acq Immune Defic Synd 3: 403–412

Poulsen A G, Kvinesdal B B, Aaby P et al 1992 Lack of evidence of vertical transmission of human immunodeficiency virus type 2 in a sample of the general population in Bissau. J Acq Immune Defic Synd 5: 25–30

Public Health Laboratory Service AIDS Centre 1991 The unlinked anonymous HIV prevalence monitoring programme in England and Wales: preliminary results. Communicable Disease Report 1: R69–R76

Regevik N, Sen P, Raska K et al 1992 Cervical HPV in women infected with HIV and its correlation with immune status and papanicolaou smear abnormalities. VIII International Conference on AIDS, Amsterdam, Abstr TuB 0528

Rothenberg R, Woelfel M, Stoneburner R et al 1987 Survival with AIDS. N Engl J Med 317: 1297–1302

Sacks H, Szabo S, Miller L H et al 1992 Gender differences in the natural history of HIV infection. VIII International Conference on AIDS, Amsterdam, Abstr MoC0030

Saimot A G, Coulaud J P, Mechali D et al 1987 HIV-2/LAV-2 in Portugese man with AIDS (Paris, 1987) who had served in Angola in 1968–1974. Lancet 1: 688

Sawanpanyalert P, Ungchusak K, Thanprasertsuk S et al 1991 Seroconversion rate and risk factors for HVI-1 infection among low class female sex workers in Chiang Mai, Thailand. VII International Conference on AIDS, Florence, Abstr WC3097

Siraprapasiri T, Thanprasertsuk S, Rodklay A et al 1991 Risk factors for HIV among prostitutes in Chiangmai, Thailand. AIDS 5: 579–582

Tappin D M, Girdwood R W A, Follett E A C et al 1991 Prevalence of maternal HIV infection in Scotland based on unlinked anonymous testing of newborn babies. Lancet 337: 1565–1567

Temmerman M, Mohamed Ali F, Ndinya-Achola J et al 1992 Rapid increase of both HIV-1 infection and syphilis among pregnant women in Nairobi, Kenya. AIDS 6: 1181–1185

Turner B J, Markson L E, McKee L et al 1991 Survival patterns of women and men with AIDS: impact of health care use prior to AIDS. VII International Conference on AIDS, Florence, Abstr TUD 112

Ungchusak T, Thanprasertsuk S, Sriprapandh S et al 1990 First national sentinel seroprevalence survey for HIV-1 infection in Thailand, June 1989. VI International Conference on AIDS, San Francisco, Abstr FC99

Vanichseni S, Wright N, Akarasewi P 1989 Case control study of HIV positivity among male intravenous drug addicts (IVDA) in Bangkok. V International Conference on AIDS, Montreal, Abstr WGP19

Vanichseni S, Sakuntanaga P et al 1990 Results of three seroprevalence surveys for HIV in IVDU in Bangkok. VI International Conference on AIDS, San Francisco, Abstr FC105

Wangroongsarb Y, Weniger B G, Wasi C et al 1985 Prevalence of HTLV-III/LAV antibody in selected populations in Thailand. Southeast Asian J Trop Med Public Health 16: 517–520

Weedon J, Allen M, Hutchison S et al 1992 Immunologic and hematologic changes during pregnancy in HIV seropositive and high risk seronegative women. VIII International Conference on AIDS, Amsterdam, Abstr PoC4374

Weniger B G, Limpakarnjanarat K, Ungchusak K et al 1991 AIDS in Thailand. AIDS 5: S71–85

World Health Organization 1992a: OMS PRESS communiqué OMS/9, 12 février 1992

World Health Organization 1992b Update: AIDS cases reported to SFI, 1 July 1992 In: VIII International Conference on AIDS, Amsterdam, conference summary report

2. Counselling around HIV testing in women of reproductive age

Lorraine Sherr

Curiously the underlying assumption in most of the literature on procreation is that reproductive decision-making is solely a women's issue. Clearly this is inaccurate. Women may carry the greater burden, may experience the pregnancy and birth, and are often the only care-givers of an infant. In some definitions an 'orphan' is a child who is defined by losing a mother only. Yet reproduction is also a very male issue. Conception cannot occur without a male partner – be he fleeting or permanent. The desire to reproduce and parent is prevalent among women and men (heterosexual and gay – Sherr & Hedge 1989). The fact that the greatest literature on reproduction and childbearing decision-making focuses on women simply reflects the limitations on research which tends to concentrate on women, question them at clinics and rarely study or interview their male counterparts (Barbour 1990). In a text on women and HIV the challenges of reproductive decision-making will be examined from a woman's perspective, but readers should bear in mind the direct role and interaction this has within the partnership.

HIV and AIDS occurred at a time when there was a growing debate in reproductive decision-making generally (Chalmers et al 1989). The problems of HIV and AIDS should not be divorced or viewed in isolation of this debate.

This chapter will examine psychological issues surrounding reproductive decision-making with an attempt to provide comprehensive evaluation of the growing data set as it currently stands and to integrate such findings into the reality of clinical management and the broader reproductive literature. Counselling around HIV testing is not simply aimed at the decision to test, but must involve the whole of pregnancy care with a thorough exam-

ination of ongoing counselling if a test proves positive, as well as the role of such counselling in behaviour change and infection prevention. Any screening policy which does not work hand in hand with prevention is limited and short-sighted. HIV testing as an issue affects not only women of reproductive age, but their wider families and their care-givers.

The chapter looks at these issues in four sections. The first section addresses the problems of HIV and AIDS in reproduction. The second provides an in-depth examination of HIV testing as a screening tool with its strengths and weaknesses, specifically applied in the context of general antenatal care. The third is a detailed discussion of counselling in all areas of reproduction ranging from preconception through pregnancy continuation/interruption and parenting. The final section presents a specific elaboration of the psychological impact of HIV and AIDS on this population.

HIV AND AIDS AS A REPRODUCTIVE ISSUE

Heterosexual and vertical transmission have been well established and are accounting for a growing number of HIV infections. The majority of worldwide HIV infections (71%) are heterosexual in origin (Mann 1992). In Pattern I countries (where spread is highly prevalent within the gay community) there is a dramatic increase in heterosexual spread (Novello 1991, CDR 1992). As the increase in other groups slows down (e.g. 17% in the UK gay community, CDSC 1992), there is a sharp contrast with heterosexual and female infections which are showing alarming rises in spread (47% and 28% respectively, in the UK for the same period). There is a direct parallel between female infection and paediatric infection rates.

Maternal–child vertical transmission is well established (Peckham & Newell 1990) but the mechanisms are still exceedingly elusive. The rate of vertical transmission is unclear. Studies vary from 12.9% in good prospective long-term follow-up investigations (European Collaborative Study 1991) to as high as 40% in other centres. The reasons for this are unclear and may relate to background health status, virus strain, length of exposure to the virus, host factors or even couple factors although the latter have never been studied. When risks for infection are studied from the child perspective over 80% in sub-Saharan Africa are infected via vertical transmission. In the UK, current figures show 68% of children infected perinatally. As the rate of infections through contaminated blood or blood factor treatment declines, the role of vertical transmission will become central throughout the world. Yet to date nosocomial infection accounts for the biggest risk factor for children with AIDS identified in Europe (emerging mostly from Romania).

Timing of infection is not understood. Such knowledge would assist counselling and decision-making greatly. It appears that the virus can cross the placenta from early on in conception, during labour itself (exacerbated by invasive procedures such as fetal scalp electrodes and episiotomy) and after delivery via breast-feeding (Dunn et al 1992). There is knowledge of how timing of infection differentially affects the infant or disease course.

Many studies are designed to understand paediatric infection. As the focus of such studies is child-centred, they may overlook some of the maternal (and particularly paternal) issues. For example there is much coverage of pregnancy variables and how they relate to outcome (Hira et al 1989, Ippolito et al 1990, ECS 1991). Yet once the baby has been born, outcome measures tend to include 'head circumference, weight, body length', with few studies examining such variables as postpartum trauma, psychological adjustment, labour satisfaction, increased (or decreased) medical interventions, maternal infant interaction, mood, anxiety or parenting perceptions.

HIV testing enters the reproductive arena

As HIV can cross the placenta and infect the baby, there are those who argue that HIV status should be known for all pregnant women. Given the high emotional cost of such knowledge and the limited intervention avenues, others argue that the situation is not that simple. This leaves a wide range of policies whereby HIV testing is considered for all or for a selected few, for those possibly exposed to higher risk situations or to those connected to 'high risk groups', varying according to background infection rates in a given centre and testing facilities available. This is all set against a background of growing concern as the epidemic increases, often fuelled by large-scale anonymous seroprevalence studies which clearly indicate a growing prevalence of infection among parturent women (Chrystie et al 1992).

The strategies for counselling vary considerably, dependent on whether or not HIV has already been identified. Initially it was felt that much of the reproductive counselling would centre around women of known HIV infection who are either contemplating a pregnancy or who are currently pregnant. Yet this provides a limited view in the light of the widespread antenatal HIV testing programmes (Larsson et al 1990, Moatti et al 1990, Barbacci et al 1991, CDSC 1991). Such programmes put HIV on the agenda of a much broader range of women, invariably when they first appear at antenatal clinics for routine checks. In the UK, for example, a variety of centres have adopted strategies for HIV screening ranging from whole population screening to selective screening. In the USA similar strategies have been reported. Few studies report on pretest counselling. When the process has been monitored, clear evidence has been gathered that HIV testing is a potentially stressful procedure for pregnant women (Stevens et al 1989), decision-making is often not well thought through and HIV testing decisions can be greatly influenced by the views of the carer more than the views of the client or her risk behaviours (Meadows et al 1990). In Africa widespread testing is often reported (see Sherr 1991 for a review) with low refusal rates. In some studies, although compliance is high (over 95%), failure to return for results is often noted. Perhaps this indicates that truly informed consent was not present, or simply that women feel unable to cope with the results and choose avoidance as an option.

Many women are first identified as HIV-positive during antenatal care (Sherr et al in press, Beavor in press). Yet Tappin and colleagues (1991) show that with the passage of time this is less so in Scotland. Johnstone and associates (1989b) reported on a study where testing was offered after counselling and with informed consent. A total of 436 women were tested of which 79 were known to be positive. There was little change over time of the number tested, but a decline in those first knowing of HIV from such a test with a simultaneous increase in those referred already knowing they were HIV-positive was noted. HIV status was known in only 1.6% of all pregnancies.

Ades and co-workers (1992) reported that when comparisons were made between anonymous screening of phenylketonuria (PKU) samples and known HIV infections from the Obstetric/Paediatric surveys in London, only 20% of cases were aligned. Thus, in London at least, 80% of HIV-positive pregnancies are unidentified as such during antenatal care. Such findings are probably true in many centres where AIDS in pregnancy probably reflects accurate incidence, but HIV figures probably reflect testing policy rather than prevalence.

THE HIV TEST

HIV testing should never be undertaken without due thought and consideration, whatever the circumstances. HIV testing in pregnancy is no exception and perhaps carries with it additional burdens. The major questions surrounding testing should relate to limitations of the test, reasons for screening, the population to be screened, screening protocols, ethics and rights, and the opinions of the pregnant women themselves.

Limitations of the HIV test

Every test has its strengths and limitations. The HIV test itself is limited in that, although it can tell whether a person has been exposed to the virus and made antibody, it does not provide insight into how the person was so exposed, when the person

contracted HIV, the stage of illness, whether they will become ill, what kind of opportunistic infections they will get or any predictions about survival. It may also miss newly acquired infection as it takes up to 12 weeks on average for sufficient antibody to be present for a positive test to register. This is particularly problematic during pregnancy which lasts 9 months, during which time many women continue to have sexual intercourse, rarely protected. Indeed, newly infected women are more likely to transmit HIV infection to their babies (van de Perre et al 1991), probably as they are viraemic during the early stages of infection.

The costs of the test are high in terms of anxiety, coping demand, stigmatization and discrimination. As no cure for HIV is yet available, interventions are limited to early treatment regimens and prophylactic treatments with uncertain long-term effects on morbidity and mortality of both the mother and the developing fetus. Termination of pregnancy is the major option under current debate, yet many women do not consider the procedure for themselves and in many countries this is still not available either directly through legislation or indirectly through the lack of expertise, facilities or finance.

Reasons for screening

The rationale for HIV testing ought to be clear. The overriding reason why any procedure should be carried out is for the *benefit* of the recipient (WHO 1988). Some centres are eager to test for epidemiological data gathering. This is fraught with problems. Epidemiology is vital for planning. Infection rates will vary according to background population infection levels and representativeness of the sample, and can only provide data on pregnant women rather than heterosexual women in general, from whom they differ systematically. Sometimes the cost of the study exceeds the available funding for subsequent service provision. Funding for screening must allow for counselling provision and follow-up – not simply cover the cost of the test. Staff training may also be a budgetary requirement.

Some staff would like to test as a result of their personal (misdirected) fears of infection from positive patients. This is not helpful as it often implies the hidden conditions that staff would refuse to treat a woman found to be positive. Staff who are anxious about their own health should not be dismissed, but should be given education to allay and address such concerns without the need to subject women to unnecessary procedures.

Population to be screened

The targeting of HIV testing is unclear. Countries vary in their approaches. Policies vary with different institutions. Some promote testing, some target testing, some incorporate HIV counselling into the general running of the clinic and some, still uncertain, revert to haphazard policies usually at the whim of individuals.

Counselling prior to antenatal HIV testing is often simply not available. Few studies report on the procedures, and those which do have varying strategies. Some rely on routine information packs whilst others delegate a few minutes of discussion to the obstetrical health care worker. Written information is rarely a substitute for interactive counselling and should be seen as an adjunct to counselling rather than a substitute (Sherr & Hedge 1990).

Specifically constructed antenatal counselling programmes are few and far between. Sunderland and colleagues (1992) describe such a programme where women were counselled in a non-directive way, exploring risks, costs and benefits of the test with their clients. Berrier and associates (1991) examined pre- and postintervention questionnaire data when comparing a control group ($n = 98$) who did not receive information and an intervention group ($n = 515$) who received full information. An educational programme did increase the level of general knowledge, but failed to support the hypothesis of a positive effect on attitudes around testing and an increase in desire for voluntary testing. The hypothesis that women reporting more risk behaviours would be more likely to agree to HIV antibody testing was only partially supported. Wenstrom and Zuidema (1989) examined antenatal patients with 34% requesting testing after counselling ($n = 349$). A total of 849 women admitted to labour wards (without counselling) were queried about risk factors and tested; 19.1% of the antenatal group

and 9.6% of the women in labour reported risk factors. Higher HIV prevalence was found in the group without counselling. The authors conclude that risk factor identification without counselling is less efficient. However, they may not have taken into account the difficulties labouring women may have when asked to discuss HIV risks during contractions!

Clearly, testing policies should be planned and not reactive. Such planning will then allow for training of staff prior to testing programmes which will maximize good practice and minimize unnecessary trauma and suffering (Sherr 1987). Such policy decisions should be made in the face of demand, population characteristics, background infection rates, facilities, treatment options available and a flexibility to change over time with the growing levels of insight.

Screening protocols

Screening protocols should provide a clear statement backed up with adequate facilities. They should set out who is to be considered with regard to HIV testing, who is to do the counselling, what training/support should be available, timing of the test within the reproductive process, handling of test results and, most importantly, continued follow-up in the event of a positive test, raised concerns or continued risk exposure.

Scarce debate is available on timing of the test. Testing at booking clinics, if prior to 12 weeks' gestation, would be ineffective in identifying any woman who has become infected by the same encounter at which she conceived (clearly not a protected sexual encounter) or any sexual encounters thereafter. Continuous testing may be unreasonable and impractical – but may be the only accurate way of monitoring antibody status over time.

Ethics and rights

Few workers examine the ethics of HIV testing studies and the rights of the women. For example Barbacci and colleagues (1991) examined prevalence of HIV in women who agreed to testing and compared such prevalence with women who specifically refused testing. Clearly in this study such refusal was overridden in the pursuit of academic insights.

Women suffer from the unique problem that their antibodies are present in someone else's blood. Thus any blood sample taken from their baby for many months after birth will give a clear indication of maternal HIV antibody status. Numerous epidemiological studies of this nature have been carried out (e.g. Ades et al 1992). Although every effort is made to protect the anonymity of such samples, there remains an ethical question of antibody scrutiny without consent. Indeed, infants themselves are incapable of consent and this doubly confounds the problem.

Testing which may exclude women from treatment if found to be positive must also be unethical.

Opinions of the pregnant women themselves

HIV testing in pregnancy when offered, has varied uptake. Specific factors may account for this such as institution bias (Meadows & Catalan 1991), national policy (Larsson et al 1990), fear of identification (Barbacci et al 1991) and limited choice. Generally the majority of studies show that pregnant women endorse the offer of HIV testing, but are uncertain about personal uptake (Stevens et al 1989). This study also revealed a high proportion of women who would 'mind' if their blood was used for anonymous testing. Where informed counselling has preceded testing with optimal, open choice, uptake is low. When such counselling is missing and large percentages 'accept' testing, return for results is low.

Meadows and Catalan (1991) examined this question in depth. They found that pretest counselling was having an effect on the number of women who had decided to have the test and were actually going ahead with it. Midwives did not appear to be offering accurate pretest counselling in many cases. Only $\frac{1}{3}$ were completely satisfied with the counselling that they received. Those in recognized risk groups were neither counselled nor tested. Much misinformation, especially amongst ethnic minorities, was identified.

Testing in the context of general antenatal care

HIV testing cannot simply be added to the battery of antenatal testing without examining current views on such batteries and the extent to which HIV testing is similar to or different from these procedures. There is a comprehensive data set on the limitations of many mass antenatal screening procedures (Chalmers et al 1989), on the psychological costs of such screening (Farrant 1980, Reading & Cox 1982, Sherr 1984, Marteau et al 1989, Garcia et al 1990, Toxoplasmosis working party 1992) and the efficacy of such procedures (Hall & Chng 1982). HIV testing cannot be viewed as simply another screening test as it not only reflects possible life-threatening illness to the baby, but it also marks maternal (and possibly paternal) infection.

The procedures and processes of the batteries of antenatal tests may pose psychological trauma for pregnant women. Tests are often not explained, consent is lacking, informed choice is limited, feedback and results are haphazard and decision-making around test outcome is fraught (Sherr 1989, Garcia et al 1990)

When HIV testing in pregnant women is studied (e.g. Ciraru Vigneron et al, 1988 ($n = 60$), Sunderland et al 1988 ($n = 177$), Barbacci et al, 1989 ($n = 89$), Holman et al 1989 ($n = 27$), Selwyn et al 1989a ($n = 64$), Selwyn et al 1989b ($n = 191$), Wiznia et al 1989 ($n = 22$), Cowan et al 1990 ($n = 146$), Irion et al 1990 ($n = 47$), Johnstone et al 1989a ($n = 163$), Kiragu et al 1990 ($n = 108$), outcome measures usually centre around test uptake and termination of pregnancy with a paucity of literature on test handling, result handling, emotional consequences, behaviour change and psychological adjustment. A few (e.g. Kiragu et al 1990) look at condom use and some at subsequent reproduction (e.g. Temmerman et al 1990, Sunderland et al 1992).

Women attending antenatal clinics, especially on their first visit, may be exceptionally vulnerable (Oakley 1979). The environment is strange, the experience may be new, the woman may be subjected to many confusing and humiliating procedures (Cartwright 1979), she is concerned for the well-being of herself and her baby (Kumar &

Robson 1978) and may have little say in the process of care (Garcia 1982). Choice may be difficult. Truly informed choice is reliant upon comprehensive and correct knowledge and the subsequent ability to be assertive with her decisions.

Emotional effects of testing are varied, depending on the tests under discussion and the results. The majority of test procedures are associated with negative feelings (Reelick et al 1984, Posner & Vessey 1988, Quilliam 1989, Booth et al 1990). Problems such as false-positive or -negative results can have long-term effects on women, even if in the end accurate results are obtained (Farrant 1980, Marteau et al 1988). False diagnosis has been documented, in other areas, to lead to relationship strain, parenting difficulties and family disruption even when subsequent negative results have been identified (Tymstra 1986). Feedback can reduce such trauma and may have the added advantages of adjusting other maternal behaviours which may be potentially harmful such as alcohol and tobacco consumption (Reading & Cox 1982). Often practitioners overlook the reassuring role of negative results and omit or overlook such feedback. They rely on the notion of 'no news is good news' (Robinson et al 1984). Weinstein (1984) cautions that lack of explanation around negative results may reinforce negative life-styles and promote a sense of invulnerability. This may have the general impact of failure to pursue adequate test follow-up in the future. In the area of HIV it may have potential ramifications in the failure to avoid risk exposure situations.

The questions and myths surrounding HIV testing

HIV testing is often adopted as an immediate panic measure when systems are faced with growing HIV and AIDS cases and limited knowledge on how to react or control the epidemic. Testing must be seen in context, in that it is part of a total strategy and not an end in itself. Often the frightened and numbed first reactions in many world-wide centres have been to attempt to resolve the HIV problem by widespread testing (Sherr 1993a). Such reactions are usually at a price and are often based on the belief of the myths surrounding HIV testing rather than on sound academic or empirical data. These myths include the following.

Does HIV testing reduce risky behaviour in women of reproductive age?

There is little evidence of this, mainly because it is not measured. One of the few studies (Temmerman et al 1990) showed that HIV-positive women who were tested and counselled subsequently showed a higher desire to conceive a subsequent child. Clearly the desire for an uninfected baby was worth the risk for these women. Pregnancy incidence in women who have received counselling and HIV testing does not seem to vary between groups who know they are HIV-positive and those who know they are HIV-negative (Sunderland et al 1988, Selwyn et al 1989a, Cowan et al 1990 and Kiragu et al 1990). Few studies examine sexual behaviour change in pregnant women. Indeed, in a recent overview of the impact of HIV testing and counselling on behaviour change, Higgins and colleagues (1991) examined 11 studies of pregnant women from the USA, Scotland, France, Switzerland and Nairobi. They examined termination as the main outcome measure rather than sexual behaviour change (as was monitored in gay men, heterosexuals, drug users, haemophiliacs and all other groups reviewed). They concluded that serostatus did not affect termination decisions yet they did not control for factors such as how much a baby was wanted in the first place. All the US women were in antenatal clinics suggesting their commitment to the pregnancy. Only a Nairobi study looked at condom use and found no significant effect between seropositive and seronegative women.

Does HIV testing result in termination of pregnancy?

There appears to be no evidence in the literature to support the notion that HIV would be a predictor of termination of pregnancy. Yet a consistent minority do opt for termination and thus a special section in this chapter will consider this topic in detail (see Table 2.3).

Sunderland and co-workers (1988) found that primary prevention of HIV was to be emphasized in the first instance. They found that many seropositive women continued their pregnancy and often presented with subsequent pregnancies. They found the need to examine a broad range of input covering contraception advice, involvement of the index woman and her partner, and help in examining self-fulfilment avenues for women who often find child-bearing as their primary self-fulfilment role and thus any decisions against pregnancy had to incorporate viable alternative life experiences for women.

Workers are often ready to equate HIV and pregnancy with termination. Few examine the corollary of the issue. HIV, at a psychological level, may represent a slur on sex for women. Pregnancy is endorsed and validated by society. Women may actively seek out pregnancy in the presence of HIV to encompass a positive view of their sexuality. HIV itself may represent death or a meaningless future. The search for meaning is a common theme in survival (Marcus & Rosenberg 1989), especially in those who have had their life threatened (e.g. concentration camp survivors). Procreation – the creation of new life – may be one solution which could provide such meaning. Thus there is every possibility that HIV infection in a woman's life may prompt her to actively seek out a pregnancy and new life to provide or enhance meaning to her own existence rather than to end such life.

Does HIV testing impede routine antenatal care?

Fear of imposition of HIV testing may turn women away. Some women have primary risk factors for HIV (such as drug use, poverty, prostitution) which may in themselves be factors which would impede early and regular seeking of antenatal care (Caspe et al 1990). Whalen and associates (1990) found a significant prevalence of HIV in women who were late attenders or first appeared during labour. This study points out the importance of flexibility in programmes where targeted input may need to be incorporated into the postpartum phase.

The US data suggest that drug use which is currently highly associated with HIV infection in parturants may be a barrier to routine antenatal care. This highlights the need to examine policies beyond those of HIV testing, especially those surrounding care and support of drug-using women who account, directly or indirectly, for many of the HIV-positive and pregnant.

Does HIV testing provide reassurance if negative?

Stevens and colleagues (1989) showed significantly lower reassurance provided by HIV tests compared to other antenatal tests. Foldspong and co-workers (1989) studied 779 women in Denmark who were counselled by midwives. They examined the ethical and practical aspects of the test, but provided no follow-up. They recorded test acceptance by 95 women and noted that the effects of the test were a combination of feelings of ambiguity and anxiety. Literature from other areas must be applied to this element of care. Such literature would suggest that test feedback and explanation is important in obviating psychological trauma generally and in addressing problems around invulnerability and entrenched behaviours specifically.

Does HIV testing affect the rates of vertical transmission?

There seems to be little evidence that infant infection is being prevented by protocols of HIV testing. This is hardly surprising given the lack of any intervention or therapeutics. The use of antiviral therapy during pregnancy is now under debate. AZT has been shown to cross the placenta but it is unclear to what extent, both short- and long-term, this affects the developing baby and whether it prevents vertical infection.

LaGuardia (1991) points out that many of the studies now mounted to investigate HIV in pregnancy have the primary aim of protecting the fetus and reducing perinatal transmission with little focus on reducing maternal morbidity and mortality.

Does HIV testing identify HIV infection?

The literature clearly shows that testing can identify some women, but others are missed. Testing itself should not be seen as an end-point but part of a process of care. The rush to screen women has often been ill thought out with more concentration on HIV identification than patient handling.

Barbacci and associates (1991) examined 2724 pregnant women in the USA and compared HIV rates in those who were selectively offered screening to those who were routinely offered screening. They found that routinely offered screening was more likely to identify HIV-infected women. They subsequently examined blood from women who did not volunteer for testing and found that only 53% of HIV-infected women had acknowledged risk factors. Based on these findings the authors advocate routine screening for HIV in antenatal clinics. However, there are some problems with these data. Their rationale for the benefits of knowing HIV status may be open to question. They claim it allows for identification before 20 weeks' gestation which would allow for termination. Many studies have shown a low uptake of termination. Indeed Barbacci's own study shows that of the 81 women identified as HIV-positive, only three terminated – one of which proceeded to a subsequent pregnancy to term. Another benefit claimed is 'preventing subsequent pregnancies'. However, there are scant data to support this. Indeed Sunderland and colleagues (1992) showed a steady group of HIV-positive women with multiple pregnancies. Another benefit claimed by this study was the ability to 'prevent breast-feeding'. This is currently an issue under debate and the dialogue can occur irrespective of knowledge of HIV status. The counselling cost and implications of routine screening may be enormous or simply prohibitive.

Larsson and co-workers (1990) showed in Sweden that universally offered screening led to almost total population uptake. In other centres the focus has been on the counselling and the role of HIV infection in pregnancy and subsequent sexual behaviour rather than simply as an identification technique. In such centres uptake tends to be lower when women consider their individual risks and their emotional preparedness to undergo testing. Long-term behaviour change has not been monitored systematically in any such groups.

Lindsay and colleagues (1991) studied 23 432 women (95% consented to testing and risk behaviour profiles). HIV prevalence was 3.5 per 1000 in 1987 and rose to 5.3 per 1000 in 1989 and 1990. Crack use emerged as the most useful predictor of infection. The majority of HIV-infected women

did not self-acknowledge risk factors and would not have been identified if screening had been targeted. This is one of the few studies which outlines the timing of pretest counselling, which took on average 30 minutes and was supplemented by written material. Counselling was conducted within groups (five to seven participants) which may have hindered individual discussion, clarification or disclosure.

What is the cost of HIV counselling/testing in antenatal care?

The cost is an important factor in all testing protocols which should be initiated as a result of a clear cost–benefit analysis (for the staff, the baby and the mother). The greatest potential cost of an unwanted test is alienation of a client, fear of testing which may result in women not coming for good antenatal care or coming late, or loss of trust, especially if tested without knowledge or consent. Doctors who are uncertain of their ability to do pretest counselling were more likely to refer women (whether of low or high obstetric risk) from GP antenatal care to hospital (Sherr et al 1992).

The specific role of the information given should not be underestimated. Marteau (1989) showed that framing of information affected subsequent decisions. Sherr and co-workers (in preparation) showed that negatively framed information (there is a 25% chance of your baby being vertically infected) was significantly more likely to prompt pregnant women to opt for termination of pregnancy than the same information framed positively (there is a 75% chance of your baby being virus-free).

COUNSELLING

Counselling is a broad term which covers a wide range of activities. Counselling should be optional and some women do not want it or cannot use it. Counselling cannot be imposed on an unwilling recipient. It can operate at four broad levels:

- Communication
- Model of care
- Options
- Therapy.

The notion of counselling has been incorporated into many aspects of HIV and AIDS work ranging from counselling surrounding HIV testing, ongoing counselling for the HIV-positive, and intensive counselling for disease management and adjustment (Green & McCreaner 1989, Miller & Bor 1989, Bor et al 1992). Specific emotional reactions to AIDS-related conditions (such as anxiety, depression, panic, obsessive reactions, relationship trauma, life changes) have been amenable to counselling input.

In the context of HIV testing, pre- and post-test counselling have become accepted adjuncts to the procedure in most Western societies. Studies of gay men are more likely to acknowledge the role of counselling and indeed carry out the process prior to testing. In pregnant women this is often overlooked or poorly reported. Some workers do not distinguish between simply information-giving, informed consent procedures and counselling. Pre-test counselling presumes that the decision to test has not already been made, that women have the option to be tested or not and that no discrimination will be based on the test outcome. If these criteria are not met, then counselling simply has not occurred (Sherr et al 1992). Counselling sessions may need to involve a variety of strands, including patient education and informed consent. Studies which report on 'counselling *for* HIV testing' are deceptive as they reflect the bias of the aims of counselling. If counselling is used to persuade clients to be tested, again true choice may be an elusive concept, and there may be elements of coercion or subtle persuasion which affect whether women proceed to HIV testing. Counselling must involve a process whereby options are examined and a client comes to a personal decision. This is no mean task, especially given the power imbalance often found between doctor and patient.

Counselling around reproductive decision-making prior to pregnancy

Couples who are HIV-positive may well want to think through reproduction generally, and pregnancy specifically. This is especially true with discordant couples where conception may not only pose a possible threat to the fetus but also to the uninfected partner. Indeed, many ethical dilemmas have been raised concerning protocols for handling such couples (Smith et al 1990).

Barbour and colleagues (1989) studied uptake of AIDS counselling and testing at a Scottish family planning clinic over a 3-month period. They found low demand, but a steady request for advice and information from male and female patients. Advertising and awareness was promoted by use of written information (posters, information bookmarks and information cards in all condom packs). There were 17 requests over a 3-month period and seven of these did not proceed to have a test; 14 of the 17 were counselled and three were given information only.

Many couples decided, actively, to proceed with a pregnancy in the presence of known HIV infection. Given that it may take up to 2 years before the serostatus of the infant will be known with certainty, such a couple may need ongoing support for the duration of the pregnancy and the subsequent 2 years.

Counselling around reproductive decision-making once pregnant

Meadows and associates (1991) examined 88 London antenatal attenders. Counselling was carried out by the midwife at the booking appointment. The refusal rate was 83%. Only one-third were satisfied with their counselling.

In some countries HIV infection has been associated with higher risk behaviours such as IV drug use, or sex in the presence of haemophilia and bisexuality. Obviously good history-taking is important if such behaviours are to be addressed. Testing may be targeted if such risk behaviours are prevalent. In other countries no such pointers exist and HIV infection is widespread. Considerations for pretest counselling are summarized in Table 2.1.

Counselling around subsequent reproductive decision-making

Counselling around HIV testing should extend beyond the index pregnancy. Sunderland and colleagues (1988) examined women who learned of their HIV-seropositive status while pregnant, but

Table 2.1   Pretest counselling

Basic factual phase
Risk factors – explore risk exposures
HIV factors – explore whether known, unknown
Opinions – is a pregnancy planned/desired/undesired
Social factors – is she supported, housed, working
Relationship factors – is she alone or in a relationship
Knowledge factors – does she understand the full implications
  of HIV, vertical transmission, pregnancy

Risk assessment
Is she HIV + ve/− ve/or unknown
If − ve or unknown explore risk (sexual/partners/drug
  use/residence/transfusion history etc.)
If + ve explore current medical status, presence or absence of
  opportunistic infections

HIV test
Discuss decision, courses of action, limitations and benefits of
  the test; time of the test

Decision-making
Decision-making is a process, not an event. Talk through all
  alternatives (desired and undesired, positive and negative,
  contemplated and not contemplated)

Thinking through
In the safety of the room, explore possible outcomes and their
  ramifications

Coping
Examine coping strategies for positive and negative outcomes
Explore coping techniques and back-up

Conflict
Discuss conflicts prior to irreversible decisions
Within person – these are dilemmas where a woman may be
  torn between two sets of beliefs (e.g. I do not want to have
  a baby if I am HIV-positive – but I do not believe in abortion)
Between persons – differences of opinion with partner are
  common

Telling
Prior to testing discuss who to tell, when, how and where. This
  allows women to think the problems through rationally prior
  to results. Decision-making immediately after a positive test
  result may be ill thought out

Deciding
Decisions about testing/termination/continuation/medication
  and so on need to be made
Despite the time restraints in pregnancy, make sure the woman
  is not rushed, can think it through and has a gap between
  decision and action for changes and rethinking

Pacing
Woman and her partner need to be clear about the pacing of
  procedures, protocol for handling results, feedback/interim
  structure for any waits or delays

Follow-up
HIV testing and related decisions need long-term follow-up

in time for a legal abortion (legal limit in New York was 24 weeks' gestation) and a second group who conceived a subsequent pregnancy after HIV-positive status had been established. Essentially they found that three out of 18 women elected to terminate their pregnancy, with 15 continuing. Of the 11 who became pregnant after knowledge of HIV status, nine chose to continue their pregnancy. Of note was the fact that in this study one subject avoided hospital or medical staff until after 24 weeks gestation for fear of having to discuss the termination issue. The lesson from this study is to ensure that women realize that termination is not the only option for seropositivity in pregnancy.

Temmerman and associates (1990) studied a group of 1507 mothers in Kenya and 94 HIV-positive women were identified (no refusal rate was given). A control group was gathered from consecutive subsequent deliveries. One-year follow-up was available for 57% of the HIV-positive and 59.6% of the control group. Condom use was low for both groups and no significant differences between the HIV-positive women and the control group were noted despite counselling. Of the HIV-positive women, 15 (62%) expressed a desire to have many more children to ensure that some were healthy. The pregnancy rate at 1 year follow-up was 16.7% (4/24) of the HIV-positive women and 18.2% (6/33) for seronegative women. Furthermore, only 37% informed their partner of their HIV status.

Batter (Zaire) studied 365 HIV-positive women and reported that 30% did not tell their partners. For 68% of the HIV-positive women, HIV disease and allied risks would not prevent future pregnancy plans.

Counselling around fertility and gynaecological investigations

In some clinics couples facing infertility treatments are requested to undergo HIV testing prior to treatment. Semen donors are also required to undergo HIV testing since HIV can be transmitted during artificial insemination by donor treatments. Women undergoing such procedures need to understand possible risks and to be informed of the local procedures to protect against such infection.

Gynaecological problems may be possible complications of HIV disease. Such problems do not constitute AIDS-defining illness but this is a question currently under debate. Gynaecological manifestations may hinder fertility and, until the natural history of HIV infection in women is known, clear counselling and treatment may be difficult to deliver. Whatever the cause, failure to conceive a desired pregnancy may be traumatic and such couples may require support and help.

Counselling challenges for staff

More and more counselling is being incorporated into the working life of health care workers who do not have mental health training. Counselling is often challenging and difficult for such individuals. Short-term training can be effective in increasing competence and skills (Sherr & McCreaner 1989) but may be limited in terms of deeper level interventions (Sherr et al 1991). The counselling issues surrounding HIV in pregnancy may be particularly challenging for midwifery, obstetrical and general practice personnel (Sherr et al 1992, Sherr 1987).

As HIV testing becomes more widespread, training will become vital. Such training may not be limited to HIV pre- and post-test counselling. It may need to extend to address the fact that many HIV issues concentrate around drug use (Mulleady 1992), sexuality (Ostrow 1990) or haemophilia (Miller & Bor 1989). HIV itself can cross the blood–brain barrier and cognitive impairment, though uncommon, is documented (Maj 1990). Clearly, counselling a cognitively impaired individual or one under the influence of drugs or alcohol (Plant 1993) adds an additional dimension to the skill levels required.

Counselling around termination of pregnancy

HIV testing is often offered on the basis that the woman will consider terminating the pregnancy if found to be positive. Studies examining the endorsement of this notion show that medics endorse it highly (Sherr et al 1992), pregnant women without HIV infection endorse it somewhat (Buckett et al 1988) and pregnant women with HIV endorse it the least. Overall studies have shown that pregnancy in the presence of known

HIV may lead to termination, but this is not inevitable and for the most part women continue their pregnancies. Of those who do terminate, many proceed to a subsequent pregnancy at some later stage. Although HIV has not been found to be a predictor of termination, it may be cited as a reason. In some studies where it has been associated with termination of the index pregnancy it has not correlated with subsequent fertility. The best predictor of termination to date has been the presence of a previous termination of pregnancy. Numerous studies examining this question are summarized in Table 2.2.

Sunderland and colleagues (1992) report on one of the few studies which gives details of the counselling protocols which provided for extensive pre- and post-test counselling, with a policy of no directive recommendations. During follow-up after index pregnancy, 19 of 101 HIV-negative (18.8%) and 20 of 87 HIV-positive (23%) women had one or more live births. Overall they concluded that HIV knowledge was insufficient to prompt termination or not to contemplate subsequent pregnancy. Behaviour change was noted in other areas, as pregnancy was shown as an incentive to stop drug-taking.

Johnstone and co-workers (1990) noted that termination was common in his sample irrespective of HIV status and noted that 44 women were aware that they were HIV-positive when they became pregnant (21 of whom went on to have a termination). Thus, knowledge of HIV was not even an effective trigger for contraception. Decisions were rarely altered from the original intention, especially when pregnancy was desired. Factors associated with continuation of pregnancy were studied in the 38 women who continued their pregnancies in the presence of HIV. These included:

— current good health
— desire to have a child
— feelings against termination
— normative judgments based on knowledge of women who had babies.

It is commonly assumed that termination of pregnancy, whatever the circumstance, is associated with considerable emotional reactions. There are few prospective studies which have systematically evaluated this and no such studies for HIV-positive

Table 2.2   Termination of pregnancy in the presence of HIV

Study	Place	n	Gestation (% term)	Comments
Sunderland et al 1988	New York	177		No significant differences between HIV + ve and − ve women
Sunderland et al 1992	New York	108 − ve 98 + ve	2.9% 18.8%	23% of positives subsequently had a pregnancy
Selwyn et al 1989a	New York	64		No significant differences in termination rates
Johnstone et al 1990	Edinburgh	163	12.9%	9/21 stated HIV as a main reason (4 had AIDS); Of 10 who terminated in HIV + ve well identified in pregnancy, 9 had previous termination
Barbacci et al 1989	Baltimore	89	20%	16% became pregnant after informed of HIV
Ciraru Vigneron et al 1988	Paris	60	38% (n = 23)	
Kiragu et al 1990	Nairobi	108		
Irion 1989	Geneva	47	28%	
Holman et al 1989	New York	27	15%	
Wiznia et al 1989	New York	22	27%	Proportion of these went on to subsequent pregnancy
Lindsay et al 1990		57	17.5% (n = 10)	Over 3 years' study
Goldberg et al 1992	Scotland	Antenatal terminations		0.13% HIV + ve 0.85% HIV + ve
Stratton et al 1990	USA 49 centres	—	15%	
Griscelli 1989	France	843	45%	
Irion et al 1990	Switzerland	'low'		HIV knowledge no influence on pregnancy decisions

women. The general literature on termination with follow-up has shown that short-term psychological reactions were common but severe long-term difficulties were unusual. Few long-term problems have been identified (Greer et al 1976, Illsley & Hall 1976, Donnai et al 1981). Scant attention is paid to possible psychological benefits from termination. Shusterman (1979) found some women expressing relief after termination. For many women, emotional crisis surrounds decision-making and short-term follow-up, which is when counselling and support should be optimum.

Marcus (1979) found that counselling prior to termination was beneficial although on follow-up subsequent contraception and termination problems were still apparent. Few women have longer-term problems but it is unclear to what extent this is as a result of prevention, failure to report, or the limited length of follow-up in the studies. The proportion of problems seems to be in the region of one in ten. No studies of long-term follow-up of HIV-related terminations have yet been done. HIV and AIDS may pose an extra factor which may affect such findings. Dunlop (1978) and Shusterman (1979) have recounted risk factors for sub-

sequent problems which may well apply to HIV-positive women. These are summarized in Table 2.3.

Thus, social support, supportive decisions of others and the opportunity to discuss and reflect are advantageous ingredients to buffer against future emotional disruption. The counselling literature at the time of termination would highlight the importance of opportunities to examine:

— the current pregnancy
— future safe sex
— future contraception
— future conceptions.

Once the decision to terminate has been taken, the literature on surgical procedures and psychological preparation may ease the passage for the HIV-positive women. There is a common association between anxiety and surgery before, during and after admission (Johnston 1980). Preoperative emotional state (including anxiety, cognitive preparation and satisfaction) may interact with postoperative outcome (Janis 1970, Johnston & Carpenter 1980). Interventions have shown the beneficial impact of information in a variety of

Table 2.3 Risk factors for subsequent problems in termination

Pressure	termination decisions surrounded by pressure or coercion from a variety of sources such as medical, family, spouse or peers
Psychiatric history	previous psychiatric history (which highlights the importance of good medical and psychiatric history for all)
Medical problems	Dunlop noted that terminations prompted by 'medical reasons' may create future problems either caused by the stress of facing up to the medical problem or stress if it recurs. HIV infection which is an infection for life and deteriorates over time may well have similar effects
Pregnancy reaction	negative emotional reaction on discovering the pregnancy has been a predictor of subsequent distress
Social support	low social support, poor relationships and low partner intimacy have been associated with poor prognosis. Long-term problems may be associated with the termination itself, the relationship difficulties or both. Social support factors are particularly relevant in the case of HIV where an ill partner or a bereaved partner may have reduced social and emotional support directly because of AIDS
Regret	Shusterman (1979) recorded that regret with termination decision was a predictor of poor outcome. This would suggest that coercion is counter-productive, and time for reflection and decision turn-around should be incorporated into care packages

forms (Ley 1988 review). It may be hard to extrapolate from this literature to HIV circumstances, as studies have failed to utilize systematic input measures (which have included instruction booklets, written information, verbal information, communications, brief psychotherapy, counselling, instructions, role-play, sensitization and procedural information); have investigated considerably differing operative procedures (gynaecological surgery (Johnston & Carpenter 1980), laparoscopy (Wallace 1984), ultrasound scanning (Reading & Cox 1982) and labour (Enkin 1982 review)); and looked at varied outcome measures (including pain ratings, satisfaction, analgesia intake, length of hospital stay, psychological well-being, anxiety, medication and psychosocial adjustment). Despite such short-comings the general findings show an overall beneficial impact of intervention (Matthews & Ridgeway 1981), which is enhanced if they are tailored to meet individual coping styles (Mangan 1983, O'Sullivan & Steptoe 1986).

Continuation of pregnancy

Counselling around HIV testing in pregnancy must extend to the provision of support for those who test positive and decide to continue with their pregnancy. This should address the general emotional needs of a pregnancy and the added special demands (if any) imposed by the knowledge of HIV and AIDS.

There is a wide psychological, sociological and medical literature on the impact of pregnancy which is of particular relevance to a pregnancy in the presence of HIV. Pregnancy has often been viewed as a time of stress yet Elliott (1984) charts some of the positive mental health aspects associated with pregnancy which are often overlooked. To many women pregnancy is an enjoyable experience and may have particular personal, societal and cultural meanings – no less so in the presence of HIV infection.

When psychological problems are catalogued for pregnancy, these include intense levels of anxiety and depression. These problems are often correlated with previous obstetric abnormalities (Davids 1961, McDonald 1963, Crandon 1979) and with previous miscarriage (Kumar & Robson 1978). As HIV may present such stressors, such psychological difficulties may well present so carers need to be aware and available. Antenatal anxiety has been unrelated to labour complications (Beck 1980, Astbury 1980). Crandon (1979) described links between antenatal anxiety and birth outcome. However, this was a poorly controlled study and it seems possible that the anxiety was related to medical conditions which were responsible for the poor outcome rather than the anxiety in isolation. Again, as HIV may possibly result in vertical transmission, such problems may be present for HIV-positive women. Some studies have shown poorer outcome for HIV-positive babies who are born prematurely. Although cause and effect cannot be ruled out, it certainly does point to the need for high-level antenatal care.

Postpartum follow-up should provide support for physical and mental health needs of the mother together with the added trauma of a child who may be possibly infected or ill. The early years are surrounded by extensive uncertainty which cannot be resolved until clear HIV status is confirmed, illness emerges or new techniques (such as polymerase chain reaction tests) can ascertain infection status. There is a wide range of problems which an HIV-positive mother may face (Sherr et al 1992). These include how and when to tell the child and/or the family, the trauma of continued HIV testing and living with uncertainty, distress at infant infection/illness and some of the day to day difficulties involved in parenting in the face of parental or infant illness. These may be small-scale, such as difficulties with medication adherence or constant hospital visits, or they may be enormous involving facing up to bereavement, death or dying. In all of this, whatever the outcome for the child, the mother and father will need to address planning for the future of their child or children when their own health deteriorates. Counselling issues include the following.

Labour/delivery

Preparation for labour and delivery in the presence of HIV should be made. These include a dialogue on a variety of issues such as pain management, infection control (Minkoff 1989), emotional support (Sherr et al 1992) and routine care (Brierly 1987).

Feeding

One of the first decisions a new mother has to confront is mode of feeding – breast or bottle. There is a growing literature, which at times may be confusing. A psychological model of decision-making fits in well with such dilemmas. Here the mother needs to understand the basic factual information to date (some of which is in itself unclear), to explore the possible decisions she could make, the effects of these and to finally decide on a pathway which is acceptable to her. The factual information is changing rapidly as new studies come to the fore. Counsellors need to be updated.

HIV has been isolated in breast milk (Thiry et al 1985, Ruff et al 1992). The implications in breast-feeding are less clear (Baumslag 1987). Early studies were confined to case descriptions where HIV-negative status during pregnancy could be established as well as subsequent HIV exposure during lactation. The studies were few (about 10 world-wide – Ziegler et al 1985, Lederman 1992) and were problematic (small sample size, unusual circumstances and, of most importance, a newly infected and thus viraemic mother). No corresponding data on postnatally infected mothers who did not transmit HIV to their babies exist and data for the HIV-positive well mother have only been systematically gathered very recently. Dunn and colleagues (1992) have provided a comprehensive review, but the issue is still far from resolved. Medical opinion based on changing data may conflict with emotional factors on which women may base their feeding decisions.

Dunn and associates (1992) calculated that on the four studies of postnatal acquisition the estimated risk of vertical transmission was 29%. These figures are of limited use in the counselling situation given that new infection cannot be picked up on current tests. Of the five studies of prenatal infection, additional risk of transmission over and above in utero or delivery exposure was calculated at 14%.

The few prospective studies do give cause for concern. Hira and associates (1990) identified 19 mothers who were tested HIV-negative at delivery and HIV-positive at 1 year postpartum follow-up as part of a large cohort of 1720 mothers in a prospective study. Three children from the 19 women also tested HIV-positive. Van de Perre and colleagues (1991) studied 212 mothers in Kigali who were HIV-negative at the birth of their index baby. Of those tested and providing 3-monthly stored samples, six mothers converted before 3 months and 10 from 3 to 18 months. At 36-month follow-up after maternal conversion. five out of nine babies converted. The additional· role of breast abscesses cannot be ignored (van de Perre et al 1992), and the possible infection by the mother from her baby during breast-feeding has also been documented (Pokrovsky et al 1990). Other small-scale studies have come up with similar findings. These are summarized in Table 2.4.

Table 2.4 Breast-feeding and HIV risk

Author	Location	Findings
ECS 1992	Europe	32% transmitted if fed, 14% if never
Hutto et al	Miami USA	28% if ever, 33% if never
Blanche et al	France	44% if ever, 17% if never
Kind et al	Switzerland	15% if ever, 16% if never
Ryder et al	Zaire	20% if ever, 0% if never
	Australia	50% if ever, 17% if never

The studies are few and it seems that the risk is additional. Decision-making must be made in the context of background infection, alternative feeding methods, maternal wishes, mother–baby factors and informed decisions.

Multiple births

Some pregnancies will be multiple. Parents may need preparation for possible dual infection, and also the possibility of one twin born HIV-positive and another virus-free. Factual knowledge on twins is being gathered in the multicentre twin study which is showing an increased risk of infection for the first-born twin (Dulliege 1992).

Literature on multiple birth and bereavement should be brought in. Parents may need preparation for handling an ill sibling and a well one. Some early data (Harris 1990) have documented the effects on siblings in terms of behaviour. Datta (1991) has shown an exposure effect (not repeated in other studies). Developmental difficulties may arise directly as a virus effect, or indirectly as an environmental effect due to limitations imposed (economic, social and the like) in the presence of an ill mother, and perhaps compounded in the presence of an ill sibling.

Parenting in the face of HIV

Longer-term counselling may be focused on help with the many parenting problems encountered in the presence of HIV and AIDS in the family (Gibb & Duggan 1992). The issues are multiple and include:

- Uncertainty of the future
- Illness and the distress of loss of developmental milestones
- Separation through hospitalization or death
- Hospitalizations and their associated disruption and trauma
- Bereavement and its long-term (often multiple) ramifications
- Death and dying
- Telling others of HIV and AIDS
- Social support which is often limited in the aura of secrecy which surrounds AIDS
- Guilt over vertical transmission
- Treatment dilemmas
- Multiple infection within one family
- Economic/social strain
- Orphans

Counselling around HIV testing and the issue of safe sex

Counselling around HIV testing is not simply about whether to take the test or not, but also has a clear prevention role. As such, whether the woman proceeds to test or not, the counselling may raise a number of sexual behaviour and risk involvement issues. Reproductive decision-making extends beyond the simple notions of pregnancy and termination. It involves a wider ability to reproduce and regulate fertility; it should ensure safe passage through pregnancy; and sexual relationships should be enabled with freedom from fears of unwanted pregnancies and disease (WHO 1988). Thus the notions of safe sex enter the arena of reproductive counselling for HIV.

Unprotected sex, itself a risk for HIV transmission, is the very mode of conception. After pregnancy few women are counselled on safer sex techniques and it is rare for women to report usage of condoms while pregnant. Little counselling is given to postpartum women. In some societies there is a prohibition on sex during lactation, whilst in others this does not exist. Some condone extra-marital sex during lactation and some women see lactation as a contraception and do not consider alternatives whilst breast-feeding.

Information and availability may be a necessary but not sufficient precondition for condom use. From early on in the epidemic, women found it difficult to persuade their partners to initiate and sustain condom use, whether it was with sexual

Table 2.5 Psychological effects of HIV

Trauma of testing	decision to test, wait for results, receipt of results
Anxiety	concerns about: life threats/the unknown/uncertainty/failing health/others finding out
Depression	low mood; question the meaning of life/poor (inevitable?) prognosis lack of cure life changes imposed by HIV inward anger, guilt, despair or disappointment
Panic	sudden uncontrollable attacks body checking/obsessive compulsive behaviour misreading panic symptoms as AIDS symptoms
Suicide	suicide in pregnancy is very rare (Kleiner & Greston 1984) no HIV/pregnancy suicides have been documented predictors in HIV populations are usually previous suicidal history and medical decline attempts are more common than completions suicidal thoughts are common and should be discussed which will be reassuring
Psychosexual problems	common ranging from abstinence, rejection, loss of libido, fear of infecting loved one, powerless rape may be implicated in infection
Psychosocial problems	coping and adjustment should be seen in the light of possible economic hardship, social deprivation, refugee or migrant problems and low social support
Drug use	highly prevalent in European and American samples directly through use or indirectly through sexual partner
Cognitive impairment	low incidence usually a late-stage complication fear of cognitive impairment often acute mood variables may hinder cognitive functioning
Gynaecological problems	must be monitored and checked frequently examinations are embarrassing and difficult for many women

partners who were paid (Mann et al 1987) or with regular partners (Glaser et al 1989). Kamenga and colleagues (1991) showed that with discordant couples, condom use could be enhanced by counselling, but the detailed examination of the statistics showed higher use when the male was uninfected (and thus at risk of infection) than when the female was uninfected and possibly at risk.

PSYCHOLOGICAL EFFECTS OF HIV

Finally, any discussion on HIV testing for women of reproductive age must consider the psychological effects of HIV infection generally (Miller 1990). These encompass not only the test procedure, but also the long-term ramifications of HIV and AIDS. Such psychological effects have been monitored in general without specific study of women of reproductive age. Yet there is no evidence that they should not experience similar effects, often enhanced by the presence of a pregnancy, a baby, or multiple infection. Psychological factors are summarized in Table 2.5 which sets out the range of emotional factors associated with HIV infection. These factors cover the trauma of HIV testing, anxiety, depression and panic. Suicide is a theme under constant review with HIV-positive individuals, as are psychosexual and psychosocial problems, drug use and AIDS-associated cognitive impairment (AIDS dementia). The role of gynaecological problems has been studied and there is a growing database on this topic.

CONCLUSION

This overview has attempted to highlight the complexity of HIV as an issue for women of reproductive age. There are no corresponding data on fathers, who undoubtedly play a role but who are simply overlooked in the empirical and theoretical studies. HIV testing in women of reproductive age is a complex issue. There are many unanswered questions surrounding the way such testing should be carried out, the counselling demands surrounding the test itself, and the wide ramifications of HIV if identified at this stage. As social stigma decreases, medical interventions increase and prophylax is becomes more established, HIV testing may well increase. This is all the more reason to take into account the counselling issues. These should be integrated into holistic care policies, they should anticipate the positive as well as the negative outcomes, and should not function in isolation from reproductive care generally.

REFERENCES

Ades A, Parker S, Cubitt D, Davison C, Holland F, Berry T, Hjelm M, Wilcox A H, Peckham C 1992 Two methods for assessing the risk factor composition of the HIV 1 epidemic in heterosexual women southeast England 88–91. AIDS 6: 1031–1036

Astbury J 1980 Labour pain – the role of childbirth education information expectation. In: Peck C, Wallace M (eds) Problems in pain. Pergamon Press, Oxford

Barbacci M, Chaisson R, Anderson J et al 1989 Knowledge of HIV serostatus and pregnancy decisions. V International Conference on AIDS, Montreal, Abstr BMP 10

Barbacci M, Quinn T, Kline R et al 1989 Failure of targeted screening to identify HIV + ve pregnant women. Presented at V International Conference on AIDS, Montreal, Abstr MBP5

Barbacci M, Repke J T, Chaisson R 1991 Routine prenatal screening for HIV infection. Lancet 337: 709–711

Barbour R, Macintyre S, McIlwaine G, Wilson E 1989 Uptake of AIDS counselling and testing at a Scottish family planning clinic. Br J Fam Planning 15: 61–62

Barbour R S 1990 Fathers – the emergence of a new consumer group. In: Garcia J, Kilpatrick R, Richards M (eds) The politics of maternity care. Clarendon Press, Oxford

Beavor A 1993 AIDS Care 5(2): (in press)

Beck A, Rush A, Shaw B, Emery C 1979 Cognitive therapy of depression. Wiley, Chichester

Berrier et al 1991 HIV/AIDS education in a prenatal clinic: an assessment. AIDS Educ Prev 3(2): 100–117

Blanche S, Rouzioux C, Guhard Moscato M L et al 1989 A prospective study of infants born to women seropositive for human immunodeficiency virus type 1. N Engl J Med 320: 1643–1648

Boomslag N 1987 Breast feeding and HIV infection Lancet 2: 401

Booth C, Safer M, Leventhal H 1990 Use of physician services following participation in a cardiac screening programme. Public Health Rep 101: 315–319

Bor R, Miller R, Goldman E 1992 Theory and practice of HIV counselling – a systemic approach. Cassell Publishers, London

Brierly J 1987 Human immunodeficiency virus. The challenge of a lifetime. Midwives Chronicle Nursing Notes II Sup x–xiii

Buckett W M Conlon M H, Luesley D M, Lawton F G 1988 Attitudes of a multiracial antenatal population to HIV screening Br Med J 296(6622): 643

Cartwright A 1979 The dignity of labour. Tavistock, London

Caspe et al 1990 VI International Conference on AIDS, San Francisco, Abstr SC 667

CDSC 1991 Centres for Disease Surveillance and Control, Colindale

CDSC 1992 Centres for Disease Surveillance and Control, Report 1992

CDR reports, Centres for Disease Surveillance and Control, Colindale UK 1992

Chalmers I, Enkin M, Keirse M J 1989 Effective care in pregnancy and childbirth Oxford University Press, Oxford

Chrystie I, Palmer S, Kenney A, Banatvala J 1992 HIV seroprevalence among women attending antenatal clinics in London. Lancet 339: 364

Ciraru Vigneron N et al 1988 (Ciraru-Vigneron N, Nguyen R, Tan Ung et al 1987) Prospective study for HIV infection among high risk pregnant women. Presented at III International AIDS Conference Abstr 4627

Cowan J E, Kotloff K, Alger L, Watkins C, Johnson J 1990 Reproductive choices of women at risk of HIV infection. Sixth International Conference on AIDS, San Francisco, Abstr SC 708

Crandon A J 1979 Maternal anxiety and obstetric complications. J Psychosomatic Res 23: 109–111

Datta P 1991 Presented at the 7th Int AIDS Conference, Florence, Italy, Abstr THC 611

Davids A 1961 Anxiety, pregnancy and childbirth abnormalities. J Cons Psychol 25: 76–77

Donnai P, Charles N, Harris R 1981 Attitudes of patients after genetic termination of pregnancy. Br Med J 282: 621–622

Dulliege 1992 International AIDS Conference, Amsterdam

Dunlop J Z 1978 Counselling patients requesting an abortion. Practitioner 220: 847–855

Dunn D, Newell M, Ades A, Peckham C 1992 Risk of HIV type 1 transmission through breastfeeding. Lancet 340: 585–588

Elliott S A 1984 Pregnancy and after. In: Rachman S (ed) Contributions to Medical Psychology Pergamon Press, Oxford, vol 3

Enkin M 1982 Antenatal classes. In: Enkin M, Chalmers I (eds) Effectiveness and satisfaction in antenatal care. Spastics International Medical Books, London

European Collaborative Study 1991 Children born to women with HIV-1 infection. Natural history and risk of transmission. Lancet 337: 253–260

European Collaborative Study 1992 Risk factors for mother to child transmission of HIV 1. Lancet 339: 1007–1012

Farrant W 1980 Stress after amniocentesis for high serum alphafeto-protein concentrations. Br Med J 2: 452

Foldspong et al 1989

Garcia J 1982 Women's views of antenatal care. In: Enkin M, Chalmers I (eds) Effectiveness and satisfaction in antenatal care. Spastics International Medical Publications/Heineman Medical Books, London, p 81–92

Garcia J, Kilpatrick R, Richards M 1990 The politics of maternity care. Clarendon Press, Oxford

Gibb D, Duggan C 1992 AIDS and children (editorial). GU Med

Glaser J, Strange J, Rosati D 1989 Heterosexual HIV transmission among the middle class. Arch Intern Med 149: 645–649

Goldberg D, MacKinnon H, Smith R, Patel N, Scrimgeour J, Inglis J, Peutherer J, Urquhart G, Emslie J, Covell R, Reid D 1992 Prevalence of HIV among childbearing women and women having termination of pregnancy multi steering group study. Br Med J 304: 1082–1085

Green J, McCreaner A 1989 Counselling in AIDS and HIV Infection. Blackwell Scientific Publications, Oxford

Greer H S, Lal S, Lewis S C et al 1976 Psychosocial consequences of therapeutic abortion. Kings termination study II. Br J Psychiatry 128: 74–79

Griscelli C (1989) Diagnosis of HIV in infants. V International Conference on AIDS, Montreal, Abstr TBO 20

Hall M, Chng P K 1982 Antenatal care in practice. In: Enkin M, Chalmers I (eds) Effectiveness and satisfaction in antenatal care. Spastics International Medical Publications/Heineman Medical Books, London

Harris A 1990 Treating the non infected sibling: an AIDS dilemma. VI International Conference on AIDS, San Francisco, Abstr THD 123

Higgins D, Galavott C, O'Reilly K, Schnell D, Moore M,

Rugg D, Johnson R 1991 Evidence for the effects of HIV antibody counseling and testing on risk behaviors. JAMA 266 (17): 2419–2429

Hira S K, Kamanga J, Bhat G J, Mwale C, Tembo G, Luo N, Perine P L 1989 Perinatal transmission of HIV I in Zambia. Br Med J 299: 1250–1252

Hira S, Mangrola U, Mwale C et al 1990 Apparent vertical transmission of HIV type 1 by breast feeding in Zambia J Pediatr 117: 421–424

Holman S, Sunderland A, Berthard M et al 1989 Prenatal HIV counselling and testing. Clin Obstet Gynecol

Hutto C, Parks W, Lai S et al 1991 A hospital based prospective study of perinatal infection with HIV 1. J Pediatr 118: 347–353

Illsley R, Hall M H 1976 Psychosocial aspects of abortion: a review of issues and needed resarch. WHO Bull 53: 85–105

Ippolito G, Stegagno M, Angeloni P, Guzzanti E 1990 Anonymous HIV testing on newborns. JAMA 263: 36

Irion O 1989 Despistage systematique des anticorps contre le VIH chez la femme enceinte: seroprevalence, acceptation et utilite. WHO Paris conference, J1

Irion O, Rapin R, Taban F, Beguin F 1990 Voluntary screening for HIV infection in all pregnant women. 6th Annual International AIDS Conference, San Francisco

Johnston M 1980 Anxiety in surgical patients Psychol Med 10: 145–152

Johnston M, Carpenter L 1980 Relationship between pre operative and post operative state. Psychol Med 10: 361–370

Johnstone F, McCallum L, Brettle R, Burns S, Peutherer J 1989a Testing for HIV in pregnancy – 3 years experience in Edinburgh City. Scot Med J 34: 561–563

Johnstone F, Brettle R, MacCallum L, Mok J, Peutherer J, Burns S 1989b Women's knowledge of their HIV antibody state – its effect on their decision whether to continue the pregnancy. Br Med J 300: 23–24

Kamenga M, Ryder R, Jingu M, Mbuyi N, Mbu L, Behets F, Brown C, Heyward W 1991 Evidence of marked sexual behaviour change associated with low HIV 1 seroconversion in 149 married couples with discordant HIV 1 serostatus – experience at an HIV counselling center in Zaire. AIDS 5: 61–67

Kind C, Brindle B, Wyler C et al 1992 Epidemiology of vertically transmitted HIV 1 infection in Switzerland: results of a nationwide prospective study. Eur J Pediatr 151: 442–448

Kiragu D, Temmerman M, Wamola I, Plummer F, Piot P 1990 Counselling of women with HIV infection – effect on contraceptive practice and pregnancy. Presented at the Sixth International Conference on AIDS, San Francisco

Kleiner G, Greston W M 1984 Suicide in pregnancy. John Wright Publishers, Bristol

Kumar R, Robson K 1978 Neurotic disturbance during pregnancy and the puerperium. In: Sandler M (ed) Mental illness in pregnancy and the puerperium. Oxford University Press, Oxford

La Guardia K 1991 AIDS and reproductive helath: women's perspectives. In: Chen L, Amor J S, Segal S J (eds) AIDS and women's reproductive health. Plenum Press, New York

Larrsson G, Spangberg L, Lindgren S, Bohlin A B 1990 Screening for HIV in pregnant women – a study of maternal opinion. AIDS Care 2 (3): 223–228

Lederman S 1992 Estimating infant mortality from HIV and other causes in breast feeding and bottle feeding populations. Pediatrics 89: 290–296

Lindsay M K, Peterson H B, Feng T I, Slade B A 1989 Routine antepartum human immunodeficiency virus infection screening in an inner city population. Obstet Gynecol. (1): 289–294

Lindsay M, Peterson H, Willis M et al 1990 Incidence and prevalence of HIV infection in a prenatal population undergoing routine voluntary HIV screening 1987–90

Lindsay M, Adefris W, Peterson H, Williams H, Johnson J, Klein L 1991 Obstetric and gynecological determinants of acceptance of routine voluntary HIV testing in an inner city prenatal population. 78 (4): 678–680

McDonald R L 1963 The role of emotional factors in obstetric complications. Psychosom Med 30: 22–24

Maj M 1990 Organic mental disorders in HIV 1 infection. AIDS 4: 831–840

Mann J 1992 Plenary address, International AIDS Conference, Amsterdam

Mann J, Quinn T C, Piot P 1987 Condom use and HIV infection among prostitutes in Zaire. N Engl J Med 316: 345

Mangan 1983

Marcus R J 1979 Evaluating abortion counselling. Dimensions in Health Service, August 16–18

Marcus P, Rosenberg A 1989 In: Sherr L (ed) Death dying and bereavement. Blackwell Scientific Publications, Oxford, p 122–145

Marteau T M 1989 Framing of information – its influence upon decisions of doctors and patients Br J Soc Psychol 28: 89–94

Marteau T, Kidd J, Cook R et al 1988 Screening for Downs syndrome. Br Med J 297: 1469

Marteau R T, Johnston M, Shaw R, Michie S, Kidd J, New M 1989 The impact of prenatal screening and diagnostic tests upon the cognitions, emotions and behaviour of pregnant women. J Psychosom Res 33: 7–16

Matthews A, Ridgeway V 1981 Personality and surgical recovery: a review. Br J Clini Psychol 20: 243–260

Meadows J, Catalan J 1991 Who consents to HIV antibody testing and why? Presented at the London Conference of the British Psychological Society, City University

Meadows J, Jenkinson S, Catalan J, Gazzard B 1990 Voluntary HIV testing in the antenatal clinic: differing uptake rates for individual counselling midwives. AIDS Care 2: 229–234

Miller D 1990 Diagnosis and treatment of acute psychological problems related to HIV infection and Disease. In: Ostrow D (ed) Behavioural aspects of AIDS. Plenum Press, New York, p187–204.

Miller R, Bor R 1989 AIDS: a guide to clinical counselling. Science Press, London.

Minkoff H 1989 AIDS in pregnancy. Curr Probl Obstet Gynecol Fertil, Nov: 206–227

Moatti J P, Gales C, Seror V, Papiernik E, Henrion R 1990 Social acceptability of HIV screening among pregnant women. AIDS Care 2 (3): 213–222

Mulleady G 1992 HIV and AIDS in drug users. Blackwell Scientific Publications, Oxford

Novello A C 1991 Women and HIV infection. JAMA 265: 1805

Oakley A, 1979 Becoming a mother. Martin Robertson, Oxford

Ostrow D 1990 Behavioral aspects of AIDS. Plenum Medical, New York

O'Sullivan J, Steptoe A 1986 Monitoring and blunting coping styles in women prior to surgery. Br J Clin Psychol 25 (2): 143–144

Peckham C Newell M L 1990 HIV-1 infection in mothers and babies. AIDS Care 2 (3): 205–212

Plant M 1993 Alcohol and AIDS. In: Sherr L (ed) Heterosexual AIDS. Harwood Publications (in press)

Pokrovsky V V, Kuznetsova I, Eramova I 1990 Transmission of HIV infection from an infected infant to his mother by breast feeding. VI Int AIDS Conference, Abstr TH C 48

Posner T, Vessey M 1988 Prevention of cervical cancer: the patient's view. King Edwards Hospital Fund for London, London

Quilliam S 1989 Positive smear. Penguin, London

Reading A, Cox D 1982 The effects of ultrasound examination on maternal anxiety levels. J Behav Medi 5: 237–247

Reelick N, De Haes W, Schuurman J 1984 Psychological side-effects of the mass screening on cervical cancer. Soc Sci Med 18: 1089–1093

Robinson J, Hibbard B, Laurence K 1984 Anxiety during a crisis – emotional effects of screening for neural tube defects. J Psychosom Res 28: 163–169

Ruff A, Coberly J, Burnley A et al 1992 Prevalence of HIV in breast milk. VIII International Conference on AIDS, Amsterdam, July, Abstr TH C 1523

Ryder R, Manzila T, Baende E et al 1991 Evidence from Zaire that breast feeding by HIV 1 seropositive mothers is not a major route for perinatal HIV 1 transmission but does decrease morbidity. AIDS 5: 709–714

Selwyn P A, Carter R J, Schoenbaum E E et al 1989a Knowledge of HIV antibody status and decision to continue or terminate pregnancy among intravenous drug users. JAMA. 261: 3567–3571

Selwyn P A, Schoenbaum E E, Davenny K et al 1989b Prospective study of HIV infection and pregnancy outcomes in intravenous drug users. JAMA 261: 1289–1294

Sherr L 1984 Role of information and feedback in anxiety and satisfaction. York Conference, Society for Neonatal and Reproductive Psychology, British Psychological Society

Sherr L 1987 The impact of AIDS in obstetrics on obstetric staff. J Reprod Infant Psychol 5: 87–96

Sherr L 1989 Anxiety and communications in ante-natal care. Unpublished PhD Thesis, Warwick University

Sherr L 1991 HIV and AIDS in mothers and babies. Blackwell Scientific Publications, Oxford

Sherr L 1993a Ante-natal testing. In: Squire C (ed) The psychology of women and AIDS. Sage Press (in press)

Sherr L 1993b Counselling challenges for women with HIV infection and AIDS. In Moorey S, Hodes M (eds) Psychological treatment in human disease and illness. British Journal of Psychiatry, Gaskell Publications (in press)

Sherr L, Hedge B 1989 On becoming a mother – counselling implications for mothers and fathers. WHO Paris conference D 17

Sherr L, Hedge B 1990 The impact and use of written leaflets as a counselling alternative in mass antenatal HIV screening. AIDS Care 2 (3): 235–245

Sherr L, McCreaner A 1989 Summary evaluation of the national AIDS counselling training unit in the UK. Couns Psychol Q 2 (1): 21–32

Sherr L, Davey T, Strong C 1991 Counselling implications of anxiety and depression in AIDS and HIV infection. A pilot study. Couns Psychol Q 4(1): 27–35

Sherr L, Jefferies S, Victor C 1992 GP ante-natal care: the challenges of HIV. AIDS Patient Care 6(2):

Sherr L, Melvin D, Petrak J, Glover L, Hedge B 1993 The

psychological trauma of HIV for women. Couns Psychol Q (in press)

Shusterman L R 1979 Predicting the psychological consequences of abortion. Soc Sci Med 96: 683-

Smith J R, Reginald P W, Forster S M 1990 Safe sex and conception: a dilemma. Lancet 335: 359

Stevens A, Victor C, Sherr L, Beard R 1989 HIV testing in antenatal clinics: the impact on women. AIDS Care 1(2): 165–171

Stratton P et al 1990 VI International Conference on AIDS, San Francisco, Abstr SC 665

Sunderland A, Moroso G, Berthaud M, Holman S, Landesman S, Minkoff H et al 1988 Influence of HIV infection on pregnancy decisions. Presented at IV International Conference on AIDS, Stockholm, Sweden, June

Sunderland A, Minkoff H, Handte J, Moroso G, Landesman S 1992 The Impact of HIV serostatus on reproductive decisions of women. Obstet Gynecol 79 (6): 1027–1031

Tappin D, Girdwood R, Follett E, Kennedy R et al 1991 Prevalence of maternal HIV infection in Scotland based on unlinked anonymous testing of newborn babies. Lancet 337: 1565–1567

Temmerman M, Moses S, Kirau D, Fusallah S, Wamola I A, Piot P 1990 Impact of single session post partum counselling of HIV infected women on their subsequent reproductive behaviour. AIDS Care 2 (3): 247–252

Thiry L, Spencer Goldberger S, Jonckheer T et al 1985 Isolation of AIDS virus from cell free breast milk of three healthy virus carriers. Lancet 2: 891–892

Toxoplasmosis Working Party 1992 Findings published by the Royal College of Obstetrics and Gynaecology, London

Tymstra T 1986 False positive results in screening tests – experience of parents of children screened for congenital hypothyroidism. Family Pract 3: 92–96

van de Perre P, Simonon A, Msellati P et al 1991 Postnatal transmission of HIV type 1 from mother to infant: a prospective cohort study in Kigali, Rwanda. N Engl J Med 325: 593–598

van de Perre P, Hitimana D, Simonson A et al 1992 Postnatal transmission of HIV 1 associated with breast abscess. Lancet 339: 1490–1491

Wallace L 1984 Psychological preparation for gynaecological surgery. In: Broome A, Wallace L (eds) Psychology and gynaecological problems. Tavistock Publications, London, p161–188

Weinstein N D 1984 Why it won't happen to me: perceptions of risk factors and susceptibility. Health Psychol 3: 431–457

Wenstrom K D, Zuidema L J 1989 Determination of the seroprevalence of HIV infection in gravidas by non anonymous versus anonymous testing. Obstet Gynecol 74 (4) 558–561

Whalen L et al 1990 VI International Conference on AIDS, San Francisco, Abstr THD 85

Wiznia A, Bueti C, Douglas C et al 1989 Factors influencing maternal decision making regarding pregnancy outcome in HIV infected women. V International AIDS Conference, Montreal, Abstr MBP 7

WHO 1988 World Health Organization, Geneva

Ziegler J, Cooper D, Johnson R, Gold J 1985 Postnatal transmission of AIDS associated retrovirus from mother to infant. Lancet 1: 896–897

3. Counselling HIV-infected women and families

Riva Miller and Eleanor Goldman

INTRODUCTION

This chapter will focus on HIV-infected women and their families. It is written from a family therapist's perspective. A woman is defined as a female aged 16 or over, and families are either those of origin (both nuclear and extended), or those of choice or affiliation through marriage, sexual relationship or friendship. The connections between women and families of origin are there even if they are separated by distance, beliefs, stage of life, life-style or death. How women react to the diagnosis of HIV, subsequently live with the infection, and deal with the terminal stages of illness are moderated by the part they play in their families and vice versa. The family, in most cases, is the primary and most powerful system to which a person belongs.

As the heterosexual spread of HIV increases, not only more women but also more children will be infected and affected by HIV disease. The response of a woman and her family to HIV illness depends on the nature of the family organization, beliefs about illness, attitudes to medical treatment and relationships with the community. All these should, in turn, influence the HIV care that is offered to women.

HIV infection affects relationships, bringing into sharp focus issues related to those in the past, present and future. Relationships of closeness and distance between family members are important especially as women become ill and need the support of those closest to them. Some close family relationships may enable women to share knowledge of the diagnosis and their concerns. In other cases this closeness might make it more difficult. Distant relationships might inhibit women from discussing HIV. HIV can affect the way a woman negotiates this distance and closeness of family relationships.

Family issues for infected women can be complex, whether they are parent-child, mother-child or sexual partner and marital configurations. For most women there is a combination of all these. The problems for each HIV-infected woman will differ depending on her stage in life and HIV infection, socio-economic status, cultural and religious beliefs, and the role she plays in her family. Concerns will vary from family to family, and will change over time as the HIV disease progresses. Some issues for HIV-infected women in relation to their families, and counselling approaches to specific situations, such as telling the family, child-bearing and child rearing, family conflicts and role reversals in families will be discussed in this chapter.

ISSUES FOR WOMEN AND FAMILIES

Relationships within families can facilitate or complicate issues for women. Some recurring issues may cut across cultural and religious traditions, and others are culturally determined.

Source of HIV infection

The source of HIV infection cuts across cultural and religious boundaries and can have a bearing on which issues arise for women in relation to their families, especially at the time of testing and diagnosis. At later stages of HIV illness the source of infection may become of less importance in family relationships as other issues about child care, death and loss become more prominent.

Intravenous drug use

The diagnosis of HIV through injecting drugs may reveal to family or sexual partner a past or current hidden habit. For the woman whose family is aware of her drug use, HIV may bring renewed recriminations. Guilt due to feelings of failure for not doing more to prevent the behaviour that led to infection may resurface for parents, siblings or other family members. Drug use may have weakened links with families of origin. As HIV disease progresses, links with family may of necessity or choice be resumed, especially in the terminal phase. Women who have children may have an increased need to rely on parents, siblings or other extended family members for help during acute phases of HIV illness, and for future care of their child or children. The continued dependency on drugs for some women has to be accepted and dealt with by families and health care workers.

Transfusion-associated infection

Prior to HIV testing of donors, or in countries where blood screening is not yet fully operational, transfusion may have been the source of infection. Some women may have, or have had a pre-existing medical condition making transfusion itself life saving and affecting family relationships. For women who have remained asymptomatic, unforeseen or undetected infection could have been transmitted to sexual partners and children. HIV diagnosis brings to the fore not only issues about transmission but fears of stigma and the stresses of dealing with an incurable medical condition for the whole family. The stigma associated with HIV may kindle suspicion about life-style and past relationships.

Heterosexual transmission

Heterosexual transmission is rapidly becoming the major transmission risk in the developed world, as it is in developing countries, such as Africa. The popular association of AIDS with social deviance, such as drug use and homosexuality, prevents recognition of the high risk of heterosexual exposure. Personal and family relationships can be affected, whether the infection is transmitted from woman to man or man to woman. The responsibility of preventing transmission can provoke a personal,

family and economic crisis. Even if a woman suspects she is at risk, in many instances she may take no steps to protect herself as she is conditioned socially and culturally to acquiesce to the man's sexual demands. Discussion of measures to reduce or prevent transmission between women and men may be an unfamiliar and unacceptable prelude to sexual intercourse. Some women are dependent on prostitution for a living to support children and other family members. 'Sex work' or prostitution remains stigmatized. HIV transmission may result because clients refuse to use condoms. Drug users may need the finances from prostitution to support their habit. Heterosexually infected women's relationships with family will be affected by HIV and be influenced by pre-existing patterns of relating. Relationship patterns can change as previous liaisons and life-style are revealed, either bringing people closer, or creating rifts between them. Some women may turn to family members for help after years of independence. This may not be possible in all circumstances, such as when the pre-existing socio-economic situation led to drug use and prostitution.

The family response to HIV diagnosis, illness and the need for care

Many women come for HIV testing and medical care late in their HIV disease, often at a stage of acute illness, when there is less that can be done to improve their outlook and quality of life. They may be afraid that the diagnosis will reveal past secrets to family leading to the re-emergence of conflicts and disagreements, and the risks of being rejected and isolated when they most need support.

The nature of HIV illness makes long-range planning difficult for the woman and her family because of the often rapidly changing medical condition with periods of acute illness followed by periods of reasonable health. Families may be called upon to respond to crises, and then have to readjust to periods when women can resume control themselves. The nature of HIV with its opportunistic infections, increasing debility and sometimes disabling effects from severe damage to vision, mobility or brain functioning, leads to more physical and psychological dependence, which may be on the family. This dependence is influenced by past patterns of relationships.

The fear of stigma may retard or prevent new patterns of relationships developing between a woman and her family in response to the acute and chronic phases of illness. Past patterns may re-emerge, such as over-protection and anxiety on the part of both or either of the parents. Some women may hide their illness to protect the family or themselves from these responses. Women may be reluctant to discuss HIV with sexual partners and older children. In other families the crisis of prolonged illness may lead to reorganization, reconciliation and family unity.

Place in the family

The place an HIV-infected woman holds in her family has a bearing on the stresses which might arise. These vary from individual to individual, and family to family and include being:

- a daughter
- a sibling
- a sexual and/or marital partner
- a mother
- a child-bearer and child rearer
- a carer of nuclear and extended family
- a breadwinner.

Some women may occupy combinations of these roles. If a woman is making decisions about having or not having a child, the greatest stress may come from her sexual partner and the extended family. Future care of children might be the greatest concern for mothers. An only child or breadwinner with dependent children or adults may have fears about who else to turn to for her own and their future care and financial support.

Role reversal

HIV infection with its asymptomatic phases alternating with illness may necessitate various role reversals for women and families. A woman who has been the 'protector' of parents may be reluctant to inform them of her concerns and practical needs as she becomes ill. In some circumstances this protective role continues through the terminal stage of illness, creating additional stresses as the woman feels unable to reveal her need for support.

The role change from being a sexual partner to being a possible source of infection and an ill person not only has the potential to upset the family pattern, but has implications for continuation of the family. This disruption can lead to break-up of the nuclear family and dependence on older or younger generations of family including parents, grandparents and older children.

In many cultures women are traditionally looked upon as 'carers' of the home, the children, and elderly or sick family members. Reversing this key role through HIV can upset pre-existing patterns of relationships, but also the ability of the family unit to function and survive economically and socially. Parents or outside carers may be brought in to help if both the mother and her child are infected. Social service agencies may of necessity become involved with those women who have become isolated from families through choice or circumstances.

The balance of being 'carer' and being 'cared for' may vary over time and at different phases of HIV disease. Grandparents, parents, siblings and older children may become the prime carers, changing the family organization patterns and disrupting the 'normal' order of life events.

Having children and the wish to create a family

In most societies a woman's place is defined by her ability to have children and create a family. The emphasis placed on this varies from individual to individual, culture to culture, and at different stages in the woman's life. Pressures to marry and have children are greatest during early sexual maturity and increase again as the child-bearing age reaches its end. For HIV-infected women the pressure to procreate and continue the family may be personal, from family or from sexual partners. The infectious and incurable aspects of HIV come into direct conflict with this desire.

Unresolved conflicts

HIV infection may bring forth unresolved conflicts between women and families of origin or families of choice, particularly if relationships have been strained in the past and if there are issues of child care, economic factors or sexual relationships that are at stake. The emotions generated by HIV can reactivate past tensions. Guilt about relationships in and outside the family, drug use or life-style may surface for the woman, parents and siblings. In some instances, particularly during the terminal phase of illness, family members may dedicate themselves to attempting to save the wife, daughter or sibling after all reasonable avenues of medical treatment have been exhausted, sacrificing their own needs and future. In other instances family may abandon the woman in an attempt to avoid confronting the problems. Either situation can be stressful for the dying woman. On the other hand, HIV infection may provide an opportunity for the family to address and resolve past conflicts.

Stigma

In the 1990s there is still stigma attached to HIV infection, particularly for women, due to beliefs about acceptable behaviour, roles and position in the family and 'society'. Fears of repercussions of stigma extend to the family and can deter HIV-infected women from involving close relatives in their care. Such fears can inhibit mothers telling older children about HIV in case they pass on the information to a 'best friend' resulting in private concerns being made public. Families may also fear the effect of being associated with the infected woman. HIV fears may sever the ties of the family from their vital natural network of neighbours, friends and even social service agencies. The isolation, resulting from stigma and discrimination, can compound and intensify family difficulties. Research efforts, media information and treatment regimens have concentrated on identified 'risk groups' such as homosexuals, drug users, hae-mophiliacs and people infected by blood transfusion, all of whom have suffered from stigma. There are still people who disbelieve the existence of heterosexual transmission of HIV. Those disbeliefs can extend to women themselves and their families.

Secrets and boundaries

HIV changes family boundaries if the secret of the diagnosis is shared with some and not others. This includes sexual partners, children, siblings, parents, grandparents and other extended family members. Coalitions are created between the woman and those who know about the diagnosis. Caretaking for single women with children may force changes in who is told. Boundaries between the family and community may become more rigid as the woman tries to maintain secrets from either or both. Those women with fragile or non-existent family ties may rely more heavily on health care workers to replace the family, which can be stressful for the workers if they have not been trained to cope with such pressures.

Diminished choices

Choices over a wider range of issues may appear to be diminished for HIV-infected women and can be facilitated or made more difficult by family pressures or support. The main decisions affected by family relationships are:

- How, when and whether to involve family in decisions about the HIV test and its results
- Disclosure to sexual partners or spouses
- Whether or not to have children and the implications for the woman, sexual partner, and relationship with nuclear and extended family
- Whether or not to tell dependent family members and those who may be a source of support
- Decisions about hospital attendances and other treatment facilities are made more difficult if they are endeavouring to hide the infection from the family
- Acceptance or rejection of conventional medical treatment may be influenced by family beliefs and upbringing, particularly for young women who may have little experience of illness
- Disclosure of the diagnosis may be forced by practical needs requiring family involvement, such as for transport, child-minding, and financial support.

Maintaining balance

Maintaining a balance between leading a 'normal' life and accepting the realities of HIV infection and illness is a major challenge for women and their families. A balance has to be found between attending to the physical and psychological needs of infected women whilst enabling the family as a whole and its individual members to continue daily tasks and reach developmental milestones. For example, children must attend school and meet with peers, some level of sexual satisfaction must be achieved for couples, and the needs of elderly parents cannot be ignored.

Death and the family

The death of a daughter, sexual partner or wife, mother, or sibling forces changes in family organization. This is accentuated if the woman is young, and the death is 'out of phase' in the expected life cycle of the family. The legacy of guilt may complicate reactions to bereavement. Families may be unable to share their grief and loss due to fears of stigma and rejection. Fears for their own safety may arise for family members who have taken on an intimate caring role, and for sexual partners who may or may not be infected. The question of testing contacts has to be considered. The future care of orphaned children has to be organized, sometimes without prior preparation or adequate consideration of the rights and best interests of those children. The needs of other family members who may have been neglected during the woman's illness, such as siblings and other children, may come to the fore, complicating the bereavement and grieving process. Some families make contact only at the time of terminal illness and death, or may even approach health carers some time after the death of the woman. The family as a whole and its individual members have to regroup and reorganize patterns of relationships after death.

Health care system, woman and family

Health care workers have on the whole continued to make assumptions about the HIV status of women who present at family planning clinics, general practitioner surgeries, antenatal and gynaecology clinics. Attention has focused on those perceived to be 'at risk' for HIV. Those working closely with families such as health visitors, social workers, family planning doctors, family therapists and general practitioners have remained reluctant to raise the issues of HIV in a routine way. This reluctance may delay diagnosis in some cases and ultimately has prolonged the stigma, and prevented HIV being considered an issue for the whole family.

INHIBITORS TO LOOKING AT THE FAMILY

Several factors might account for health care workers' reluctance to address family-related HIV issues for women. These include:

1. The identified patient is the target of intervention in traditional medical and psychological care. The confidential doctor–patient relationship can inhibit developing approaches to the 'wider system', such as the patient's family. Conflicting interests of the woman, her sexual partner, child, parents and siblings can further inhibit approaching family issues.
2. Beliefs about 'intruding' may inhibit asking questions which could open discussion of family relationships.
3. The overwhelming number of overlapping issues for HIV-infected women can make difficulties appear insuperable, especially those relating to family interactions.
4. Dealing with the reactions and issues for more than one person in a session can be intimidating. The woman's fears that 'things will get out of control' may compound the fears of the health care worker and inhibit family sessions.
5. Personal views, ethical issues and the influence of religious, family and cultural pressures that women experience may make it difficult to assume a neutral stance and to avoid colluding with different family members.
6. A mother's fears that her child will be 'taken into care' or anxiety about breaches of confidentiality may inhibit adequately assessing how the family as a 'caring' unit can best be helped.

7. Working alone without consultation, supervision or a team.

8. Lack of training and experience to incorporate a family perspective.

GUIDELINES FOR WORKING WITH FAMILIES

Some approaches can be developed to deal with the complex relationships of women and their families more effectively in settings that are primarily for medical care and treatment. These include the following methods.

Having a theoretical model

Developing a 'systemic view' and acquiring some specific counselling skills facilitate addressing family issues for HIV-infected women effectively. This means seeing the patient in the context of a network of relationships. The systemic approach takes into account the reciprocity of relationships and sees the family as the unit of intervention. All behaviour is seen as an interactive process, whether at home, at work or in the context of illness. The system may be the HIV-infected woman and her family of origin or choice, or the woman and the health care system in the context of HIV infection. Women can be assessed in relation to their families even if other family members are not present at the session. The use of hypothetical questions about views and beliefs is an effective way of doing this; for example, 'If your mother knew about your dilemma about telling her that you are HIV-positive, what do you think she would say?'

A systemic perspective crosses cultural boundaries and takes into account religious and social beliefs. HIV cuts across familiar, well defined, entrenched patterns of communication between women, their families, sexual partners and children as issues of transmission and prevention emerge. Infected women can be helped to make more informed choices about family relationships through using existing links and past events to stimulate ideas and new patterns of decision-making. For example, 'You say that you are reluctant to tell your mother how unwell you are because she gets so anxious. From your past experience, was she more anxious when she actually had to face a problem or before it happened? If she does get anxious now, who do you think she would turn to for help?'

Systemic counselling helps women and families to consider the resources they have and to think about those that they might seek out to help them cope. Asking how they have coped with difficulties in the past and how they might cope in the future will link them with others and enable them to acquire a different view of their situation. The systemic approach can help women to keep the panorama of issues in perspective, to identify and rank problems and reduce them to manageable proportions.

Working as a team

Working as a team makes it easier to deal with difficult issues. This can be achieved by seeing women and families with a colleague, or having pre- and post-session discussions. In this way skills are shared and neutrality is more likely to be maintained, which is essential when working with more than the index patient. Team-work provides the essential support for individual workers to avoid the stresses of taking on too many burdens. Failing to explore whether family resources exist for infected women may leave health carers playing a major role in the woman's life and they may find themselves in coalition against the patient's family who must ultimately take over responsibility.

Defining aims of family counselling

Having aims helps to structure family sessions. These include:

- Making no assumptions
- Having small goals
- Identifying and ranking concerns
- Reducing anxiety for women and families to manageable proportions
- Avoiding dependency
- Setting boundaries
- Maintaining neutrality
- Helping the woman and other family members to get closer in order to discuss issues that they might otherwise find difficult, or which might need resolution, and enabling them to deal with

unfinished business, such as wills, care of dependent children, and wishes about death and burial
- Obtaining appropriate services
- Preparing the family for bereavement
- Co-ordinating the multiple services and views to reduce the risk of duplicating, which increases the complication and multiplication of the problems that are being addressed.

Achieving the aims of family counselling

The following steps can help to achieve the aims of family counselling:

- Make an hypothesis about the problem based on any available information including:
  - Stage of life the woman has reached; for example, there are different pressures about having children at age 20 and 45
  - Stage of HIV infection
  - Position in family
  - The source of referral
- Decide whether to see the woman alone or with significant others
- Decide whether to counsel alone or with a team
- Start the session by introducing yourself, defining the time limits, and explaining the particular setting
- Elicit and give information by:
  - Asking questions, correcting misinformation, and filling in the gaps in the person's knowledge
  - Using a genogram, which is a format for drawing the family tree, to map the family structure, record family information and delineate family relationships over generations. It is an effective way of engaging women in exploring family connections; clarifying who is available in the family network; revealing past ways of coping; and integrating medical and social history
- Identify concerns and wishes
- Keep a focus to the session by using questions to help family members to be specific and rank concerns
- Analyse the information gained in the session by taking into account the following:
  - What has been seen as well as what has been heard during the session

- The resources the woman has to help with the HIV illness
- Any problems there may be in medical compliance
- Family stresses which may intensify the difficulties
- Past coping abilities and how she sees herself coping in the future
- Ending the session
  - An intervention must be made which will summarize what has been seen and heard, and allow the woman and her family to see the resources available in the family and any possible barriers that have prevented them from being used
  - Follow-up sessions, encouraging the woman to come with whomever she wishes to bring from her family system, should be offered

CASE EXAMPLES

Telling the family about HIV

Jane, aged 21, was found to be HIV-positive after having donated blood at work. The result was a shock to her as she had not perceived herself to be at risk. The counsellor, who told her the diagnosis, helped her to think about who to tell and the possible place of this news in the patterns of her family and other important relationships. Whilst discussing the family connections the counsellor used a genogram to map out the relationships. (Fig 3.1)

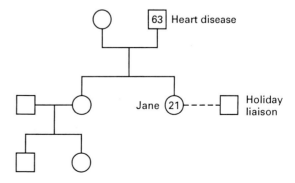

Figure 3.1 Genogram demonstrating relationships in Jane's family

She had an older married sister and parents, both in their 60s, who relied on her for help from time to time as her father has coronary heart disease. Jane's understanding of the result, its implications for her future health and the possible source of infection were established. She had had a holiday 'fling' with a man thought to have used drugs in the past.

> *Counsellor*: What is your greatest concern right now?
>
> *Jane*: My parents. I cannot ever tell them.
>
> *Counsellor*: If you did decide to tell them what might be their reaction?
>
> *Jane*: I couldn't. My father is recovering from a bad heart attack. It would make him ill again and might kill him.
>
> *Counsellor*: Have you ever kept secrets from your family before?
>
> *Jane*: Not really. I can talk to my mother about most things but not this.
>
> *Counsellor*: Does your mother know about your holiday romance?
>
> *Jane*: No.
>
> *Counsellor*: Are you more worried about yourself or your parents?
>
> *Jane*: Right now I'm worried about them, but I am scared for myself also. I need their support.
>
> *Counsellor*: If you became ill who would you turn to for this support?
>
> *Jane*: Not my sister because her husband would never let me near the children. He is very conventional. So no-one.
>
> *Counsellor*: You say you are very close to your mother. If she heard this conversation what do you think she might say to you? Would she feel upset that you couldn't tell her?
>
> *Jane*: I hadn't thought of it that way. Maybe in time I will be able to tell her. I'll begin to think about how I might do it.

The counsellor, despite the difficulties, has posed some hypothetical questions to help Jane think more realistically about how and when she might tell her family, and has found ways to explore Jane's perception of her mother's reactions.

Planning for the future

Sally, 24, was approached by the paediatrician who was puzzled by the symptoms of her 15-month-old baby who had had several admissions to hospital with symptoms of 'failure to thrive'. He wanted to do an HIV test on the baby. The father of the child was a Nigerian law student; they were living together and were hoping to marry (Fig. 3.2). This extract from two interviews demonstrates how the paediatrician and physician identified the main concerns of the couple and the influence of family on all of these.

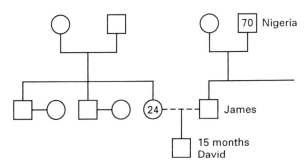

Figure 3.2   Genogram demonstrating relationships in Sally's family

> *Paediatrician*: Sally, as you know we have not been able to establish a diagnosis to help us treat David. I would like to do an HIV test. Do you know what that is?
>
> *Sally*: Yes I do. If my baby has AIDS I just couldn't go on.
>
> *Paediatrician*: Do you think that there is any risk?
>
> *Sally*: I don't know and I don't want to know.
>
> *Paediatrician*: Would you consider being tested?
>
> *Sally*: I suppose so, but I'm petrified.

The paediatrician hypothesizes that family pressures are a main concern and that, until these are openly discussed, pursuing HIV testing would only create more stress for Sally.

> *Paediatrician*: Can you tell me what most petrifies you?
>
> *Sally*: My family knowing. They never wanted me to be with James anyway.

Paediatrician: Who do you mean by family?

Sally: My Mum, Dad and two brothers, and their wives.

Paediatrician: What about James? What is your relationship with him?

Sally: We are not married, but we have been together 5 years. He is David's father. You see, he is Nigerian and my Dad never liked it.

The conflicts between family of origin and choice are becoming apparent, as are the family members whom the paediatrician knows may prove to be the main source of support for Sally, James and their baby. He tries to remain neutral by using questions to help Sally look at her dilemmas from different points of view.

After a long discussion Sally agreed to be tested. She was found to be anti-HIV-positive. Although it was possible for the baby to have maternal antibodies rather than being infected himself, it was decided to assume he was infected and treat him with special medicines. She was seen again some weeks later with James, whose test was positive. Neither of them seemed surprised by the result. Several months later she had still not told her parents. Sally and James had been referred to a specialist HIV physician. The two teams liaised to achieve co-ordinated care for the whole family unit. The HIV physician was concerned to arrange more support for them.

Physician: James, how do you think Sally has been coping these last months?

James: Not bad. But very tense and snappy with me.

Physician: Sally, do you agree that you have been snappy with James?

Sally: I suppose he sees it like that, but it isn't because of him.

Physician: James you've heard what Sally said. Who do you think it really is?

James: Her family.

Physician: Is that right, Sally?

Sally: Yes.

Physician: Sally, we'll come back to your family, but first tell me how do you think James has been managing?

Sally: As usual. He just doesn't worry about anything and we've all been OK.

Physician: Sally, if he had any concerns what do you think might be the main one?

Sally: That he might not see his family again.

Consultant: Is that right, James?

By questioning each of them on their view of how the other is coping and checking whether they agree with each other's views, the physician gains rapid understanding of relationships and beliefs. Neutrality is maintained as the physician has not aligned himself with Sally or James. He has to choose which aspect to follow in order to find more support for the family unit should all or any become ill. He voices his concern so that the couple will not feel that they are expected to cope alone, and allows them to explore the resources they might have.

Physician: James, I have a concern. You are all well at present, but what if one or all of you became ill? How do you see yourselves coping, and who might you turn to for help?

James: Well really, the only person is Sally's Mum, but we can't tell her about the HIV.

Physician: Sally, who do you see as helping?

Sally: The only person is my Mum. I'm not used to keeping things from her.

A new idea is introduced to help them think differently about their dilemma. The physician pushes the couple to find solutions for themselves.

Physician: What makes you think that she doesn't know that something is wrong?

Sally: Well, she does keep asking questions about David.

Physician: How do you answer the questions?

James: Sally just changes the subject. It only makes things worse.

Physician: Which of you would most want to tell Sally's family?

Sally: I would, but they would blame me for being with James.

Physician: Just suppose you decided to tell her and she blamed James. How would you cope with that?

Sally: Like I always have. I would do what I think is best and stick to my choices.

Physician: Is that how you see Sally coping?

James: Yes, I suppose so. Actually Sally's Mum and I get on well now.

Physician: Did you know that James thinks he gets on well with Mum now?

Sally: I didn't know he felt that, but I suppose she does really like him.

Physician: If you told Dad what might be his reaction?

Sally: He'd explode!

Physician: How long would the explosion last?

Sally: He actually gets over things quickly.

Physician: Have you ever seen Sally's Dad explode?

James: Often. It doesn't frighten me any more.

Physician: Who might help Sally to tell her family, James?

James: I think her sister-in-law. They are very close and see each other a lot. I think she has guessed something is up with us.

Physician: What do you think of James' idea, Sally?

Sally: I hadn't thought about telling her first, but maybe I could. She handles my Dad well.

The physician has started to achieve the aims of the session and decides to end here, leaving further decisions to the couple. Too much discussion can remove the tension and blur the issues. The counsellor tries to balance avoiding the creation of anxiety with helping them to accept the reality of the whole family being infected with a life-threatening incurable condition. False reassurance is not given.

Physician: We have talked for some time now. I can see that all three of you are quite well at present and both of you are managing. My concern is that it is possible that you might not always be well. I have heard that although you have not yet told your family, Sally, you are beginning to think how you might do so. Although you are afraid of your parents' reactions, from past experience you are able to handle them, and have your sister-in-law to help.

Family and cultural beliefs

The following excerpts from two interviews with Mr J and his wife illustrate:

- Engaging the family through the index patient

- Crossing cultural boundaries because of HIV
- Conducting an interview with more than one person.

Mr J, who comes from a culture with strong religious beliefs and a tradition of arranged marriages, has haemophilia and HIV infection. His marriage was arranged before he knew that he was HIV-positive. His parents did not tell his prospective parents-in-law about haemophilia as they feared that the knowledge of disability in the family would ruin not only his chances of marriage but also those of his two unmarried sisters. The index patient initially came along for medical care. The counsellor's concerns and responsibilities were:

- To ensure that Mr J had sufficient information to enable him to make informed decisions about the risks of HIV transmission to wife and children
- To engage the couple
- To overcome traditional cultural and family traditions which might prevent them from taking the precautions needed to reduce the risk of HIV transmission.

The following is an extract from an interview where the counsellor has already given some general information about HIV.

Counsellor: As you now understand the risks of passing on this infection to your future wife, how do you plan to prevent it happening?

Mr J: I will do as you say and use condoms, but I cannot the first time as it will need discussion and this is impossible.

Counsellor: It is not easy to talk about these things, but I have to be sure that you understand that the first time could be very risky as there is likely to be bleeding.

Mr J: Even so. I must marry and only tell afterwards.

Counsellor: If you told her before, how do you think she would react?

Mr J: I can't tell her. She would tell her parents and then mine would hear about HIV. My parents wouldn't understand and would be very angry with me. They have arranged a big family wedding.

Counsellor: How will you manage between you if she gets infected?

Mr J: I can't think about that now. We don't talk about these things between men and women. We must have a child quickly whilst I am well.

Counsellor: If you and your new wife decided not to have a child would that be a problem?

Mr J: Yes, her parents would be dissatisfied with me as a son-in-law, and my parents would be upset for us not to have a son.

The counsellor is becoming overwhelmed with the number of issues and the complexity of the situation. He also knows that he cannot do more to prevent consummation of the marriage in the traditional way. He decides to deal with the most urgent issue of avoiding infection and postulates the worst scenario: the wife and offspring could be infected with HIV. Mr J says that he will tell her in his own way very soon after marriage. An appointment is to be arranged as soon as possible after he has revealed his HIV infection to his wife so that the counsellor can ensure that she understands the risks.

Counsellor: Mrs J, has your husband told you why I asked him to bring you today?

Mrs J: (Looks at her husband to answer, and is reluctant to talk).

Mr J: I have told her everything.

Counsellor: (Tries again to get Mrs J to reply as he is anxious to know from her what she understands). Mrs J, I know it is not the custom to talk in this way and that your husband usually answers the questions, but I need to know from you what you understand.

Mrs J: (Looks again at her husband).

Counsellor: Please ask your wife to answer for herself.

The counsellor takes control. Mrs J responds and says she understands about her husband having HIV, and something about the risks to her.

Counsellor: Mr J, do you think your wife has any worries?

Mr J: No. We are using condoms now.

Counsellor: Mrs J, is it right that you have no worries?

Mrs J: I am worried about my husband. He will die and I want children.

Counsellor: Mr J, which of those do you think she worries about most?

Mr J: Having children. She keeps on asking me how soon we can have one and I wanted you to tell her about the problems.

Counsellor: Mrs J, is your husband right?

Mrs J: (Nods).

The counsellor then offers the following three scenarios:

1. Mrs J could become infected, but have an uninfected child who could be left an orphan.
2. Mrs J could conceive without becoming infected, but could become a single parent.
3. Mrs J and the child could be infected.

They are asked how they would cope with the possible consequences of any of these situations. If they decide that any risk would be unacceptable, the possibility of artificial insemination by screened donor could be suggested, although for many people this might be difficult. If they are determined to have a child in spite of the risk, they should be offered an ovulation kit and advised to abandon barrier contraception only at the time of ovulation in an attempt to reduce the amount of exposure to infection.

CONCLUSIONS

The complex issues that HIV-infected women face are addressed in this book. The family remains the most fundamental source of support, but it may also be a source of pressure and stress to women because of the special tensions surrounding HIV. Families of infected women also have special needs. In addition to supporting the woman, preparing for bereavement and possibly taking on the responsibility of caring for her children, they may have fears for themselves.

In most medical systems there is a one to one relationship with the patient and counselling would be organized in the same way. Interventions sometimes become redundant and care fragmented because the focus rarely concentrates on the co-ordination of services and using the resources of the family–patient system. This is frustrating to those caring for women, as well as to women themselves. Without co-ordination of services, practical assistance and counselling have little effect. A family systems approach is one way of overcoming these problems.

Acquiring a family perspective, increasing skills in dealing with families, and working in a team facilitate effective approaches to complex issues. Training, observation and practice are ways of acquiring and enhancing skills.

BIBLIOGRAPHY

Arras JD 1990 1. HIV and childbearing. 2. AIDS and reproductive decisions: having children in fear and trembling. Milbank-Q 68(3): 353–382
Barbacci M, Dalabeta G, Repke J et al 1990 Human immunodeficiency virus infection in women attending an inner-city prenatal clinic: ineffectiveness of targeted screening. Sexually Transmitted Diseases 17: 122–126
Bor R, Miller R, Goldman E et al 1989 The impact of AIDS/HIV on family: themes emerging from family interviews. Practice 1: 42–48
Bor R, Miller R, Goldman E 1992 Theory and practice of HIV counselling: a systemic approach. Cassell, London
Bradbeer C 1989 Women and HIV Br Med J 298: 342–343
Carter B, McGoldrick M 1989 The changing family life cycle, 2nd edn. Allyn and Bacon, Boston
Cosmi E, Falcinelli C, Anceschi M et al 1992 Perinatal AIDS. Eur J Obstet Gynecol Reprod Biol May 13 44(3): 165–173
Eyster M, Ballard J, Gail M et al 1989 Predictive markers for the acquired immunodeficiency syndrome (AIDS) in haemophiliacs: persistence of P24 antigen and low T4 cell count. Ann Int Med 110: 963–969
Goldman E, Miller R, Lee CA 1992 Counselling HIV positive haemophiliac men who wish to have children. Br Med J 304: 829–830
Holman S 1992 HIV counseling for women of reproductive age. Baillieres Clin Obstet Gynaecol Mar 6(1): 53–68
Levine C, Dubler N 1990 1. HIV and childbearing. 2. Uncertain risks and bitter realities: the reproductive choices of HIV-infected women. Milbank Q 68(3): 321–351
McGoldrick M, Gerson R 1985 Genograms in family assessment. W W Norton, New York
Mason J, Preisinger J, Sperling R et al 1991 Incorporating HIV education and counseling into routine prenatal care: a program model. AIDS Educ Prev Summer 3(2): 118–123
Miller R, Bor R 1988 AIDS: a guide to clinical counselling. Science Press, London
Novick B, Rubinstein A 1987 AIDS: the paediatric perspective. AIDS 1: 3–7
Selvini-Palazzoli M, Boscolo L, Cecchin G et al 1980 Hypothesizing, circularity, neutrality: three guidelines for the conductor of the session. Family Process 19: 3–12
Selwyn P, Carter R, Schoenbaum E et al 1989 Knowledge of HIV antibody status and decisions to continue or terminate pregnancy among intravenous drug users. JAMA Jun 23–30 261(24): 3567–3571
Sherr L 1991 HIV and AIDS in mothers and babies: a guide to counselling. Blackwell Publications, Oxford
Walker G 1991 In the midst of winter: systemic therapy with families, couples, and individuals with AIDS infection. W W Norton, New York

4. Testing and screening programmes

C. A. Carne

INTRODUCTION

Programmes for testing and screening for HIV infection may have various aims often depending on the setting. The design of such programmes is governed by their aims and by technical, ethical and legal considerations. In this chapter, the feasibility of achieving these aims will be examined in the light of relevant research findings and the technical, ethical and legal considerations; various types of programmes will be reviewed; and situations where clinicians should think about counselling for testing will be suggested. First, however, it is necessary to define the terms to be used.

DEFINITIONS

The World Health Organization (WHO 1987) has defined testing and screening for HIV infection as follows:

Testing is a serologic procedure for determining the HIV antibody (or antigen) status of an individual person.
Screening is the systematic application of HIV testing to whole populations; and donors of blood products and cells, tissues or organs.

Approaches to testing have been defined as follows by The Department of Health's Working Group (UK) on the monitoring and surveillance of HIV infection and AIDS (DHSS 1988):

Compulsory testing is the process of determining HIV antibody status without the individual's consent, and with legal sanctions to enforce compliance.

Involuntary testing is the process of determining HIV antibody status without obtaining the individual's consent.
Voluntary testing is the process of determining HIV antibody status with the individual's consent.

Approaches to screening have been defined as follows by the 'Committee on Prenatal and Newborn Screening for HIV Infection' (1991) in the USA:

Mandatory screening means that all individuals within a defined population are tested without an opportunity for refusal.
Voluntary screening with right of refusal means that each individual within a defined population is informed that the test will be performed unless he or she explicitly refuses.
Voluntary screening with specific informed consent means that each individual within a defined population is informed that the test is available but that it will be performed only with a person's specific informed consent.

These approaches can either be named or unnamed, defined as follows by the Health Education Authority in the UK (Carne & Kapila 1988): in *named testing*, the individual's identifying details remain with the sample. In *unnamed testing* any details which could lead to the blood sample and its results being traced back to the individual are removed. In the UK, this is commonly called anonymous (or anonymized) testing. (In the US literature, the term anonymous has a different meaning, implying that the sample and person are identifiable only by a personal number or other code.) To avoid confusion this will be referred to as anonymized testing or Screening.

THE AIMS OF TESTING AND SCREENING

These aims can be viewed from the perspective of the woman being tested or screened, or from the public perspective. The woman's perspective is that there are potential advantages (and disadvantages) in knowing her HIV status: it may help her and her partner decide on their sexual practices; it may allay unnecessary anxiety about HIV; it may influence the decision on whether to become pregnant or continue with a pregnancy; it may influence decisions on whether to breast-feed; it may lead to improved medical care in both the symptomatic and asymptomatic HIV-positive woman and in the HIV-positive baby.

The potential disadvantages of discovering one's HIV status are: the psychological distress which may result from receiving a positive result; the possible rejection by partner, family and friends; problems at work, at school or in housing; difficulty in obtaining life insurance and mortgages, even sometimes as a consequence of being tested despite the result being negative; the possibility of being lulled into a false sense of security about the risk of acquiring HIV if high-risk behaviour is continued.

The balance between the potential advantages and disadvantages varies from woman to woman, and may vary over time. For instance, a pregnant woman may decide to opt for the test although she had not sought one prior to her pregnancy. The aim of most testing programmes is simply to allow women the option of having the test.

The public health perspective is: that there may be benefits in lessening the spread of HIV if it is true that knowledge of an HIV result encourages behaviour change (see later); that the practice of partner notification resulting from any woman identified as HIV-positive may lessen the spread of HIV (see later); that knowledge acquired about seroprevalence of HIV will aid forecasting of the course of the epidemic and hence allow improved service planning, allocation of appropriate resources, and better targeting and evaluation of health promotion programmes.

The question of whether HIV antibody testing and counselling influences risk behaviours was examined in 66 studies published or presented between January 1986 and July 1990. Higgins and colleagues (1991), on reviewing these studies concluded:

'All longitudinal studies of homosexual men reported reductions in risky behaviour among both tested and untested men, and a few reported greater decreases among seropositive men than among seronegative men and those untested or unaware of their serostatus. For intravenous drug users in treatment, we found reductions in intravenous drug use and sexual risk behaviours regardless of counseling and testing experience. We found little evidence for the impact of counseling and testing on pregnancy and/or pregnancy termination rates for either seropositive or seronegative high-risk women. We noted substantial risk reduction among heterosexual couples with one infected partner. Findings among other heterosexuals at increased risk were scanty and mixed.

A Lancet editorial (Editorial 1991) expressed the view on partner notification that, 'For society it is probably the most cost-effective method of identifying new cases of infection in low-risk groups in which large-scale screening programmes are lacking, and therefore of controlling the spread of disease.' More recently (Landis et al 1992), the effectiveness of partner notification has been examined in a randomized trial comparing provider referral and patient referral. A total of 74 subjects (31% women) were randomly assigned to one of two groups. In the provider referral group counsellors successfully notified 78/157 partners (50%) as compared to only 10/153 (7%) successfully notified by patients in the patient referral group. Of the partners notified by the counsellors, 94% were not aware that they had been exposed to HIV.

TECHNICAL CONSIDERATIONS

The usefulness of a test, especially when used for screening, depends on sensitivity, specificity and predictive value. Sensitivity is the ability of a test to detect the condition of interest in those individuals who truly have that condition. Specificity reflects the ability of a test to exclude those who do not have the condition. The predictive value of a test reflects false-positive and false-negative results. The predictive value of a positive test is the probability that an individual is infected, given that the test result is positive (the positive predictive value); the predictive value of a negative test is the probability that an individual is not infected, given that the test is negative (the negative predictive value). The predictive value of any test varies according to the prevalence of the condition in the population being studied. The positive predictive value diminishes with declining prevalence; i.e. the proportion of positive test results which are falsely positive tends to rise.

Currently, tests for HIV antigens lack sufficient sensitivity for routine application in testing and screening programmes. A variety of different methods for HIV antibody testing exists. The most commonly employed are the various types of ELISA (enzyme-linked immunosorbent assay). In order to minimize the problem of false-positive results laboratories generally insist on: repeat tests of same type on an apparently positive serum sample, confirmatory testing by one or more different methods, and confirmatory testing on a second serum sample from the patient. It has been estimated that HIV antibody testing using two different ELISAs with two repeats has a theoretical false-positive rate of less than one in a million (Mortimer 1988a). A high degree of specificity can be achieved even when only a single specimen is available if several assays by different methods are employed (Ranki et al 1987).

False-negative results occur during the window period, i.e. the time between initial infection with the virus and the development of detectable levels of antibodies. Currently it is normal practice in most centres to test adults at 3 months after a possible exposure to HIV. An unknown (but small) proportion of people will take longer than this to develop detectable antibodies. However, the testing procedure in current use in the UK (and elsewhere) is sufficiently sensitive to ensure that 'once seroconversion has occurred, simple antibody assays will detect HIV infection whatever the immunological competence of the subject' (Mortimer 1988b).

ETHICAL AND LEGAL CONSIDERATIONS

The design of testing and screening programmes needs to comply with ethical and legal guidelines. In the UK, guidelines for HIV testing have been drawn up by the General Medical Council (1988) and the British Medical Association (1984).

Central to these is the principle that the doctor/patient relationship 'is founded on mutual trust, which can be fostered only when information is freely exchanged between doctor and patient on the basis of honesty, openness and understanding.' The two central issues to be considered in the context of HIV testing and screening are confidentiality and consent.

Broader ethical guidelines on confidentiality apply also to HIV testing and screening (BMA 1984). These require the doctor to preserve secrecy on all that he knows, with five exceptions where a breach of confidentiality is permissible: when the patient gives consent; when it is undesirable on medical grounds to seek a patient's consent, but it is in the patient's own interest that confidentiality be broken; when the doctor's duty to society overrides his duty to the patient; for the purposes of medical research, when approved by an appropriately constituted ethical committee; and when the information is required by due legal process.

There is, as always, considerable difficulty in drawing a clear line between a doctor's duty to society and his duty to the patient. Where there is a potential conflict this can often be resolved by open and full discussion with the patient as encouraged by the General Medical Council. Should the patient not wish the doctor to disclose his or her positive HIV antibody test result to a health care worker involved in their care (e.g. the general practitioner) or to their sexual partner or spouse, this issue should be fully discussed between patient and doctor. If the issue cannot be satisfactorily resolved the General Medical Council (1988) advises that the doctor may consider breaching confidentiality in the belief that his professional duty to protect others overrides his duty to his patient. In such a situation the doctor must be prepared to justify his decision.

The ethical guidelines on confidentiality are sometimes backed up by law. In the UK the National Health Service (Venereal Diseases) Regulations 1974 are applicable to HIV testing and require employees of regional and district health authorities to preserve confidentiality except for the purpose of informing a medical practitioner or his employee. 'But, a general practitioner or private doctor or other person not employed by a regional or district health authority is subject only to the common law duty of confidentiality which is subject to a general public interest exception' (Medical Defence Union 1988).

The issue of consent is especially pertinent to the design of testing and screening programmes. Broader guidelines on consent are applicable to HIV testing and screening: 'The patient's trust that his consent to treatment will not be misused is an essential part of his relationship with his doctor. For a doctor even to touch a patient without consent may constitute an assault' (BMA 1984). Consent is only valid when it is freely given by a patient who understands the nature and consequences of what is proposed; i.e. informed consent requires adequate pretest discussion of these issues. Assumed consent or consent obtained by undue influence is valueless. The General Medical Council (1988) has stated that the need to obtain consent 'is particularly important in the case of testing for HIV infection, not because the condition is different in kind from other infections but because of the possible serious social and financial consequences which may ensue from the mere fact of having been tested for the condition'.

The special issue of anonymized screening has been considered by an Institute of Medical Ethics working party. It concluded that anonymized HIV screening for epidemiological purposes is to be welcomed, given certain safeguards. It also approved voluntary screening with right of refusal in the antenatal clinic provided that adequate briefing was available (Boyd 1990).

There are conflicting legal opinions on the need for consent for HIV testing. The General Medical Council guidelines in the UK are based on the opinion of Michael Sherrard QC that 'testing for HIV antibody without the consent of the patient will, save in the rarest cases, expose the medical practitioner to the risk of criminal and/or civil liability at law'. A conflicting opinion from Leo Charles QC, stated that unless the patient specifically asks, it is up to the doctor's clinical judgement whether he tells the patient that the test is for HIV. The extent of disclosure of information to the patient depends on what is acceptable medical practice. This conflict may be resolved if and when a case is brought in the courts.

TESTING AND SCREENING IN DIFFERENT SETTINGS

Women in general, and some groups of women in particular, may benefit from testing and screening programmes designed to meet their specific needs. One issue that may influence the setting and the context of programmes is that women whose sexual relationships take place in a social context of male dominance may have particular difficulty in insisting on safer sex (Holland et al 1990), a problem which may be ameliorated by appropriate training in assertiveness and communication skills. Pregnant women and women contemplating pregnancy have specific issues to discuss related to the possible effect of pregnancy on HIV infection, the risk of vertical transmission and the advisability or otherwise of breast-feeding. Prostitutes may encounter judgmental attitudes and ignorance among services offering HIV testing. Women drug users and partners of drug users may also encounter prejudice and also have difficulty in being assertive in protecting themselves against HIV.

In the USA nearly all visits by women to publicly funded services for HIV counselling and testing occurred in either sexually transmitted disease (STD) clinics (29%), HIV counselling and testing sites (29%) or women's (family planning and prenatal) clinics (28%). Drug treatment centres accounted for 4% of all tests. The seropositivity rate among tests from drug treatment centres (3.7%) was higher than tests from other sites (counselling and testing sites 3.0%, STD clinics 2.2% and women's clinics 0.7%) (CDC 1991). The authors advise that counselling and testing sites that serve women in areas with high prevalence of HIV seropositivity should routinely offer all clients HIV counselling and testing. In areas with low prevalence of HIV seropositivity, standardized, thorough risk assessments may assist in identifying a person's risks for HIV infection, and recommendations for HIV testing can be made based on the results of each assessment.

Planning of local services for HIV testing and screening depends on local epidemiology which can best be examined by anonymized screening. In Scotland a study was designed to determine the prevalence of HIV among pregnant women, in particular those deemed to be at 'low risk' of HIV infection. The prevalence of HIV in Dundee among antenatal clinic attenders and women having termination of pregnancy was 0.13% and 0.85%, respectively. In these two settings those assessed as 'low risk' by virtue of their behaviour and their partner's behaviour had rates of 0.11% and 0.13%. It was therefore concluded that a policy of selective testing of only those assessed to be at 'high risk' was inappropriate (Goldberg et al 1992). No system of voluntary testing is likely to identify all seropositive women. This has been shown in studies where anonymized screening and named testing programmes have been run in parallel, such as in a public prenatal and family planning centre in Los Angeles. Only 14% (96/685) of clients offered HIV testing chose to accept and none of the four women who tested positive on the anonymized screening chose named testing (Fehrs et al 1991). In an inner city area of Baltimore, USA, only 57% of pregnant women with HIV would have been identified by screening directed at groups with acknowledged risk factors. However, by offering counselling and HIV testing to all pregnant women the detection rate was raised to 87%. The authors conclude that routine screening should be offered to all pregnant women.

If the motivation for universal screening is better control of spread of HIV, this has to be measured against the cost-effectiveness of other strategies. Currently, however, there is a lack of reliable evidence on the effectiveness of alternative approaches for promoting sexual health (Godfrey et al 1992). In the absence of such evidence Goldberg and Johnstone (1992) have suggested that voluntary named testing (of pregnant women) should be performed on a selective basis in settings where unlinked anonymized testing has shown a low prevalence of HIV (perhaps less than 0.1%). Where the prevalence of HIV is greater, voluntary named testing on a universal basis should be strongly considered. Women undergoing termination of pregnancy often have a higher risk of HIV infection than those continuing with the pregnancy (Goldberg et al 1992); they may, however, be less inclined to have an HIV test as it is not going to influence the decision about termination (Meadows et al 1991).

An ambitious programme of anonymized screen-

ing has been in operation in New York State since mid-1987 in an effort to determine the prevalence, distribution and trends of HIV infection in the state (New York State HIV Seroprevalence Project 1991). Six populations were selected as 'windows' on the epidemic: newborns, homeless adolescents in a New York shelter, prisoners, and clients of family planning, STD, and drug treatment clinics. The authors argue that, 'Seroprevalence determinations of human immunodeficiency virus are essential for design and implementation of preventive strategies. By demonstrating the severity of HIV infections within communities, New York State surveys have spurred preventive interventions, including information to the public and health care providers and increased counseling and testing of women of reproductive age.'

Premarital testing for HIV has been advocated in some areas. In New Jersey two anonymized HIV serosurveys were conducted on premarital blood specimens taken for syphilis serology. The first survey was in the year starting September 1987, the second was in the spring of 1989. The prevalences found were 0.49% and 0.62%, respectively. The results were held to support a recommendation in New Jersey of voluntary HIV-1 counselling and testing for marriage applicants (Altman et al 1992). Mandatory premarital testing in Illinois, however, was associated with an abrupt decrease in the number of marriages in Illinois (and an increase in 'crossover' marriages in states bordering Illinois) followed by a rebound when the law was repealed (McKillip 1991).

SCREENING FOR OTHER INFECTIONS

A decision has to be made for each testing and screening programme as to whether screening for other infections should be incorporated. When an HIV blood test is being taken it is simple enough (though more costly) to test homosexual/bisexual men also for hepatitis B and syphilis, and injecting drug users (IDUs) for hepatitis B and C and maybe syphilis. It is more difficult outside the setting of STD clinics to screen for *Chlamydia trachomatis* and other STDs which require the taking of swabs. There is evidence, however, that these tests may often be worthwhile in other settings. A study of

1245 injecting drug users (mean age 27.5 years) in Sydney, Australia showed that over one-third of IDU men and over half of IDU women reported at least one STD in their lifetime (Ross et al 1991). The association between prostitution and injecting drug use (van den Hoek et al 1989) further emphasizes the potential risk of IDUs carrying other STDs. Much has also been written on the role of other STDs in facilitating HIV transmission. Clearly there are benefits in preventing morbidity from identification of other STDs, but the extent of the impact on the HIV epidemic of STD control programmes has yet to be determined. In each setting a decision has to be made on whether screening for other STDs is warranted based on their prevalence, either measured or estimated.

SAME-DAY TESTING

Undergoing HIV testing is usually stressful whatever the outcome. Anecdotally there are people who are put off seeking testing because of the stress of awaiting the result. Programmes for same-day testing are popular (Squire et al 1991) and are becoming more common. Often it is impossible, however, to incorporate testing for other STDs into a same-day testing programme. Further evaluation is therefore needed to assess the impact on the public health; however, it is clear that from the individual's perspective such programmes meet a demand. From the author's own experience they also have the potential advantage of bringing into contact with helping agencies some of those at high risk of HIV infection, e.g. homeless IDUs who would not otherwise seek contact.

WHO TO TEST?

Testing as opposed to screening implies some selection as to who should be tested. The decision on whether to raise the subject of HIV testing will usually rest with the doctor. A survey in a midwestern US state found that only 11% of doctors at a teaching hospital routinely asked about high risk behaviours (Ferguson et al 1991). While most of the doctors had received training in human sexuality, most had not received training in substance abuse screening. Those trained felt more confident in addressing these areas. More training

in these areas is required to aid doctors in correctly identifying who should be offered testing. In some settings a handout may be appropriate. A report from the Royal College of Obstetricians and Gynaecologists (1987) recommended that 'all antenatal patients should be given information on the current categories of HIV risk groups and invited to declare themselves if they are in a high risk group'. It may be preferable to use such a handout but emphasize that women may request counselling with or without HIV testing whether or not they believe themselves to be at high risk. In December 1992, the UK Department of Health offered guidance 'that in areas of known or suspected higher prevalence of HIV, women receiving antenatal care should be offered a test on the basis that they may not perceive that they have been at risk'.

There may be clinical manifestations which raise the doctor's index of suspicion. One survey showed that genital infection, persistent generalized lymphadenopathy, and general malaise were the commonest clinical presentations among women with HIV (Kell et al 1991). Again, as doctors become better educated about the clinical manifestations of HIV infection, so targeting of testing will improve.

CONCLUSION

The design of testing and screening programmes has to take account of technical, ethical, legal and other considerations as well as the individual and public health perspectives. Technical considerations limit the usefulness of screening in very low prevalence populations as the ratio of false-positive to true positive results becomes unacceptably high. Ethical guidelines emphasize the need for informed consent in named testing and screening programmes although there is also support for voluntary screening with right of refusal in the antenatal clinic provided that adequate briefing is available. There is conflicting legal advice in the UK, but programmes which follow current ethical guidance meet the legal requirements. Women in general and some groups of women in particular require testing and screening programmes in settings other than STD clinics and counselling and testing sites in order to meet specific needs. Depending on the prevalence of other STDs, testing programmes should consider incorporating other relevant tests. A doctor's decision to initiate discussion on HIV testing is based on communication skills surrounding possible risk factors, and clinical skills and knowledge. Greater training in these areas will improve the targeting of testing. In some settings the use of written information about HIV risk behaviours may be useful in stimulating women to request counselling about the HIV test.

Same-day testing programmes are popular and appear to meet the needs of some women who would not otherwise seek testing. The public interest aim of gathering data for planning services is best met by anonymized screening programmes. The public interest aim of curbing the spread of HIV is much more difficult to meet and further work is required to determine the most cost-effective use of resources when planning testing and screening programmes.

REFERENCES

Altman R, Shaheid S I, Pizzutti W et al 1992 Premarital HIV-1 testing in New Jersey. J AIDS 5: 7–11

Boyd K M 1990 HIV infection: the ethics of anonymised testing and of testing pregnant women. J Med Ethics 16: 173–178

British Medical Association 1984 The handbook of medical ethics. BMA, London

Carne C, Kapila M, 1988 Testing and screening for HIV infection. AIDS Programme Paper 2. London, Health Education Authority

Centers for Disease Control 1991 Characteristics of, and HIV infection among, women served by publicly funded HIV counselling services – United States 1989–1990. Morbid Mortal Weekly Rev 40: 195–197, 203–204

Committee on Prenatal and Newborn Screening for HIV Infection 1991 HIV screening of pregnant women and newborns. In: McHardy L (ed) Screening of pregnant women and newborns. National Academy Press, Washington DC, pp 19–23

Department of Health and Social Security 1988 Report of a working group on the monitoring and surveillance of HIV infection and AIDS. DHSS, London

Editorial 1991 Partner notification for preventing HIV infection. Lancet 338: 1112–1113

Fehrs L J, Hill D, Kerndt P R et al 1991 Targeted HIV screening at a Los Angeles prenatal/family planning health center. Am J Public Health 81: 619–622

Ferguson K J, Stapleton J T, Helms C T 1991 Physicians

effectiveness in assessing risk for human immunodeficiency virus infection. Arch Intern Med 151: 561–564

General Medical Council 8 August 1988 HIV infection and AIDS: the ethical considerations. Letter to all doctors

Godfrey C, Tolley K, Drummond M 1992 The economics of promoting sexual health. In: Curtis H (ed) 'Promoting sexual health'. BMA Foundation for AIDS, London, pp 55–64

Goldberg D J, Johnstone F D 1992 HIV testing programmes in pregnancy. In Bailliere's Clin Obstet Gynaecol 6: 33–51

Goldberg D J, MacKinnon K, Smith R et al 1992 Prevalence of HIV among childbearing women and women having termination of pregnancy. Br Med J 304: 1082–1085

Higgins D L, Galavotti C, O'Reilly K R et al 1991 Evidence for the effects of HIV antibody counseling and testing on risk behaviours. JAMA 266: 2419–2429

Holland J, Ramazanoglu C, Scott S, Sharpe S, Thomson R 1990 Sex, gender and power: young women's sexuality in the shadow of AIDS. 12: 336–350

Kell P D, Barton S E, Hawkins D A, Marwood R, Howard L C 1991 The clinical presentation of women with human immunodeficiency virus infection. Br J Obstet Gynaecol 98: 103–104

Landis S E, Schoenbach V J, Weber D J et al 1992 Results of a randomized trial of partner notification in cases of HIV infection in North Carolina. N Engl J Med 326: 101–106

McKillip J 1991 The effect of mandatory premarital HIV testing on marriage: the case of Illinois. Am J Public Health 81 (Suppl): 650–653

Meadows J, Catalan J, Gazzard B 1991 Attitudes of parturient women to HIV antibody testing in antenatal clinics. Proceedings of the Seventh International Conference on AIDS, Florence. Abstr MC 3330

Medical Defence Union 1988 AIDS: medico-legal advice. MDU, London

Mortimer P P 1988a Screening for HIV. N Engl J Med 318: 379

Mortimer P P 1988b Test for infection with HIV: slandered goods. Br Med J 296: 1615–1616

New York State HIV Seroprevalence Project 1991 Am J Public Health 81 (Suppl): 3–63

Ranki A, Valle S-L, Krohn M et al 1987 Long latency precedes overt seroconversion in sexually transmitted human immunodeficiency virus infection. Lancet 2: 589–593

Ross M W, Gold J, Wodak A, Miller M E 1991 Sexually transmissible diseases in injecting drug users. Genitour Med 67: 32–36

Royal College of Obstetricians and Gynaecologists, October 1987. Report of the Royal College of Obstetricians and Gynaecologists Subcommittee on problems associated with AIDS in relation to obstetrics and gynaecology. Royal College of Obstetricians and Gynaecologists

Squire S B, Elford J, Tilsed G et al 1991 Open access clinic providing HIV-1 antibody results on day of testing: the first twelve months. Br Med J 302: 1383–1386

van den Hoek J A R, van Haastrecht H J A, Scheeringa-Troost B, Goudsmit J, Coutinho R A 1989 HIV infection and STD in drug addicted prostitutes in Amsterdam and potential for heterosexual HIV transmission. Genitour Med 65: 146–150

WHO Global Programme on AIDS 1987 Report of the meeting on criteria for HIV screening programmes. Document WHO/SPA/GLO/87.2

5. Prophylaxis against opportunistic infection

D. E. Mercey

INTRODUCTION

Opportunistic infections account for the over-whelming majority of AIDS-defining diagnoses in men and women with HIV infection and are a major cause of morbidity and mortality. The patterns of occurrence of major opportunistic infections in women appear to be similar to those in men of similar risk group (Benslow et al 1992) with some suggestion that oesophageal candidiasis may be more common in women (Sacks et al 1992). Opportunistic infections including *Pneumocystis carinii* pneumonia (PCP), toxoplasmosis, oesophageal *Candida* and cryptococcal meningitis have also been documented in pregnant women (Stratton et al 1992).

Primary prophylaxis is the administration of therapy in the absence of clinically apparent infection, or history of infection, in order to prevent or delay its occurrence. For some conditions primary prophylaxis probably prevents new infection (for example, PCP): for others it prevents relapse from an asymptomatic latent phase (for example, toxoplasmosis). (Secondary prophylaxis, given after treatment of an opportunistic infection will not be considered in this chapter.)

For primary prophylaxis for a given infection to be feasible, several conditions must be fulfilled:

1. The opportunistic infection must be sufficiently common, amongst those identified to be at risk, for prophylaxis to be worthwhile. This is undoubtedly true for PCP in European and American patients but may not be so in Africa.
2. The natural history of the occurrence of the infection in HIV-positive patients needs to be defined. The association between the occurrence of PCP and the patient's CD4 cell count is well documented (Phair et al 1990) but herpes zoster, for example, may occur at almost any time after seroconversion. For some infections it may be possible to identify those at greatest risk by selecting patients who have asymptomatic latent infection, e.g. using serology to detect those who have latent *Toxoplasma gondii* infection.
3. Any morbidity associated with the prophylaxis must be considerably less than that caused by the infection itself. Ideally, a suitable agent of low toxicity, easy administration and proven efficacy should be available. This is certainly not the case as yet for prophylaxis against, for example, cytomegalovirus retinitis; and indeed even for PCP where primary prophylaxis is part of standard therapy, no ideal drug exists. The more unpleasant, inconvenient or complicated the regimen the worse compliance is likely to be.

When considering primary prophylaxis during pregnancy the above considerations apply but in addition the outcome of the infection for the mother and fetus needs to be assessed and the potential value of any prophylaxis must be weighed against the possible teratogenic or fetotoxic effects of any agent used.

In this chapter we will describe prophylaxis against PCP and toxoplasmosis in some detail and then consider other possible future developments in primary prophylaxis.

PNEUMOCYSTIS CARINII PNEUMONIA

PCP is the most common AIDS-defining opportunistic infection in women in most large series (Keenlyside et al 1992), and is therefore also the most widely reported major opportunistic infection to occur in pregnant women (Stratton et al 1992). Although the early reports of fatal outcomes of PCP in pregnancy (Minkoff et al 1986) were probably subject to reporting bias and were often amongst women with little or no access to health care, the concern remains that PCP in pregnancy causes serious morbidity and possibly mortality. Primary PCP prophylaxis for immunosuppressed children was established before the first case reports of AIDS appeared (Hughes et al 1977).

It is recommended that HIV-positive patients whose CD4 cell counts fall below 200 per mm^3 should be offered primary PCP prophylaxis (Centers for Disease Control 1989). This guidance was based on the observation that 8.4% and 18.4% of men with CD4 counts of less than 200 per mm^3 at enrolment in the Multicentre AIDS Cohort Study developed PCP at 6 and 12 months, respectively. Furthermore, of those patients who developed a CD4 cell count of below 200 per mm^3 during the study, the proportions with PCP at 6 and 12 months were 13% and 24%, respectively. Patients with symptoms such as fever or oral candidiasis were noted to have an increased risk of PCP even if their CD4 cell count was greater than 200 and the authors recommended that symptomatic patients be offered prophylaxis regardless of CD4 count (Phair et al 1990). In the absence of equivalent data for women and with the emerging evidence that clinical disease presentation in women is similar to that in men it seems not unreasonable to extrapolate the guidance to women. The CDC guidelines specifically excluded pregnant women from their recommendations (Centers for Disease Control 1989); however, the well documented occurrence of PCP in pregnancy, its potential to kill both mother and thus her unborn child (Koonin et al 1989) and the availability of relatively safe and effective prophylaxes make it compulsory for the physician caring for pregnant women to at least be aware of the options and discuss these, where appropriate, with the woman herself. The final decision about the risk–benefit ratio in each individual case may then be determined by the patient and her physician. Pregnancy is known to have a small effect on CD4 cell counts (Biggar et al 1989) but to date the absence of appropriate data means that most physicians base decisions about prophylaxis on information derived from non-pregnant women or male subjects.

The first choice of agent for primary PCP prophylaxis in many centres is co-trimoxazole (trimethoprim and sulphamethoxazole) 960 mg once or twice daily or three times a week. The advantages of this agent are that it is highly effective against PCP (Fischl et al 1988) and it provides prophylaxis against the rare complication of extrapulmonary *Pneumocystis carinii* infection. It also provides cross-prophylaxis against toxoplasmosis (Schneider et al 1992). It is simple to take and it is cheap. The major disadvantage of co-trimoxazole is the higher incidence of adverse reactions amongst HIV-positive patients, frequently necessitating cessation of treatment (Martin et al 1992). No clearly superior dose has been identified as few comparative studies have enrolled sufficient patients to demonstrate minor differences. There is some suggestion that lower doses delay the onset of allergic reactions but do not prevent them.

The use of co-trimoxazole in pregnancy is theoretically contraindicated as folate antagonists may be teratogenic and sulphamethoxazole may induce haemolysis and methaemoglobinaemia and increase the risk of neonatal kernicterus. In practice, however, co-trimoxazole appears to be safe (Ocho 1976) and physicians may still choose to use this drug after full discussion with the pregnant woman. Use of co-trimoxazole during lactation is not thought to present any significant risk to the neonate.

Aerosolized pentamidine also has been shown to be effective as primary PCP prophylaxis (Hirschel et al 1991). A dose of 300 mg once a month appears better than 150 mg every 2 weeks (Leoung et al 1990). The advantages of aerosolized pentamidine include the low incidence of serious side-effects (Schneider et al 1992, Martin et al 1992). Rarely, pulmonary haemorrhage and pneumothorax have been associated (but not necessarily causally) with this treatment. Compliance is easily monitored if the treatment is administered in hospital and some patients prefer a non-systemic treatment whilst they feel themselves to be well. There are, however, disadvantages of aerosolized pentamidine. It may be less effective in preventing *Pneumocystis* pneumonia than co-trimoxazole

(Schneider et al 1992). When used as secondary prophylaxis there appears to be an appreciable risk of apical disease relapse (Abd et al 1988). It is poorly tolerated by some patients due to local side-effects of administration: a bad taste in the mouth, cough and bronchospasm (the latter two being mostly preventable by prior use of bronchodilators). Administration of aerosolized pentamidine is time-consuming for health professionals and is relatively expensive. Environmental contamination by the pentamidine and cross-infection by other pathogens amongst patients receiving pentamidine are concerns (Fischl et al 1992). It offers no prophylaxis against systemic *Pneumocystis* infections (Hardy et al 1989) and no protection against cerebral toxoplasmosis. One study has suggested less efficient absorption of a nebulized drug by women compared to men (Knight et al 1988).

The use of aerosolized pentamidine in pregnancy has a certain appeal as only small amounts are systemically absorbed (Montgomery et al 1988), but there are also concerns that due to pulmonary compression by the gravid uterus distribution of the drug might be impaired and its efficacy thus reduced. A single spontaneous miscarriage has been reported following aerosolized pentamidine administration as primary prophylaxis.

Dapsone in a dose of 100 mg once a day has also been used for primary PCP prophylaxis and has been shown to be as effective as co-trimoxazole (Blum 1992). Dapsone and pyrimethamine combinations have been shown to be more effective than aerosolized pentamidine in preventing PCP (although not conferring any survival advantage), and to have the added advantage of providing cross-prophylaxis against toxoplasmosis. However, as with co-trimoxazole, adverse reactions necessitating change of treatment are common (Girard et al 1992). Many different doses and combinations of dapsone with pyrimethamine or trimethoprim have been used but no study of sufficient size to show conclusive advantages of one regimen over another has been conducted.

Dapsone and pyrimethamine have been used in pregnancy for the prophylaxis and treatment of malaria with little reported adverse effect (Anonymous 1983), despite the fact that pyri-

methamine is a folate antagonist and has been suggested to be teratogenic (Harpey et al 1983), and dapsone has been associated with neonatal haemolysis and methaemoglobinaemia. When used for the prophylaxis or treatment of malaria in pregnant women, it is recommended that folate supplements are given.

Fansidar (pyrimethamine and sulfadoxine) has also been used as PCP prophylaxis. There are no randomized studies comparing its efficacy or side-effect profile to co-trimoxazole or aerosolized pentamidine. Despite similar potential dangers of its use during pregnancy, like dapsone it appears to be relatively safe.

Zidovudine per se has been suggested to have some effect in lowering the incidence of *Pneumocystis* pneumonia over and above any concomitant prophylaxis, but if real this effect is slight and should not be relied upon (Leoung et al 1990).

TOXOPLASMOSIS

The rate of occurrence of clinically apparent toxoplasmosis in HIV-positive patients is related to the background seroprevalence of the population under study, and most cases are thought to be due to reactivation rather than primary infection. Neurotoxoplasmosis usually presents as a late complication of HIV infection in patients with low CD4 counts. Treatment does not always prevent mortality or irreversible morbidity. The majority of patients with neurotoxoplasmosis have evidence of prior latent infection in the form of pre-existing immunoglobulin G (IgG) antibodies to *Toxoplasma gondii*, although absence of antibody is not an absolute guarantee that the patient will never develop toxoplasmosis. Toxoplasmosis has been reported in HIV-positive pregnant women (Stratton et al 1992).

Co-trimoxazole has been shown to reduce the incidence of neurotoxoplasmosis when given as primary PCP prophylaxis (Schneider et al 1992). In patients who have evidence of latent *Toxoplasma* infection or who are from a population with a high seroprevalence, co-trimoxazole should be the first line agent for PCP prophylaxis. There is no evidence to suggest that those patients not requiring primary PCP prophylaxis would benefit from prophylaxis against neurotoxoplasmosis.

Dapsone and pyrimethamine in combination have also been shown to reduce the risk of neurotoxoplasmosis and offer an alternative for those patients unable to tolerate co-trimoxazole (Girard et al 1992).

The use of co-trimoxazole, dapsone and pyrimethamine during pregnancy is discussed above.

THE FUTURE OF PRIMARY PROPHYLAXIS

When considering the long-term administration of antimicrobials the risk of inducing resistant organisms must always be considered. This is not thought to be a problem with *Pneumocystis carinii* although the inability to culture this organism makes routine sensitivity testing impossible. Resistant strains of *Candida albicans* (Powderly 1992), herpes simplex (Safrin et al 1991), and *Mycobacterium tuberculosis* (Fischl et al 1992) are well documented in HIV-positive patients but the relative contribution of prior antimicrobial exposure and degree of immunocompromise of the patient are difficult to disentangle.

The possibility of preventing all opportunistic infections in HIV disease with easily administered non-toxic regimens remains a dream – however, progress is being made. That primary prophylaxis against systemic fungal infections such as cryptococcal meningitis and histoplasmosis may be possible is suggested by an open-label study of fluconazole using historical controls (Nightingale et al 1992). The use of rifabutin as a single-agent primary prophylactic against atypical mycobacterial disease has shown some promise (Cameron et al 1992). A trial of oral acyclovir as prophylaxis against cytomegalovirus retinitis was unfortunately not able to show any benefit in reducing cases of retinitis, but an unexpected survival advantage remains unexplained (European–Australian Acyclovir Study Group 1992).

REFERENCES

Abd A, Nierman D, Ilowite J, Pierson R, Bell A 1988 Bilateral upper lobe Pneumocystis carinii pneumonia in a patient receiving inhaled pentamidine prophylaxis. Chest 94: 329–331

Anonymous 1983 Pyrimethamine combinations in pregnancy. Lancet 2: 1005–1007

Benslow S, Melnick S, Hillman D et al 1992 Gender, HIV related clinical events and mortality: preliminary & observational data from the community programs for clinical research on AIDS (CPCRA). VIII International Conference on AIDS, Amsterdam. Abstr MoC0031

Biggar R, Pahwa S, Minkoff H et al 1989 Immunosuppression in pregnant women infected with human immunodeficiency virus. Am J Obstet Gynecol 161: 1239–1244

Blum R, Miller L, Gaggini L, Cohn D 1992 Comparative trial of dapsone versus trimethoprim sulphamethoxazole for primary prophylaxis of pneumocystis pneumonia. J Acq Immune Defic Synd 5: 341–347

Cameron D, Conaut M, Garber G et al 1992 Refabutin prophylaxis of Mycobacterium avium complex bacteraemia in acquired immune deficiency syndrome. International Congress on Drug Therapy in HIV infection, Glasgow. Abstr 0–8C.4

Centers for Disease Control 1989 Guidelines for prophylaxis against Pneumocystis carinii pneumonia for persons infected with human immunodeficiency virus. MMWR 38 (Suppl 5): 1–9

European-Australian Acyclovir Study Group 1992, Placebo controlled trial of high dose acyclovir for the prevention of cytomegalovirus disease in advanced HIV disease. International Congress on Drug Therapy in HIV Infection, Glasgow. Abstr 0–16.2

Fischl M, Dickinson G, La Voie L, 1988 Safety and efficacy of sulphamethoxazole and trimethoprim chemoprophylaxis for Pneumocystis carinii pneumonia in AIDS. JAMA 259: 1185–1189

Fischl M, Uttamchandani R, Daikos G et al 1992 An outbreak of tuberculosis caused by multidrug-resistant bacilli among patients with HIV infection. Ann Intern Med 117: 177–183

Girard P M, Landman R, Gaudebout C et al 1992 Dapsone, pyrimethamine vs aerosolized pentamidine for primary prophylaxis of pneumocystis and neurotoxoplasmosis. VIII International Conference on AIDS, Amsterdam. Abstr WeB1017.

Hardy D, Northfelt D, Drake T 1989 Fatal, disseminated pneumocystosis in a patient with acquired immunodeficiency syndrome receiving prophylactic aerosolised pentamidine. Am J Med 87: 329–331

Harpey J-P, Darbois Y, Lefebvre G 1983 Teratogenicity of pyrimethamine (letter). Lancet 2: 399

Hirschel B, Lazzarin A, Chopard P et al 1991 A controlled study of inhaled pentamidine for primary prevention of Pneumocystis carinii pneumonia. N Engl J Med 324: 1079–1083

Hughes W, Kuhn S, Chaudhary S et al 1977 Successful chemoprophylaxis for pneumocystis carinii pneumonitis. N Engl J Med 297: 1419–1426

Keenlyside R, Phillips A, Johnson A, Evans B, Barton S, Brettle R 1992 HIV infection and AIDS in women in the United Kingdom. VIII International Conference on AIDS, Amsterdam. Abstr PoC4740

Knight V, Yu C, Gilbert B, Divine G 1988 Estimating the dosage of ribavirin aerosol according to age and other variables. J Infect Dis 158: 443–448

Koonin L, Ellerbrock T, Atrash H et al 1989 Pregnancy associated deaths due to AIDS in the United States. JAMA 261: 1306–1309

Leoung G, Feigal D, Montgomery B et al 1990 Aerosolized pentamidine for prophylaxis against Pneumocystis carinii pneumonia. N Engl J Med 323: 769–775

Martin M, Cox P, Beck K, Styer C, Beall G 1992 A comparison

of the effectiveness of three regimens in the prevention of
Pneumocystis carinii pneumonia in human
immunodeficiency virus infected patients. Arch Intern Med
152: 523–528

Minkoff H, Haynes de Regt R, Landesman S, Schwarz R 1986
Pneumocystis carinii pneumonia associated with acquired
immunodeficiency syndrome in pregnancy: a report of three
maternal deaths. Obstet Gynaecol 67: 284–287

Montgomery A, Deks R, Luce J et al 1988 Selective delivery
of pentamidine to the lung by aerosol. Am Rev Resp Dis
137: 477–478

Nightingale S, Cal S, Peterson D et al 1992 Primary
prophylaxis with fluconazole against systemic fungal
infections in HIV positive patients. AIDS 6: 191–194

Ocho P 1976 Trimethoprim and sulphamethoxazole in
pregnancy. JAMA 217: 1244

Phair J, Muno A, Detels R, Kaslow R, Rinaldo C, Saah A
1990 The risk of Pneumocystis carinii pneumonia among
men infected with human immunodeficiency virus type 1.
N Engl J Med 322: 161–165

Powderly W 1992 Letter to the editor. AIDS 6: 604–605

Sacks H, Szabo S, Miller L et al 1992 Gender differences in
the natural history of HIV infection from the VIII
International Conference on AIDS, Amsterdam. Abstr
MoC0030

Safrin S, Crumpacker C, Chatis P et al 1991 A controlled trial
comparing foscarnet with vidarabine for acyclovir resistant
muco-cutaneous herpes simplex in the acquired immuno
deficiency syndrome. N Engl J Med 325: 551–555

Schneider M, Hoepelman I, Danner S et al 1992 Efficacy of
aerosolized pentamidine and low dose co-trimoxazole for
primary prevention of pneumocystis carinii pneumonia. VIII
International Conference on AIDS, Amsterdam. Abstr WeB
1018

Stratton P, Mofenson L, Willoughby A 1992 Human
immunodeficiency virus infection in pregnant women under
care at AIDS clinical trials centres in the United States.
Obstet Gynaecol 79: 364–368

6. Antiviral therapy

Ian Williams

INTRODUCTION

The optimum therapy for HIV infection has yet to be defined but considerable research has been undertaken to identify and evaluate specific therapeutic strategies. These can be broadly divided into those which inhibit viral replication and those which stimulate or activate the immune system against HIV. Various sites within the replication cycle of HIV have been identified (Table 6.1) as possible targets for antiviral drugs. Some of these remain theoretical interventions but for others, drugs have been developed for clinical use and are under current evaluation. In particular, the efficacy and toxicity of nucleoside analogues which inhibit viral DNA polymerase (reverse transcriptase) have been assessed in clinical trials and open observational studies.

Zidovudine (3-azido-3-deoxythymidine) was the first (Yarchoan et al 1986) and is now used extensively in clinical practice within the developed world. Clinical trials are ongoing to assess other nucleoside analogues comparatively or in combination with zidovudine, and at various stages in the natural history of the disease. As the majority of HIV infection in the developed world to date has occurred in homosexual/bisexual men, they have formed the core population taking part in clinical trials. However, unless pharmokinetic and safety profiles are substantially different, it is unlikely that gender will greatly influence clinical efficacy of a particular drug. In this chapter the current clinical evidence for the use of antiviral drugs in the management and treatment of HIV infection will be outlined.

Table 6.1 Anti-HIV agents; targets within the replication cycle and anti-HIV agents currently undergoing in vitro and clinical evaluation

Target in replication cycle	Agents
Viral binding and adsorption	recombitant soluble CD4 analogues neutralizing antibodies
Reverse transcriptase	deoxynucleoside analogues, e.g. zidovudine, didanosine non-nucleoside analogues, e.g. TIBO derivatives, neviraprine
Integration of DNA into the host genome	
Transcription and translation of viral genes	inhibitors of tat, e.g. RO5-3335 antisense oligodeoxynucleotides
Viral product assembly and processing	protease inhibitors glycosylation inhibitors
Viral budding	interferons

ZIDOVUDINE

Zidovudine, a nucleoside analogue which inhibits HIV DNA polymerase (reverse transcriptase), is structurally related to thymidine but differs in having an azido group (N_3) at the 3 position on the ribose ring. On entry to the cell it is phosphorylated by cellular enzymes to zidovudine triphosphate which acts by two mechanisms to inhibit transcription of viral RNA to DNA. The first is by competitive inhibition of deoxythymidine triphosphate for reverse transcriptase and the second by terminating DNA synthesis when incorporated into the proviral DNA chain (Mitsuya H et al 1985, Furman et al 1986, St Clair et al 1987). The substitution of the hydroxyl by the azido group inhibits the formation of a phospho-diester bond necessary for chain growth. The affinity of zidovudine for viral reverse transcriptase is many-fold greater than for human cellular DNA polymerases, particularly α and β, though its activity against these and γ may form the basis of its toxicity profile.

Symptomatic HIV infection

In 1987 a randomized study in 282 patients with either previous *Pneumocystis carinii* pneumonia (PCP) or symptoms of severe AIDS-related complex (ARC) reported a significant reduction in mortality and probability of developing an opportunistic infection in patients treated with zidovudine compared to those who received placebo (Fischl et al 1987). Patients within the trial had completed a median of just over 4 months on treatment when the study was terminated early following an interim analysis finding that one of 145 patients on zidovudine compared to 19 of 137 on placebo had died. In addition, in those persons receiving zidovudine there had been an improvement in symptoms, a significant though modest and transient rise in CD4 count and reduction in serum p24 antigen levels. As a result of this trial and despite the high incidence of haematological toxicity, zidovudine received a licence in many countries, even before formal publication of the trial results. Although long-term efficacy and toxicity remained unknown, clinicians felt able to extend the use of zidovudine to all patients with severely symptomatic disease.

Continued follow-up of the original participants in the trial showed that the overall survival at 12 months of those patients who received zidovudine was 84.5%, higher than expected from historical controls (Fischl et al 1989). Similar 1-year survival rates have been reported in uncontrolled observational studies (Creagh-Kirk et al 1988, Williams et al 1989, Swanson & Cooper 1990, Moore et al 1991a), and from date of diagnosis of AIDS a median survival of between 2 and 2.5 years has been reported in persons treated with zidovudine compared to between 6 and 14 months in contemporary controls who were not (Lemp et al 1990, Moore et al 1991b, Vella et al 1992). Equally, the survival of persons with AIDS has shown a marked improvement after 1987, with zidovudine use strongly associated with improved

outcome (Lemp et al 1990, Swanson & Cooper 1990, Moore et al 1991b).

Care must be taken in attributing improvement solely to treatment with zidovudine. Other factors for which zidovudine may have acted as a marker are likely to have been important and include access to medical care, the character of the initial AIDS-defining illness and better treatment and prophylaxis of opportunistic infections.

Subsequently in 1990, the efficacy of zidovudine (200 mg 4-hourly) was reported in the AGTG 016 study of 711 persons with early and mild symptomatic disease (Fischl et al 1990c). The clinical end-points were progression to AIDS or symptoms of advanced ARC with a CD4 count less than $200 \times 10^6/1$. Over a median duration of 11 months the rate of progression per 100 patient-years for those persons with a baseline CD4 count between 200 and $500 \times 10^6/1$ was 11.2 for placebo and 4.5 for zidovudine. The incidence of anaemia and neutropenia in those persons treated with zidovudine was 5% and 4%, respectively, considerably lower than the rates reported in severe symptomatic disease. The reported efficacy, low toxicity and better tolerance supported the early use of zidovudine by clinicians in patients with symptomatic disease.

The majority of persons participating in these earlier clinical trials and reported on in observational studies were white homosexual men, prompting concern of the efficacy of zidovudine in other subpopulation groups. Data from one study of 714 persons with AIDS diagnosed between April 1987 and June 1989 reported a significantly greater rate of survival at 2 years in white homosexual men compared to ethnic minorities, women and injecting drug users (Moore et al 1991b). This disparity was attributed to the preferential use of zidovudine. On further subanalysis the investigators were able to show that treatment with zidovudine was associated with a similar increase in estimated survival probability irrespective of a population group. Similarly, in an observational study of 1025 persons with AIDS or ARC treated with zidovudine for up to 2 years and following adjustment for more advanced state of disease, as evidenced by lower CD4 counts at initiation of zidovudine therapy, and the lower use of PCP prophylaxis in black and Hispanic patients, no significant ethnic/racial difference in survival was shown (Easterbrook et al 1991). The later presentation of disease and start of therapy may possibly reflect poorer access to medical resources and different attitudes to health care by minority populations.

In addition to survival, the observation that zidovudine delays progression to AIDS was found to be equally valid for Whites, Blacks and Hispanics. In a combined analysis of data from two randomized clinical trials in asymptomatic and early symptomatic infection, a similar trend was also seen in women and injecting drug users but because of smaller numbers did not reach statistical significance (Lagakos et al 1991).

It is clear from these analyses that future clinical trials need to incorporate and stratify for subpopulation groups, or that large prospective studies for each group are needed to assess treatment effect and tolerance. It is unlikely, though, that gender, race or transmission category specifically will have an independent effect on the efficacy of an antiviral treatment over and above that determined by dose and stage of disease.

The efficacy of zidovudine in HIV-related neurological disease will be difficult to establish, as treatment with zidovudine has now become standard clinical practice for patients with symptomatic disease. Anecdotally, in a small number of patients zidovudine has been reported to improve symptoms of dementia and peripheral neuropathy (Yarchoan et al 1987, 1988b; Dalakas et al 1988). In the first placebo-controlled trial of zidovudine in severely symptomatic patients, transient improvements in neuropsychometric measures were seen in the treatment group (Schmitt et al 1988). The early termination of this trial and the general improvement in the physical well-being of those treated with zidovudine meant a significant effect on neurological outcome could not be established. However, the findings that levels of p24 antigen and recovery of HIV-1 from the cerebrospinal fluid are both reduced in zidovudine-treated individuals (de Gans et al 1988), and the reports of a declining incidence of AIDS-related dementia (Portegies et al 1989) following the licensing of zidovudine, support a probable benefit in HIV neurological disease. These observations were made in patients taking relatively higher doses

of zidovudine, but more recently lower dosages have been employed and concern has been voiced over whether they will be effective in neurological disease. A recent dose-comparative study reported a trend for lower incidence of HIV encephalopathy in those patients receiving a higher dose of zidovudine (1200 mg daily) than a lower dose (400 mg daily) (Nordic Medical Research Councils' HIV Therapy Group 1992). Further evaluation of antiviral therapy in HIV neurological disease is necessary.

Zidovudine appears to have no effect on the development of Kaposi's sarcoma in patients with symptomatic disease (Fischl et al 1987), nor does it affect the natural history and clinical course of Kaposi's sarcoma when used as monotherapy (Lane et al 1989). Dependent on CD4 count, most clinicians, though, would still advocate initiating therapy with zidovudine in patients presenting with Kaposi's sarcoma as their first symptom of HIV disease.

Asymptomatic infection

Approximately 50% of persons will cumulatively progress to AIDS or 75% to symptomatic disease 8–10 years after initial infection (Moss & Bacchetti 1989, Rutherford et al 1990). This high rate of progression of toxicity in severely symptomatic disease, plus evidence that over a time viral load and replication increases, supported trials of zidovudine in patients who were asymptomatic. The ACTG 016 study (Fischl et al 1990c) reported a delayed progression to AIDS in persons who had both early manifestations of symptomatic disease and CD4 counts between 200 and $500 \times 10^6/1$. In the same year a trial (ACTG 019) in asymptomatic individuals reported clinical benefit in those randomized to receive either 1000 mg or 500 mg zidovudine daily compared to placebo (Volberding et al 1990). The trial was discontinued after a median follow-up of 55 weeks in the 1338 patients whose baseline CD4 count was between 200 and $500 \times 10^6/1$. There were too few clinical events in those persons with CD4 counts greater than $500 \times 10^6/1$ and the trial in this group is ongoing. The rate of progression to AIDS or severe ARC per 100 person-years was significantly decreased in both treatment groups (500 mg: 3.6; 1500 mg:

4.3; placebo: 7.6). The equivalent efficacy but lower rate of haematological toxicity led to the recommendation in the USA that treatment with 500 mg daily of zidovudine should be started in asymptomatic HIV-seropositive individuals with a CD4 count below $500 \times 10^6/1$.

Observational data from 2516 seropositive men who participated in a multicentre AIDS cohort provided further evidence that treatment with zidovudine favourably influenced progression to AIDS (Graham et al 1991). Significant reduction in rates attributed mainly to zidovudine was seen at 6, 12, 18 and 24 months in those participants with CD4 counts above $350 \times 10^6/1$ or less with similar but non-significant trends in those with CD4 counts above $350 \times 10^6/1$. More recently in 1992 a collaborative Australian–European randomized trial in asymptomatic individuals with CD4 counts greater than $400 \times 10^6/1$ reported that zidovudine (1 gm daily) significantly reduced the risk of progression at 2 years to symptomatic disease or a CD4 count less than $350 \times 10^6/1$ (Cooper 1992). Although the high voluntary withdrawal rate, the surrogate and soft clinical endpoints and failure to use an intention-to-treat analysis are criticisms of this trial, it adds further support for those who advocate early intervention strategies.

The optimum time to initiate zidovudine therapy with reference to CD4 count and clinical status remains controversial. There are uncertainties over the long-term toxicity of zidovudine, the influence that the development of in vitro resistance has on clinical outcome and whether early therapy ultimately improves survival. The relatively short duration of the ACTG 019 study made it impossible for the investigators to assess the effect of early therapy on survival. Subsequently, though, in a trial of zidovudine (1500 mg daily) in 338 persons with both early symptomatic disease and CD4 counts of 200–$500 \times 10^6/1$, no survival benefit over a duration of 2 years was noted in those persons randomized to receive early therapy (23 deaths occurred in this group) compared to those who initially received placebo and started zidovudine only when their CD4 count either fell below $200 \times 10^6/1$ or they developed AIDS (20 deaths) (Hamilton et al 1992). There was, however, a relatively high number of non-AIDS deaths in both groups; but analysis after a further 12 months, and after all study participants had been offered open-label zidovudine, confirmed no difference in survival (Simberkoff et al 1992).

In contrast, observational data from the multicentre AIDS cohort study found a survival benefit for persons receiving early zidovudine therapy, particularly those with CD4 counts between 200 and $349 \times 10^6/1$ (Graham et al 1992). A placebo-controlled trial of zidovudine (1 gm daily) in approximately 1800 asymptomatic individuals (in France and the UK) is due to report in the spring of 1993. As the median follow-up in this trial will be over 3 years, the long-term efficacy with respect to progression to symptomatic disease and survival may be defined more fully.

Toxicity

The most common toxicity associated with the use of zidovudine is bone marrow suppression. Approximately 45% of patients with severe symptomatic HIV disease treated with 1500 mg daily of zidovudine developed anaemia or neutropenia in the original phase II trial (Richman et al 1987). A lower incidence of toxicity occurs with dose reduction and in persons with less advanced disease (Table 6.2). In the ACTG 019 study, 1.1% of persons with asymptomatic infection receiving 500 mg daily developed an anaemia (haemoglobin < 8 g/dl) and 1.8% neutropenia ($< 0.75 \times 10^9/1$) compared to 0.2% and 1%, respectively, on placebo (Volberding et al 1990).

The mechanism of zidovudine-induced marrow suppression is not clear but is thought to involve the incorporation of zidovudine triphosphate and the competitive inhibition of thymidine triphosphate into the DNA of bone marrow progenitor cells (Furman et al 1986, Sommadossi et al 1989). Persons treated with zidovudine develop a macrocytosis but the extent of this does not correlate with the risk of anaemia (Volberding et al 1990, Fischl et al 1990a). Bone marrow findings have variably been reported to show megaloblastic and/or hypoplastic change in erythroid and myeloid cell lines (Gill et al 1987, Walker et al 1988). In some patients who develop an anaemia the mean cell volume does not rise and bone

Table 6.2 Incidence of haematological toxicity with zidovudine

Trial	Medium follow-up (months)	Population	Daily dose (mg)	Anaemia (%) (< 8.0 g/dl)	Neutropenia (%) (< 0.75 × 10⁹/l)
Richman et al 1987	4	AIDS & severe ARC	1500	24.5*	38.6
Fischl et al 1990 (ACTG 002)	25.6	AIDS (PCP)	a) 1500 b) 1200 for 4/52 then 600	39 29	51 37
Fischl et al 1990 (ACTG 016)	11	early symptomatic (CD4 > 0.2 × 10⁹/l)	1200	5	4
Volberding et al 1990 (ACTG 019)	12.75	asymptomatic (CD4 0.2–0.5 × 10⁹/l)	a) 1500 b) 500	6.3 1.1	6.3 1.8
Cooper et al 1992	24	asymptomatic (CD4 >0.4 × 10⁹/l)	1000	1	2

* < 7.5 g/dl

marrow examination reveals a pure erythroid hypoplasia (Cohen et al 1989).

Recovery from haematological toxicity usually occurs within 3–4 weeks of discontinuation of therapy, though longer suppression has been reported (Walker et al 1988). Clearly, though, the severity of HIV disease and the occurrence of opportunistic infections (*Mycobacterium avium* complex (MAC), parvovirus) and tumours (lymphoma) may influence this. When toxicity occurs, dose reduction, transfusion support, intermittent regimens and cytokine therapy have been employed in attempts to continue zidovudine treatment.

Recombinant erythropoietin has been shown to be of help in reducing transfusion dependency (Fischl et al 1990c), particularly in those patients with lower serum erythropoietin levels, and granulocyte macrophage colony stimulating factor (GM-CSF) can be of help in HIV- and drug-associated leukopenia (Groopman et al 1987). Initial studies, though, reported increased replication of HIV in macrophages/monocytes (Koyanagi et al 1988) and rising levels of serum p24 antigen with GM-CSF (Pluda et al 1990), though when used in combination with zidovudine it enhances the drug's anti-HIV effect in macrophages by facilitating entry and phosphorylation (Perno et al 1989). With availability of alternative nucleoside analogues (didanosine, ddI; and dideoxycytidine, ddC) with little haematological toxicity, there is, however, little rationale for using these agents to continue treatment with zidovudine in persons with previous haematological toxicity.

Gastrointestinal side-effects are common, particularly at higher dose and in more advanced disease, though they are a less frequent cause of permanent discontinuation of therapy than haematological toxicity. In severely symptomatic patients nausea was reported in 46% of persons randomized to receive zidovudine 1500 mg daily compared to 18% receiving placebo (Fischl et al 1987), whilst in asymptomatic individuals severe nausea was considerably less frequent – 3.3% with zidovudine 500 mg daily and 0.2% for placebo (Volberding et al 1990). Other gastrointestinal symptoms were reported more frequently, particularly in symptomatic patients, and included vomiting, dyspepsia, bloating and the more general symptoms of malaise, fatigue and insomnia. These in themselves may not be serious side-effects but they affect an individual's acceptance of and compliance with therapy.

Myalgia was originally reported as an adverse effect of zidovudine but subsequently in two trials in persons with less advanced disease, no difference was observed between placebo and zidovudine (Volberding et al 1990, Fischl et al 1990c). The incidence, though, was at considerable variance between the two studies, implying a different definition or ascertainment. Since the widespread licensure of zidovudine in treating symptomatic patients, a myopathy has been described in those who had received long-term therapy (Bessen et al 1988, Helbert et al 1988). Although both degenerative and inflammatory myopathies associated with HIV infection had previously been reported before the widespread use of zidovudine (Dalakas et al

1986, Simpson & Bender 1988), investigators have argued that there are distinctive features of zidovudine-induced myopathy. In a review of 20 HIV-positive patients with myopathy, 'ragged' red fibres indicative of mitochondrial abnormalities were found on biopsy only in the 15 persons who had been treated with zidovudine, and their number correlated with the severity of the myopathy (Dalakas et al 1990). The inhibition of γ DNA polymerase in mitochondria by zidovudine is the suggested pathogenic mechanism. There were, however, irrespective of zidovudine, common findings in these 20 patients of degenerating muscle fibres, cytoplasmic bodies and infiltrates of CD8 cells and macrophages consistent with class I major histocompatibility complex (MHC) antigens. This suggests that a T cell-mediated MHC-1 restricted cytotoxic process is the underlying mechanism for the myopathy in HIV infection, and it is unclear whether zidovudine therapy or another disease process is the main factor responsible for the development of symptoms.

The variable clinical symptoms and laboratory findings both on the presentation of myopathy and in response to discontinuation of zidovudine, and the fact that severely symptomatic patients are more likely to have been treated with zidovudine and to be living longer, make it difficult to assess how much is caused by HIV or drug use. The case for zidovudine as the cause of myopathy has been strengthened recently by the finding of a depleted content of mitochondrial DNA in zidovudine-treated patients presenting with myopathy compared to controls (Arnaudo et al 1991). Careful clinical assessment including electromyography (EMG) and muscle biopsy should be undertaken before deciding to discontinue zidovudine or determining other therapeutic options.

The number of women infected with HIV and the rising number reported with AIDS has raised concerns about the safety of zidovudine in pregnancy. Zidovudine crosses the placenta (Gillet et al 1989, Watts et al 1991) and thus, theoretically, maternal treatment might decrease the rate of vertical transmission. The risk to the fetus of toxicity is not known. Uncontrolled retrospective studies of women receiving zidovudine during pregnancy, though, have not reported any increase in major adverse effects in either the fetus or the mother

(Viscarello et al 1991, Ferrazin et al 1991). In particular, in one series (Sperling et al 1992), no teratogenic abnormalities occurred in 12 infants whose mothers took zidovudine during the first trimester. Overall, in this series of 45 infants born to 43 mothers there appeared to be no increased risk of prematurity or of intrauterine growth retardation. Although these reports are useful they do not exclude a relative risk of adverse pregnancy outcome in women receiving zidovudine, and further information is needed.

Dose

Pharmokinetic studies suggested the need for higher daily dose and frequent dosaging but the subsequent unacceptable rate of intolerance secondary to haematological toxicity made lower dose regimens in clinical practice routine. A randomized dose comparison study in patients with a previous single episode of PCP showed no significant difference in the estimated 2-year survival probabilities between those receiving 1200 mg daily reduced to 600 mg after 4 weeks, and those treated with 1500 mg daily (Fischl et al 1990b). At 18 months' therapy a survival advantage in favour of the lower dose was seen but change in CD4 count and p24 antigen was similar in both groups. Severe anaemia and neutropenia occurred more frequently and earlier on treatment with 1500 mg daily.

Equally in asymptomatic individuals treated with 500 mg daily, haematological toxicity was lower and efficacy similar to 1500 mg daily (Volberding et al 1990). In addition, open observational studies report a high incidence of toxicity and intolerance in severely symptomatic patients treated with 1200–1500 mg daily (Dournon et al 1988, Swanson et al 1990, Moore et al 1991a). Lower doses are now routinely used in clinical practice, but the optimum lower dose is not clear. In two large clinical trials in Australia and Europe of zidovudine in asymptomatic individuals, the dose employed was 1 g daily, chosen to complement US studies. In the first of these (Cooper 1992) the incidence of anaemia (< 8 g/dl) and neutropenia (< 0.75 × 10⁹/l) was 1% and 2%, respectively, in patients with CD4 counts > 400 × 10⁶/l, similar to rates reported in the

500-mg arm of ACTG 019 study. The other study, the France/UK Concorde Trial is due to report in spring 1993. A dose comparison study in persons with symptomatic disease or low CD4 counts reported no difference in survival in 474 patients randomized to receive either 400, 800 or 1200 mg of zidovudine daily over a median duration of 19 months (Nordic Medical Research Councils' HIV Therapy Group 1992). There was, however, a trend for more AIDS-defining events per person and a significantly higher number developing dementia in the 400-mg arm. The incidence of anaemia was significantly lower in the 400-mg arm but the number of patients requiring blood transfusion was similar irrespective of dose.

Although the correlation between change in surrogate markers and clinical outcome has not been fully defined, reduction in levels of p24 antigen or plasma viraemia are taken as an indicator of a drug's potential anti-HIV activity. In a pilot study of zidovudine in combination with acyclovir a fall in the levels of p24 antigen and plasma viraemia was reported equally with daily dosages of 300 mg, 600 mg and 1500 mg of zidovudine alone (Collier et al 1990). This is not to say that 300 mg daily should be advocated, as the reduction in p24 antigen is very variable between individuals and the number in this study was small.

The optimum dose for an individual may depend on drug absorption, renal and hepatic function and weight, all of which could influence serum and cellular levels of zidovudine. This together with the ability to suppress viral replication as measured by levels of viraemia needs to be set against the risk of toxicity and the occurrence of viral resistance. If surrogate markers are developed which closely correlate with clinical outcome, then a therapeutic option could be optimized to each individual.

DIDEOXYINOSINE

2',3'-Dideoxyinosine (ddI, didanosine), a purine nucleoside analogue, is phosphorylated by cellular enzymes to dideoxyadenosine triphosphate and inhibits HIV replication at the level of the viral DNA polymerase reverse transcriptase. In vitro studies confirmed inhibition of HIV replication in T lymphocytes, and showed that ddI has little

toxicity against human bone marrow progenitor cells, has anti-HIV activity in macrophages/monocytes, and in its triphosphate form has a long intracellular half-life of 12 h Ahluwalia et al 1987, 1988, Du et al 1989, Perno et al 1989). DdI, however, is unstable in acid conditions and thus needs to be given with a buffer to increase gastric pH and to be taken at least 2 h after a meal.

Phase I trials have reported increases in CD4 cell counts and reduction in levels of p24 antigen and HIV viraemia (Yarchoan et al 1989, Lambert et al 1990, Cooley et al 1990. Based on these changes in surrogate markers and before the clinical efficacy of ddI could be established the drug received a licence in October 1991 in the USA for use in patients who were intolerant to zidovudine or who had deteriorated clinically or immunologically on zidovudine therapy. Elsewhere it became available in compassionate release programmes at a dose of 250–500 mg daily or by participation in clinical trials.

The main toxicities of ddI are pancreatitis, hepatitis and peripheral neuropathy, all of which occurred more frequently at higher dose (Lambert et al 1990, Cooley et al 1990, Yarchoan et al 1990) and led to doses below 750 mg daily being employed in phase II trials. The incidence of pancreatitis in patients who are severely symptomatic has been reported to be between 0.5 and 13%, with most cases occurring within the first few months on therapy (Kahn et al 1992, Darbyshire & Aboulker 1992). Pancreatitis has been noted more commonly in patients with more advanced disease, particularly in those with disseminated cytomegalovirus infection or previous history of pancreatitis, and also in association with concomitant therapy with intravenous pentamidine. Care should be taken in these patients if treated with ddI, and in those with a high alcohol intake or prior elevation of triglyceride or amylase blood levels. A rise in serum amylase whilst on therapy occurs more frequently than, and is probably not predictive of the risk of, pancreatitis and may in some incidences be due to salivary amylase coincidental with symptoms of a dry mouth (Sweeney et al 1992). Deaths from acute pancreatitis have been reported in patients whilst on ddI.

Diarrhoea may occur and is thought to be due to the buffer contained within the preparation.

Other adverse events include nausea, confusion, headaches and convulsions (Yarchoan et al 1990, Rozencwieg et al 1990, Dudley et al 1992). One problem in assessing safety data is determining whether the underlying HIV disease progression is responsible rather than ddI in patients who are already severely symptomatic. Both pancreatitis and peripheral neuropathy can occur in HIV disease. Both phase I trials and expanded access programmes give us little information on the clinical efficacy of a drug.

Recently a trial of ddI (500 mg or 750 mg daily) in persons with AIDS or ARC who had previously tolerated at least 16 weeks of zidovudine treatment reported a significant reduction in the number of new AIDS-defining events and deaths in persons who were switched to ddI compared to those who remained on zidovudine (Kahn et al 1992). This effect was seen primarily in persons with ARC randomized to receive 500 mg ddI and was commensurate with an overall rise of CD4 count above baseline and reduction in levels of p24 antigen when compared to those persons who remained on zidovudine.

The European/Australian Alpha trial in 1775 symptomatic patients previously intolerant of zidovudine, however, showed no difference in overall survival between those persons randomized to receive 200 mg compared to 750 mg daily (Darbyshire & Aboulker 1992). This was despite a highly significant but small difference in change in CD4 count favouring the higher dose. Although an increase in CD4 count was associated with an improved survival irrespective of dose, the size of difference in CD4 response between a higher and lower dose was too small to have an impact on the overall survival between the two groups. It is unlikely, because of the size of this trial and the large number of deaths making it statistically very powerful, that any true survival difference remained undetected. In view of the much higher number of adverse events in the 750-mg arm, lower doses of ddI should probably be used in these patients with advanced symptomatic disease.

The question whether ddI is clinically effective in this group of patients remains unanswered by the Alpha trial, but other ongoing studies of ddI in single or combination regimens will hopefully provide further information on clinical efficacy.

Whether ddI has a greater and more prolonged effect than zidovudine or whether sequential or combination use is better remains to be determined.

DIDEOXYCYTIDINE

Dideoxycytidine (ddC) is a pyrimidine nucleoside analogue which in vitro has a more potent anti-HIV activity than zidovudine and less toxicity against bone marrow progenitor cells (Mitsuya et al 1986). Unfortunately, in the initial phase I studies a severe painful but reversible peripheral neuropathy developed in a high proportion of patients on doses greater than 0.09 mg/kg daily, after 3–4 months on therapy (Yarchoan et al 1988a, Merigan et al 1989). Other toxicities noted at high dose included stomatitis, rashes, arthralgia and fever. At low dosages the incidence of peripheral neuropathy was much lower but the decline in p24 antigen and rise in CD4 count was less consistent and more gradual. An alternating regimen of low-dose zidovudine and ddC resulted in a lower incidence of toxicity and sustained changes in surrogate markers in some patients (Yarchoan et al 1988a).

DdC has now moved into Phase II trials as monotherapy and in combination regimens. The results from a dose-ranging open labelled study of low-dose zidovudine (150, 300 or 600 mg daily) in combination with ddC (0.015 or 0.03 mg daily) in 56 patients with advanced HIV disease and no previous history of treatment with antiretroviral therapy showed persistent reduction in p24 antigen and increases in CD4 count above baseline for periods up to 40 weeks (Meng et al 1992). These favourable changes in surrogate markers are encouraging for the ongoing Phase II trials of combination therapy.

Since 1990 ddC has been made available through an expanded access programme to persons with asymptomatic disease or CD4 count less than $200 \times 10^6/l$ intolerant to zidovudine and ddI. Safety data from these programmes report an incidence of peripheral neuropathy of 12–19% in patients receiving either 0.375 mg or 0.75 mg over 8 h (Lieberman et al 1992, Schlech et al 1992). As with other nucleoside analogues, the incidence of severe toxicity is likely to be substantially lower in asymptomatic individuals and using lower dosages. In addition, resistant isolates have been identified in patients receiving prolonged ddC monotherapy with a mutation occurring at codon 69 on the reverse transcriptase gene (Fitzgibbon et al 1992).

RESISTANCE

The transient response in CD4 count and ongoing clinical progression in patients with symptomatic disease treated with zidovudine suggests that the efficacy of monotherapy in advanced disease is not prolonged. Toxicity, variable and incomplete suppression of HIV replication, increasing viral burden, development of toxicity at a cellular level and the emergence of a drug-resistant virus may all be possible explanations for this. Following an initial fall, serum p24 antigen levels in some patients on long-term zidovudine increase towards baseline, suggesting a loss of antiviral effect (Reiss et al 1988, Williams et al 1990). Confirmation of in vitro viral resistance was established in 1989 with a report that sensitivity to zidovudine of isolates from symptomatic patients who had received more than 6 months of therapy was up to 100-fold less than isolates from untreated patients (Larder et al 1989a). Subsequently, multiple mutations have been identified in the *pol* gene responsible for reverse transcriptase, particularly at codons 41, 67, 70, 215 and 219 (Larder et al 1989b, Richman D D et al 1991a, Kellam et al 1992). The sequence and number of mutations that occur, with those at 41, 70 and 215 the most critical, and the proportion of both wild-type and mutant sequences within a virus population, probably determine the extent of resistance (Larder et al 1989a, Boucher et al 1990, 1992b). The mechanism for resistance at a molecular level is uncertain as the reverse transcriptase from resistant isolates (Larder et al 1989a) has similar binding to and inhibition by zidovudine triphosphate as that from sensitive isolates. Furthermore, whether in light of severe immunodeficiency, increasing viral burden determines the emergence of resistant isolates, or whether the development of mutations precedes an increase in viraemia has not been evaluated, and underlines the fact that the exact mechanism and sequence of resistance is not known. However, in patients treated with the non-nucleoside ana-

logue reverse transcriptase inhibitor nevaripine, there is a close correlation between the initial decrease and rise in plasma viraemia and the development of a mutation at codon 181 (Richman et al 1991b). In patients treated with zidovudine this temporal relationship is less clear.

In persons with asymptomatic disease and higher CD4 cell counts treated with zidovudine, the emergence of resistant isolates takes longer and occurs to a lesser extent (Richman et al 1990, Boucher et al 1990). This might be expected because of the lower viral load in individuals with early disease (St Clair et al 1991), and the greater mixture of HIV isolates to which some are zidovudine-sensitive and others resistant in persons with severely symptomatic disease. Such an argument would favour earlier treatment with zidovudine – dependent, though, on the evaluation of the relationship between clinical outcome and viral resistance on therapy.

Although initial studies suggested no cross-resistance between zidovudine-resistant isolates and other nucleoside analogues that do not have a 3' azido group, a more recent study suggests that this might occur but at a low level (Mayers et al 1992). Resistant isolates have also been identified in persons treated with both ddI and ddC monotherapy (Richman R C et al 1991, Fitzgibbon et al 1992, McLeod et al 1992). Interestingly, the occurrence of a sequence change at codon 74 in patients on prolonged ddI therapy previously treated with zidovudine is associated with development of ddI resistance and re-establishment of zidovudine sensitivity (St Clair et al 1991). Combination therapy with drugs acting at different sites of replication may make it less likely for resistant isolates to develop if more complete and prolonged viral suppression is achieved. Equally, the use of convergent combination therapy that targets reverse transcriptase may induce multiple mutations that are incompatible with competent viral replication (Chow et al 1992).

Apart from genotype changes, the viral phenotype has also been implicated in determining the sensitivity of HIV variants to zidovudine. Those persons with persistent non-syncytial-inducing strains of HIV replication appear to be less likely to progress to AIDS or symptomatic disease and for HIV to be more susceptible to inhibition by zidovudine than those with syncytial-inducing variants (Tersmette et al 1989, Koot et al 1991). Furthermore, progression to AIDS on treatment with zidovudine was better correlated with the presence of a syncytial-inducing phenotype than the occurrence of zidovudine-resistant mutation (Boucher et al 1992a, St Clair et al 1992). However, an increased likelihood of clinical progression or declining CD4 counts in persons on long-term zidovudine therapy is probably associated with the development of reverse transcriptase genotype mutations, though the exact relationship may be confounded not only by the level of viral burden and immune competence of the host but also by the viral phenotype. Future studies will need to evaluate the importance of each of these, and whether any could predict the clinical response to and options for therapy in an individual.

COMBINATION TREATMENT

The failure to sustain changes in surrogate markers, and the loss of efficacy and emergence of resistant isolates in patients treated with zidovudine are strong reasons to consider combining therapy in HIV infection. Various agents including cytokines and other non-nucleoside analogues have exhibited either synergism or an additive effect with zidovudine in inhibiting HIV replication in cultures of T lymphocytes. Combining agents may provide improved activity against multiple HIV variants in vivo and in different cell types, thereby achieving more complete suppression of viral replication. In addition, such a strategy may be able to achieve a lower incidence of toxicity and restrict the emergence of resistant isolates in the absence of significant cross-resistance or similar toxicity profiles between agents. Options of which agents to employ include those which act at the same or different sites of the replication cycle and those which augment the immune response. Encouragingly, recent in vitro work reports that the use of several agents which act at the level of reverse transcriptase results in the emergence of mutations that restrict the replicative ability of the virus (Chow et al 1992).

Results of phase I/II clinical trials of zidovudine in combination with other nucleoside analogues, acyclovir and interferon-*a* have been reported. In one of these, a dose-ranging comparative study of zidovudine (150, 300 or 600 mg daily) in combination with dideoxycytidine (0.015 or 0.03 mg/kg daily), enhanced and prolonged increases in CD4 counts were seen in patients with AIDS or ARC greater than previously reported with zidovudine alone (Meng et al 1992). These increases were started with the relatively higher dose combinations, with the mean change in CD4 counts remaining above baseline levels for periods greater than 44 weeks. Toxicity was not increased and the pharmacokinetics of each drug were not altered. A daily dose of 150 mg zidovudine produced suboptimal changes in CD4 count and p24 antigen levels when compared to combination treatment. Unfortunately, no higher dose single agent regimen of either drug was incorporated into the study design and so controlled comparison was not possible.

However, similar changes in surrogate markers have been reported with a combination of zidovudine and ddI in patients who are either zidovudine-naive or had been treated for less than 3–4 months (Yarchoan et al 1992, Collier 1992). In one of these, an alternating regimen every 3 weeks of zidovudine 600 mg with ddI 500 mg daily was compared to a simultaneous treatment with zidovudine 300 mg and ddI 250 mg daily in 41 patients with CD4 counts $< 350 \times 10^6$/l. In the simultaneous group the mean CD4 count remained above pretreatment levels after 54 weeks of follow-up but had declined to baseline at 27 weeks in those persons receiving the alternating regimen (Yarchoan et al 1992). The increase in CD4 count was also enhanced with a mean increase at 18 weeks of 66 cells on simultaneous therapy compared to only 20 cells on the alternating regimen.

Currently several large phase II trials in the USA, Canada, Europe and Australia have been started to assess the clinical efficacy of zidovudine alone or in combination with ddC or ddI in patients who are either receiving antiretroviral treatment for the first time or had been tolerating zidovudine for some months previously. Apart from clinical efficacy the impact on viral load as assessed by plasma and cell viraemia, the viral phenotype and the development of drug resistance of dual therapy are being investigated.

Acyclovir has an additive effect with zidovudine

in inhibiting HIV replication in vitro (Mitsuya & Broder 1987) and, theoretically, in vivo may suppress herpes viruses (e.g. cytomegalovirus, human herpes simplex virus 6) which possibly act as cofactors for more rapid progression to symptomatic disease. However, initial studies of combination therapy reported no significant differences in changes in p24 antigen levels or CD4 count compared to zidovudine alone (Surbone et al 1988). Subsequently, a large European/Australian placebo-controlled trial of zidovudine 1 g daily with or without acyclovir 4.8 g daily reported no difference in clinical progression or survival between the two groups at 6 months of follow-up (Cooper et al 1991). A further study with the primary aim of assessing the efficacy of high-dose acyclovir in patients with a CD4 count $< 150 \times 10^6/l$ as prophylaxis against cytomegalovirus disease reported a survival benefit at 1 year for acyclovir use over placebo (Youle 1992). However, the effect was largely explained by differential zidovudine use, though after controlling for this the investigators reported a small reduction in the risk of dying with acyclovir (0.57). The probability of developing cytomegalovirus disease at 1 year was no different between the two groups (0.24 on placebo, 0.23 on acyclovir). Further information on whether acyclovir in combination with zidovudine may act by mechanisms which do not result in an enhanced CD4 count response but yet have clinical efficacy may come from an ongoing large trial in over 600 patients with early symptomatic disease (Lavelle et al 1992).

Recombinant interferon-a has been used as a single agent for treating persons with Kaposi's sarcoma with a variable clinical response (Abrahams & Volberding 1987). High-dose regimens were not well tolerated, with neutropenia, fever and flu-like symptoms common side-effects. As well as an antitumour effect, interferon-a inhibits HIV replication in vitro, possibly by interfering with viral assembly and budding. In vitro synergism with zidovudine has been demonstrated (Hartshorn et al 1987) and several clinical studies have now reported on their combined use in persons with Kaposi's sarcoma (Kovacs et al 1989, Krown et al 1990, Berglund et al 1991). Increased tolerance, reduction in p24 antigen and a clinical response in 40–50% of Kaposi's sarcoma lesions

were seen at lower doses of interferon-a than if used as a single agent. A greater anti-HIV effect in persons with higher CD4 counts was noted when interferon-a was used as monotherapy, and similarly the improved clinical outcome when combined with zidovudine was primarily seen in patients with Kaposi's sarcoma with CD4 counts $> 200 \times 10^6/l$. Combination use is currently being assessed in persons with asymptomatic HIV with CD4 counts $> 400 \times 10^6/l$ (Lane et al 1992). Preliminary results at 16 months show a non-significant trend to higher CD4 response with combination therapy but a higher rate of voluntary withdrawal due to subjective intolerance. No data on clinical efficacy were reported because of insufficient clinical end-points. The need for subcutaneous administration of interferon-a and the relatively high rate of side-effects in persons who are otherwise asymptomatic would, however, seem to preclude widespread use by most physicians.

Scope for combination therapies is immense and may lead to multiple-agent treatments. This should not be limited to antiretrovirals but strategies should explore a combined use with immunomodulators including postinfection immunization regimens that may enhance host factor responses to HIV infection. The ultimate use of any such strategy is to maintain complete viral suppression and prolong clinical efficacy without significant short- or long-term toxicity to otherwise asymptomatic patients.

NEW ANTIRETROVIRAL AGENTS

Multiple agents have undergone in vitro testing to identify those with a potent anti-HIV activity. Some are currently undergoing phase I trials to evaluate pharmacokinetic and safety profiles and their effect on virological and immunological markers. To date, agents which inhibit viral replication at the level of reverse transcriptase have received the most interest in development, particularly nucleoside analogues. In addition to those already in clinical use, a further two are likely soon to proceed from phase I to more extensive clinical trials. The first, D4T, a thymidine analogue which in vitro has similar anti-HIV activity to zidovudine on a molar basis has in initial clinical trials resulted in favourable increases in CD4 counts and falls in p24 antigen (Dunkle et al 1992). The main adverse events reported in these first 264 patients were a peripheral neuropathy, neutropenia and raised liver transaminases, particularly at high dose.

The other, 3TC (2'-deoxy-3'-thiacytidine), is a potent and selective inhibitor of HIV-1 and -2 replication (Coates et al 1992) and appears to be less toxic to lymphocytes than zidovudine in vitro (Lisignoli et al 1992). In a dose escalation study in 90 patients with a CD4 count $< 400 \times 10^6/1$, although no significant drug toxicity was reported, the most common side-effect being a headache in 10% of individuals, changes in CD4 count and p24 antigen were not large, suggesting that higher dose escalation is necessary (Van Leeuwen et al 1992).

Non-nucleoside reverse transcriptase inhibitors have also received much attention recently as alternative agents and appear in vitro to have good anti-HIV activity with minimal cytotoxicity. These compounds include derivatives of TIBO (Pauwels et al 1990), pyridinone (Goldman et al 1991), bisheteroarylpiperazine (Romero et al 1991) and nevirapine (a dipyridodiazepinone) (Koup et al 1991). Their exact mechanism of action is not known but appears to be different from the deoxynucleoside analogues. The finding that HIV-resistant isolates rapidly emerge within a few weeks in individuals receiving these agents has brought into question their role as single agent therapy. A fall in the level of p24 antigen occurs with nevirapine but rapidly rises again and is associated with the development of mutant changes at RT codon 181 (Richman 1992). The concomitant administration of zidovudine did not appear to delay resistance. Further clinical trials of these agents in combination may define a clearer role for their use in therapy.

Agents which act at alternative sites to reverse transcriptase are being evaluated. The binding of recombinant soluble CD4 to the HIV envelope protein GP120 results in inhibition of infection of both T lymphocytes and macrophages in vitro (Fisher et al 1988, Perno et al 1990). Initial clinical trials of soluble CD4, however, were disappointing with no or little in vivo antiviral activity demonstrated, though no toxicity was seen (Kahn et al 1990). Modified forms of soluble CD4 involving the attachment of immunoglobulin or *Pseudomonas*

exotoxin proteins have been developed to try and overcome the problems of short half-life and the lack of in vivo efficacy (Chaudhary et al 1988, Bryn et al 1990). Clinical trials are ongoing. More recently, inhibitors of the HIV regulation gene product tat and HIV-1 protease which is responsible for cleavage of precursor core structural proteins of gag and pol have been developed and are entering phase I trials (Sham et al 1991, Petty et al 1992).

Interest is increasing in the immunogenic potential of recombinant HIV envelope and core proteins for postinfection immunization strategies. New and enhanced humoral antibody responses have been reported in uncontrolled trials of recombinant GP160 (Redfield et al 1991, Valentine et al 1992). Their effect on CD4 counts, HIV viraemia and clinical end-points needs to be addressed in placebo-controlled trials. If these immunotherapeutic agents are to be successful, then they will need to promote new and sustainable cytotoxic T cell responses to HIV and be immunogenic against all HIV variants.

REFERENCES

Abrahams D I, Volberding P A 1987 Alpha interferon therapy of AIDS-associated Kaposi's sarcoma. Semin Oncol 14: 43–47

Ahluwalia G, Cooney D A, Mitsuya H et al 1987 Initial studies on the cellular pharmacology of 2',3'-dideoxyinosine, an inhibitor of HIV infectivity. Biochem Pharmacol 36: 3797–3800

Ahluwalia G, Johnson M A, Fridland A, Cooney D A, Broder S, Johns D G 1988 Cellular pharmacology of the anti-HIV agent 2',3'-dideoxyadenosine. In: Proceedings of the American Association for Cancer Research, New Orleans, May 25–28. Waverly Press, Baltimore; p 349 (abstract)

Arnaudo E, Dalaka M, Shanske S, Moraes C T, Dimauro S, Schon E A, 1991 Depletion of muscle mitochondrial DNA in AIDS patients with zidovudine-induced myopathy. Lancet 337: 508–510

Berglund O, Engman K, Ehrnst A et al 1991 Combined treatment of human immunodeficiency type 1 infection with native interferon-alpha and zidovudine. J Infect Dis 163: 710–715

Bessen L J, Greene J B, Louie E, Seitzman P, Weinberg H 1988 Severe polymyositis-like syndrome associated with zidovudine therapy of AIDS and ARC. N Engl J Med 318: 708

Boucher C A, Tersmette M, Lange J M A et al 1990 Zidovudine sensitivity of human immunodeficiency viruses from high-risk, symptom-free individuals during therapy. Lancet 2: 585

Boucher C, Lange J, Miedman F et al 1992a HIV 1 phenotype rather than high level AZT resistance is associated with rapid clinical progression of asymptomatic treated patients. VIIIth International Conference on AIDS, Amsterdam, July 19–24. Abstr POB3570

Boucher C A, O'Sullivan E, Mulder J W et al 1992b Ordered appearance of zidovudine resistance mutations during treatment of 18 human immunodeficiency virus positive subjects. J Infect Dis 165: 105–110

Bryn R A, Mordenti J, Lucas C et al 1990 Biological properties of a CD4 immunoadhesin. Nature 344: 667

Chaudhary V K, Mizukami T, Fuerst T R et al 1988 Selective killing of HIV-infected cells by recombinant human CD4-pseudomonas exotoxin hybrid protein. Nature (London) 335: 369

Chow Y, Hirsch M, Merrill D et al 1992 Replication in compatible and replication compromising combinations of HIV 1 RT drug resistance mutations. VIIIth International Conference on AIDS, Amsterdam, July 19–24. Abstr POA2450

Coates J A V, Cammack N, Jenkinson H J et al 1992 2'-deoxy-3'-thiacytidine as a potent, highly selective inhibitor of human immunodeficiency virus type 1 and type 2 replication in vitro. Antimicrob Agents Chemother 36(4): 733–739

Cohen H, Williams I, Matthey F, Miller R F, Machin S J, Weller I V D 1989 Short communication: reversible zidovudine-induced pure red-cell aplasia. AIDS 3: 117–118

Collier A C 1992 Effect of combination therapy with zidovudine and didanosine on surrogate markers. Recent report session, VIIIth International Conference on AIDS, Amsterdam, July 19–24

Collier A C, Bozzette S, Coombs R W et al 1990 A pilot study of low-dose zidovudine in human immunodeficiency virus infection. N Engl J Med 323: 1015–1021

Cooley T P, Kunches L M, Saunders C A, et al 1990 Once-daily administration of 2',3'-dideoxyinosine (ddI) in patients with the acquired immunodeficiency syndrome of AIDS-related complex. N Engl J Med 322: 1430–1435

Cooper D A 1992 The efficacy and safety of zidovudine therapy in early asymptomatic HIV infection. VIIIth International Conference on AIDS, Amsterdam, July 19–24. Abstr POB3718

Cooper D A, Pedersen C, Aiuti F et al 1991 The efficacy and safety of zidovudine with or without acyclovir in the treatment of patients with AIDS-related complex. AIDS 5: 933–943

Creagh-Kirk T, Doi P, Andrews E et al 1988 Survival experience among patients with AIDS receiving zidovudine. JAMA 260: 3009–3015

Dalakas D C, Pezeshkpour G H, Gravell M, Sever J L 1986 Polymyositis associated with AIDS retrovirus. JAMA 256: 2381–2383

Dalakas M C, Yarchoan R, Spitzer R, Elder G, Sever J L 1988 Treatment of human immunodeficiency virus-related polyneuropathy with 3'-azido-2',3'-dideoxythymidine. Ann Neurol 23: S92–94

Dalakas M C, Illa I, Pezeshkpour G H, Laukaitis J P, Cohen B, Griffin J L 1990 Mitochondrial myopathy caused by long-term zidovudine therapy. N Engl J Med 322: 1098–1105

Darbyshire J H, Aboulker J 1992 Didanosine for zidovudine intolerant patients with HIV disease. Lancet 340: 1346–1347

De Gans J, Lange J M A, Deriot M M A et al 1988 Decline of HIV antigen levels in cerebrospinal fluid during treatment with low dose zidovudine. AIDS 2: 37–40

Dournon E, Matheron S, Rozenbaum W et al 1988 Effects of

zidovudine in 365 consecutive patients with AIDS or AIDS-related complex. Lancet 2: 1297–1302

Du D L, Volpe D A, Murphy M J Jr, Grieshaber C K 1989 Myelotoxicity of new anti-HIV drugs (2',3'-dideoxynucleosides) on human hematopoietic progenitor cells in vitro. Exp Hematol 17: 519

Dudley G, Montaner J S Q, Rachlis A, Beaulieu R, Gill J, Schlech W, Anclair C et al 1992 Safety principal of ddI; preliminary report of results of the Canadian open ddI treatment program. VIIIth International Conference on AIDS, Amsterdam, July 19–24. Abstr POB3003

Dunkle L, Anderson R, McLaren C et al 1992 Stavudine (d4T) a promising anti-retroviral agent. VIIIth International Conference on AIDS, Amsterdam, July 19–24. Abstr WeB1011

Easterbrook P, Keruly J C, Creagh-Kirk T et al 1991 Racial and ethnic differences in outcome in zidovudine-treated patients with advanced HIV disease. JAMA 266: 2713–2718

Ferrazin A, Terragna A, Loy A et al 1991 Zidovudine (ZDV) therapy of HIV infection during pregnancy: assessment of the effect on the newborns. Presented at the 7th International Conference on AIDS, Florence, Italy, June 16–21, abstr MC 3023

Fischl M A, Richman D D, Grieco M H et al 1987 The efficacy of azidothymidine (AZT) in the treatment of patietns with AIDS and AIDS-related complex. N Engl J Med 317: 185–191

Fischl M A, Richman D D, Causey D M et al 1989 Prolonged zidovudine therapy in patients with AIDS and advanced AIDS-related complex. JAMA 262: 2405–2410

Fischl M, Galpin J E, Levine J D et al 1990a Recombinant human erythropoietin for patients with AIDS treated with zidovudine. N Engl J Med 322: 1488–1493

Fischl M A, Parker C B, Pettinelli C et al 1990b A randomised controlled trial of a reduced daily dose of zidovudine in patients with the acquired immunodeficiency syndrome. N Engl J Med 323: 1009–1014

Fischl M A, Richman D D, Hansen N et al 1990c The safety and efficacy of zidovudine (AZT) in the treatment of subjects with mildly symptomatic human immunodeficiency virus type 1 (HIV) infection. A double-blind, placebo-controlled trial. Ann Intern Med 112: 727–737

Fisher R A, Bertonis J M Meier W et al 1988 HIV infection is blocked in vitro by recombinant soluble CD4. Nature (London) 331: 76

Fitzgibbon J E, Howell R M, Haberzettl C A et al 1992 Human immunodeficiency virus type 1 pol gene mutations which cause decreased susceptibility to 2',3'-dideoxycytidine. Antimicrob Agents Chemother 36: 153–157

Furman P A, Fyfe J A, St Clair M H et al 1986 Phosphorylation of 3'-azido-3'-deoxythymidine and selective interaction of the 5'-triphosphate with human immunodeficiency virus reverse transcriptase. Proc Natl Acad Sci USA 83: 8333–8337

Gill P S, Rarick M, Brynes R K, Causey D, Loureiro C, Levine A M 1987 Azidothymidine associated with bone marrow failure in the acquired immunodeficiency syndrome (AIDS). Ann Intern Med 107: 502–505

Gillet J Y, Garraffo R, Abrar D, Bongain A, Lapalus P, Dellanmonica P 1989 Fetoplacental passage of zidovudine. Lancet 2: 269–270

Goldman M E, Nunberg J H, O'Brien J A et al 1991 Pyridinone derivatives: specific human immunodeficiency virus type 1 reverse transcriptase inhibitors with antiviral activity. Proc Natl Acad Sci USA 88: 6863–6867

Graham N M H, Zeger S L, Park L P et al 1991 Effect of zidovudine and pneumocystis carinii pneumonia prophylaxis on progression of HIV-1 infection to AIDS. Lancet 338: 265–269

Graham N M H, Zeger S L, Lawrence P et al 1992 The effects on survival of early treatment of human immunodeficiency virus infection. N Engl J Med 326: 1037–1042

Groopman J E, Mitsuyasu R T, DeLeo M J et al 1987 Effect of human granulocyte-macrophage colony-stimulating factor on myelopoiesis in the acquired immunodeficiency syndrome. N Engl J Med 317: 593

Hamilton J D, Hartigan P M, Simberkoff M S et al 1992 A controlled trial of early versus late treatment with zidovudine in symptomatic human immunodeficiency virus infection. N Engl J Med 326: 437–443

Hartshorn K L, Vogt M W, Chou T C et al 1987 Synergistic inhibition of human immunodeficiency virus in vitro by azidothymidine and recombinant alpha A interferon. Antimicrob Agents Chemother 31: 168–172

Helbert M, Fletcher T, Peddle B, Harris J R W, Pinching A J 1988 Zidovudine-associated myopathy. Lancet 2: 689–690

Kahn J O, Allan J D, Hodges T L et al 1990 The safety and pharmacokinetics of recombinant soluble CD4 (rCD4) in subjects with the acquired immunodeficiency syndrome (AIDS) and AIDS-related complex. A phase I study. Ann Intern Med 112: 254

Kahn J O, Lagakos S W, Richman D D et al 1992 A controlled trial comparing continued zidovudine with didanosine in human immunodeficiency virus infection. N Engl J Med 327: 581–587

Kellam P, Boucher C A, Larder B A 1992 Fifth mutation in human immunodeficiency virus type 1 reverse transcriptase contributes to the development of high-level resistance to zidovudine. Proc Natl Acad Sci 89: 1934–1938

Koot M, Keet I P M, Vos A H V et al 1991 Biological phenotype as a prognostic marker for AIDS in a large population of seropositive individuals. VIIth International Conference on AIDS, Florence, June 16–21, Abstr WA80

Koup R A, Merluzzi V J, Hargrave K D et al 1991 Inhibition of human immunodeficiency virus type 1 (HIV-1) replication by the dipyridodiazepinone BIRG-587. J Infect Dis 163: 966–970

Kovacs J A, Deyton L, Davey R et al 1989 Combined zidovudine and interferon-alpha therapy in patients with Kaposi sarcoma and the acquired immunodeficiency syndrome (AIDS). Ann Intern Med 111: 280–287

Koyanagi Y, O'Brien W A, Zhao J Q et al 1988 Cytokines alter production of HIV-1 from primary mononuclear phagocytes. Science 241: 1673

Krown S E, Gold J W, Buedzwiecki D et al 1990 Interferon-alpha with zidovudine: safety, tolerance, and clinical and virological effects in patients with Kaposi sarcoma associated with the acquired immunodeficiency syndrome (AIDS). Ann Intern Med 112: 812–821

Lagakos S, Fischl M A, Stein D S, Lim L, Volberding P 1991 Effects of zidovudine therapy in minority and other subpopulations with early HIV infection. JAMA 266: 2709–2712

Lambert J S, Seidlin M, Reichman R C et al 1990 2', 3'-dideoxyinosine (ddI) in patients with the acquired immunodeficiency syndrome of the AIDS-related complex. A phase 1 trial. N Engl J Med 322: 1333–1340

Lane C H, Herpri B, Banks S et al 1992 Zidovudine vs alpha interferon vs the combination in patients with early HIV infection. VIIIth International Conference on AIDS, Amsterdam, July. Abstr MOB52.

Lane H C, Falloon J, Walker R E et al 1989 Zidovudine in patients with human immunodeficiency virus (HIV) infection and Kaposi sarcoma. Ann Intern Med 111: 41–50

Larder B A, Darby G, Richman D D 1989a HIV with reduced sensitivity to zidovudine (AZT) isolated during prolonged therapy. Science 243: 1731

Larder B A, Kemp S D 1989b Multiple mutations in HIV-1 reverse transcriptase confer high-level resistance to zidovudine (AZT). Science 246: 1155

Lavelle J, Lang W, Lefhowitz C et al 1992 A randomised trial comparing zidovudine alone and in combination with acyclovir for treatment of early symptomatic HIV infection. VIIIth International Conference on AIDS, Amsterdam, July 19–24. Abstri POB3585

Lemp G F, Payne S F, Neal D, Temelso T, Rutherford G W 1990 Survival trends for patients with AIDS. JAMA 263: 402–406

Lieberman J, Nauss-Karol C, Salgo M, Kaul I, Yucailis J, Soo W 1992 Safety experience with dideoxythymidine (ddC) in an expanded population. VIIIth International Conference on AIDS, Amsterdam, July 19–24. Abstr POB3004

Lisignoli G, Facchini A, Cattini L et al 1992 In vitro toxicity of 2',3'-dideoxy-3-thiacytidine (BCH189/3TC), a new synthetic anti-HIV 1 nucleoside. Antiviral Chemother 3(5): 299–303

McLeod G, McGrath J M, Ladd E, Hammer S M 1992 Didanosine and zidovudine resistance patterns in clinical isolates of human immunodeficiency virus type 1 as determined by a replication endpoint assay. Antimicrob Agents Chemother 36: 920–925

Mayers D, Wagner K F, Ching R C Y et al 1992 Dideoxynucleoside resistance emergence during AZT therapy. VIIIth International Conference on AIDS, Amsterdam, July 19–24. Abstr POB3574

Meng T-C, Fischl M A, Boota A M et al 1992 Combination therapy with zidovudine and dideoxycytidine in patients with advanced human immunodeficiency virus infection. A phase I/II study. Ann Intern Med 116: 13–20

Merigan T C, Skowron G, Bozzette S A et al 1989 Circulating p24 antigen levels and responses to dideoxycytidine in human immunodeficiency virus (HIV) infections. Ann Intern Med 110: 189

Mitsuya H, Broder S 1986 Inhibition of the in vitro infectivity and cytopathic effect of human T-lymphotrophic virus type III/lymphadenopathy-associated virus (HTLV-111/LAV) by 2' 3'-dideoxynucleosides. Proc Natl Acad Sci USA 83: 1911–1915

Mitsuya H, Broder S 1987 Strategies for antiviral therapy in AIDS. Nature (London) 325: 773–778

Mitsuya H, Weinhold K J, Furman P A et al 1985 3'-azido-3'-deoxythymidine (BW A509U): An antiviral agent that inhibits the infectivity and cytopathic effect of human T-lymphotropic virus type III/lymphadenopathy-associated virus in vitro. Proc Natl Sci USA 82: 7096–7100

Moore R D, Creagh-Kirk T, Keruly J et al 1991a Long-term safety and efficacy of zidovudine in patients with advanced human immunodeficiency virus disease. Arch Intern Med 151: 981–986

Moore R D, Hidalgo J, Sugland B W, Chaisson R E 1991b Zidovudine and the natural history of the acquired immunodeficiency syndrome. N Engl J Med 324: 1412–1416

Moss A R, Bacchetti P 1989 Natural history of HIV infection. AIDS 3: 55–61

Nordic Medical Research Councils' HIV Therapy Group 1992 Double blind dose–response study of zidovudine in AIDS and advanced HIV infection. Br Med J 304: 13–17

Pauwels R, Andries K, Desmyter J et al 1990 Potent and selective inhibition of HIV-1 replication in vitro by a novel series of TIBO derivatives. Nature (London) 343: 470–474

Perno C-F, Yarchoan R, Cooney D A et al 1989 Replication of human immunodeficiency virus in monocytes. Granulocyte/macrophage colony-stimulating factor (GM-CSF) potentiates viral production yet enhances the antiviral effect mediated by 3'-azido-2'3'-dideoxythymidine (AZT) and other dideoxynucleoside congeners of thymidine. J Exp Med 169: 933

Perno C-F, Baseler M W, Broder S, Yarchoan R 1990 Infection of monocytes by human immunodeficiency virus 1 blocked by inhibitors of CD4-gp 120 binding, even in the presence of enhancing antibodies. J Exp Med 171: 1043

Petty B, Grunsberg R, Lewis C et al 1992 Pharmokinetics safety and tolerance of a Tat antagonist. VIIIth International Conference on AIDS, Amsterdam, July 19–24. Abstr M0321

Pluda J M, Yarchoan R, Smith P D et al 1990 Subcutaneous recombinant granulocyte-macrophage colony-stimulating factor used as a single agent and in an alternating regimen with azidothymidine in leukopenic patients with severe human immunodeficiency virus infection. Blood 76: 463

Portegies P, de Grans J, Lange J M A et al 1989 Declining incidence of AIDS dementia complex after introduction of zidovudine. Br Med J 299: 819–821

Redfield R R, Birx D L, Ketter N et al 1991 A phase I evaluation of the safety and immunogenicity of vaccination with recombinant gp160 in patients with early human immunodeficiency virus infection. N Engl J Med 324: 1677–1684

Reiss P, Lange J M A, Boucher C A, Danner S A, Goudsmit J 1988 Resumption of HIV antigen production during continuous zidovudine treatment. Lancet 1: 421

Richman D 1992 Loss of nevirapine activity associated with the emergence of resistance in clinical trials. VIIIth International Conference on AIDS, Amsterdam, July 19–24. Abstr POB3576.

Richman D D, Fischl M, Grieco M H et al 1987 The toxicity of azidothymidine (AZT) in the treatment of patient with AIDS and AIDS-related complex. N Engl J Med 317: 192–197

Richman D D, Grimes J, Lagakos S 1990 Effect of stage of disease and drug dose on zidovudine susceptibilities of isolates of human immunodeficiency virus. J AIDS 3: 743

Richman D D, Guatelli J C, Grimes J, Tsiatis A, Gingeras T 1991a Detection of mutations associated with zidovudine resistance in human immunodeficiency virus by the use of polymerase chain reaction. J Infect Dis 164: 1075

Richman D D, Shih C-K, Lowy I et al 1991b HIV-1 mutants resistant to non-nucleoside inhibitors of reverse transcriptase arise in tissue culture. Proc Natl Acad Sci USA 88: 11241–11245

Richman R C, Lambert J S, Strussenberg J, Dolin R 1991 Decreased dideoxyinosine (ddI) sensitivity of HIV isolates obtained from long-term recipients of ddI. VIIth International Conference on AIDS, Florence, June 16–21. Abstr TuB92

Romero D L, Busso M, Tan C-K et al 1991 Nonnucleoside reverse transcriptase inhibitors that potently and specifically block human immunodeficiency virus type 1 replication. Proc Natl Acad Sci USA 88: 8806–8810

Rozencwieg M, McLaren C, Beltangady M et al 1990 Overview of phase I trials of 2',3'-dideoxyinosine (ddI) conducted on adult patients. Rev Infect Dis 12: 5570–5575

Rutherford G W, Lifson A L, Hessol N A et al 1990 Course of HIV-1 infection in a cohort of homosexual and bisexual men. An 11 year follow up study. Br Med J 301: 1183–1188

St Clair M H, Richards C A, Spector T et al 1987 3'-azido-3'-deoxythymidine triphosphate as an inhibitor and substrate of purified human immunodeficiency virus reverse transcriptase. Antimicrob Agents Chemother 31: 1972–1977

St Clair M H, Martin J L, Tudor-Williams G et al 1991 Resistance to ddI and sensitivity to AZT induced by a mutation in HIV-1 reverse transcriptase. Science 253: 1557–1559

St Clair M H, Hartigan P M, Andrews J C, Hamilton J D, Simberkoff M S 1992 Matched progressor-non-progressor study of zidovudine resistance and disease progression. VIIIth International Conference on AIDS, Amsterdam, July 19-24, Abstr POB3578

Schlech W, Beaulieu R, Gill J, Montaner J, Rachlis A, Bristow M, Fauchere S 1992 VIIIth International Conference on AIDS, Amsterdam, July 19–24. Abstr POB8006

Schmitt F A, Bigley J W, McKinnis R, Logue P E, Evans R W, Drucker J L 1988 Neuropsychological outcome of zidovudine (AZT) treatment of patients with AIDS and AIDS-related complex. N Engl J Med 319: 1573–1578

Sham H L, Betebenner D A, Wideburg N E et al 1991 Potent HIV-1 protease inhibitors with antiviral activities in vitro. Biochem Biophys Res Commun 175: 914–919

Simberkoff M J, Hartigan P M, Hamilton J D, VA Co-op Study Grp 1992 Longterm follow up of VA trial comparing early vs late AZT for symptomatic HIV infection. VIIIth International Conference on AIDS, Amsterdam, July 19–24. Abstr POB3723

Simpson D M, Bender A N 1988 Human immunodeficiency virus-associated myopathy: analysis of 11 patients. Ann Neurol 24: 79–84

Sommadossi J P, Carlisle R, Zhou Z 1989 Cellular pharmacology of 3'-azido-3'-deoxythymidine with evidence of incorporation into DNA of human bone marrow cells. Mol Pharmacol 36: 9–14

Sperling R S, Stratton P, O'Sullivan M 1992 A survey of zidovudine use in pregnant women with human immunodeficiency virus infection. N Engl J Med 326: 857–861

Surbone A, Yarchoan R, McAtte N et al 1988 Treatment of the acquired immunodeficiency syndrome (AIDS) and AIDS-related complex with a regimen of 3'-azido-2',3'-dideoxythymidine (azidothymidine or zidovudine) and acyclovir. Ann Intern Med 108: 534–540

Swanson C E, Cooper D A 1990 Factors influencing outcome of treatment with zidovudine of patients with AIDS in Australia. AIDS 4: 749–757

Sweeney J, Valentine C B, Campbell M, Pinching A J, Sherwood R, Deenmamode J, Mancroft K C et al 1992 Nucleoside analogues and patterns of salivary pancreatic and total amylase in HIV positive individuals. VIIIth International Conference on AIDS, Amsterdam, July 19-24. Abstr MOB78

Tersmette M, Lange J M A, De Goede R E Y et al 1989 Association between biological properties of human immunodeficiency virus variants and risk for AIDS and AIDS mortality. Lancet 983–985

Valentine F, Katzustein D, Haslett P et al 1992 A randomized controlled study of immunogenicity of RGP160 in HIV infected subjects. VIIIth International Conference on AIDS, Amsterdam, July 19–24. Abstr TuB561

Van Leeuwen R, Boucher C, Katlama C et al 1992 A phase I/II study of 3TC in HIV positive asymptomatic or mild ARC patients. VIIIth International Conference on AIDS, Amsterdam, July 19–24. Abstr WeB1014

Vella S, Giuliano M, Pezzotti P et al 1992 Survival of zidovudine-treated patients with AIDS compared with that of contemporary untreated patients. JAMA 267: 1232–1236

Viscarello R R, DeGennaro N J, Hobbins J C 1991 Preliminary experience with the use of zidovudine (AZT) during pregnancy. Am J Obstet Gynecol 164 (suppl 248), abstr 15

Volberding P A, Lagakos S W, Koch M A et al 1990 Zidovudine in asymptomatic human immunodeficiency virus infection. A controlled trial in persons with fewer than 500 CD4 positive cells per cubic millimeter. N Engl J Med 322: 941–949

Walker R E, Parker R I, Kovacs J A et al 1988 Anemia and erythropoiesis in patients with the acquired immunodeficiency syndrome (AIDS). Ann Intern Med 108: 372–376

Watts D H, Brown Z A, Tartaglione T et al 1991 Pharmacokinetic disposition of zidovudine during pregnancy. J Infect Dis 163: 226–232

Williams I, Gabriel G, Cohen H et al 1989 Zidovudine in the first year of experience. J Infect 18(S1): 23–31

Williams I G, Gabriel G, Kelly G et al 1990 Response of serum p24 antigen and antibody to p24 antigen in patients with AIDS and AIDS-related complex treated with zidovudine. AIDS 4: 909–912

Yarchoan R, Klecker R W, Weinhold K J et al 1986 Administration of 3'-azido-3' deoxythymidine, an inhibitor of HTLV-111/LAV replication, to patients with AIDS or AIDS related complex. Lancet 1: 575–580

Yarchoan R, Berg G, Brouwers P et al 1987 Response of human-immunodeficiency-virus associated neurological disease to 3'azido-3'-deoxythymidine. Lancet 1: 132–135

Yarchoan R, Perno C F, Thomas R V et al 1988a Phase 1 studies of 2',3'-dideoxycytidine in severe human immunodeficiency virus infection as a single agent and alternating with zidovudine. Lancet 1: 76–81

Yarchoan R, Thomas R V, Grafman J et al 1988b Long-term administration of 3'-azido-2', 3'-dideoxythymidine to patients with AIDS-related neurological disease. Ann Neurol 23: S82–87

Yarchoan R, Mitsuya H, Thomas R V et al 1989 In vivo activity against HIV and favourable toxicity profile of 2',3'-dideoxyinosine. Science 245: 412–415

Yarchoan R, Pluda J M, Thomas R V et al 1990 Long-term toxicity/activity profile of 2',3'-dideoxyinosine in AIDS or AIDS-related complex. Lancet 336: 526–529

Yarchoan R, Lietgen J A, Brawley O, Ngugen B Y, Pluda J M, Wyvill K M, Broden S 1992 Therapy of AIDS or symptomatic HIV infection with simultaneous or alternating regimes of AZT and ddI. VIIIth International Conference on AIDS, Amsterdam, July 19–24. Abstr MD354

Youle M S 1992 Placebo controlled trial of high dose acyclovir for the prevention of cytomegalovirus disease in advanced HIV disease. International Congress on Drug Therapy in HIV Infection, Glasgow, November 9–12. Abstr 0–16.2

7. Clinical management of asymptomatic and symptomatic HIV infection

Marc C. I. Lipman and Margaret A. Johnson

THE CLINICAL MANAGEMENT OF ASYMPTOMATIC AND SYMPTOMATIC HIV INFECTION

Over the last few years it has become apparent that HIV infection is a chronic illness often lasting many years with a relatively short terminal period of ill health. The first reports of AIDS (CDC Los Angeles 1981) could only focus on this latter stage, though now it is clear that asymptomatic HIV infection also requires comprehensive medical care. In this review we will cover the practical management of both early asymptomatic and late symptomatic adult HIV-1 infection. HIV-2 infection (confined mainly to West Africa) appears to have a similar though rather slower clinical picture and will not be specifically addressed.

Background

It is estimated that there are 12–13 million HIV-infected adults world-wide, of which approximately 50% are in Africa. North America, South America and Asia also have large pools of infection (WHO 1991). One million adults and 500 000 children are thought to have AIDS. Approximately 40% of the infected population are women, and over 75% of infections were acquired through heterosexual intercourse. Other risks for HIV seropositivity are intravenous drug use and perinatal transmission (each accounting for 10% of the total), and the use of infected blood or blood products (responsible for 5% of all infections).

As only an estimated 10% of infected individuals have AIDS, there is a large reservoir of asymptomatic unknown infection within the community. An awareness of this issue, and the demonstration that infected individuals can benefit from early intervention and treatment has led to more voluntary HIV antibody testing. There is thus an increasing number of people with early asymptomatic HIV infection requiring medical and psychosocial care.

Laboratory markers and staging classifications of disease

The median time between infection and development of AIDS has been estimated as 10 years (Rutherford et al 1990). Over this period changes in laboratory markers can be used to predict the likelihood of developing AIDS. Currently the most useful tests are either T lymphocyte-dependent (fall in absolute and relative CD4 count, reduced CD4/CD8 ratio), or measure increased systemic viral (HIV antigenaemia) or immune activation (e.g. rising serum $\beta 2$ microglobulin ($\beta 2M$), which presumably reflects increased cell destruction, and rising serum neopterin – a marker of increased macrophage turnover). Taken together these have a relatively good predictive value (Moss & Bachetti 1989), though more accurate methods are needed – e.g. using the phenotypic properties of the HIV isolate to measure T cell reactivity, viral load or in vitro syncytium formation.

HIV antigenaemia is present early in disease in only about 15% of cases. However, its persistence increases the relative risk of progression to AIDS two – to fourfold in the common subgroup of individuals with CD4 counts $> 200 \times 10^6/1$ and $\beta 2M < 5$ mg/1 (Moss & Bacchetti 1989).

The frequency with which one measures T lymphocyte subsets, $\beta 2M$ and HIV antigen is subject to debate. The 'average' rate of decline of CD4 counts is 11% per 6 months (Aledort et al 1992), though variation can occur through stress, exercise, time of day, intercurrent infection and laboratory measurement. Thus, in an asymptomatic seropositive individual, it is probably wise to measure immune markers twice a year, though more frequently if a patient has evidence of marked immunosuppression (CDC 1992a).

Table 7.1 Centers for Disease Control classification of HIV infections (1985)

Group I	acute infection
Group II	asymptomatic infection
Group III	persistent generalized lymphadenopathy
Group IV	other disease
subgroup A	constitutional disease
	weight loss > 10% body wgt or > 4.5 kg
	fevers > 38°C
	diarrhoea > 2 weeks
subgroup B	neurological disease
	HIV encephalopathy
	myelopathy
	peripheral neuropathy
subgroup C	secondary infectious diseases
	C1 AIDS-defining secondary infectious disease
	Pneumocystis carinii pneumonia
	cerebral toxoplasmosis
	cytomegalovirus retinitis
	C2 other specified secondary infectious diseases
	oral *candida*
	pulmonary tuberculosis
	multidermatomal varicella zoster
subgroup D	secondary cancers
	Kaposi's sarcoma
	non-Hodgkin's lymphoma
subgroup E	other conditions
	lymphoid interstitial pneumonitis

Staging of HIV infection is useful as it enables one to make prognoses, select treatments and define trial end-points before clinical progression has occurred. Early classifications were based on clinical criteria (Table 7.1 – CDC classification) though there is now an increasing tendency to incorporate immune markers into HIV staging (Royce et al 1991). It is likely that by the time of publication, a CD4 T lymphocyte cell count $< 200 \times 10^6/1$ or CD4 percentage $< 14\%$ in the absence of clinical findings, pulmonary tuberculosis, recurrent bacterial infections and cervical carcinoma will also be regarded as AIDS-defining conditions (CDC 1992b).

The newly diagnosed seropositive

An HIV antibody test must always be voluntary and should be carried out with informed consent after pretest discussion (Bor et al 1991). It may be performed for a number of different reasons. These include recent or long standing 'high risk' activity, the development of symptoms attributable to HIV, or as part of routine screening, e.g. through the blood transfusion service or an insurance medical. Time must be spent with all new seropositive individuals in order to deal with the considerable psychological and social problems generated (e.g. who to tell, what to do about jobs/pensions/mortgages, and the thought of future disease and early death).

The important medical points are:

1. Every HIV antibody test must be confirmed, using different assays and checked with a second blood sample
2. Ascertaining the individual's stage of disease through history, examination and laboratory tests
3. Performing baseline screening for other potentially important diseases
4. Establishing a good rapport with the patient to encourage her to return for regular review
5. Educating the individual about risk reduction, life-style management and the role of therapeutic interventions
6. Considering issues of relevance to the individual's specific risk group (e.g. cervical smears in women or rehabilitation programmes in intravenous drug users). The help of a counsellor who can advise on social issues and benefits, as well as provide support for the individual and partner/family in the long term is essential.

Baseline investigations are summarized in Table 7.2.

Primary HIV infection

In the majority of cases primary HIV-1 infection is symptomatic but is usually not clinically recognized. A wide variety of symptoms and signs have been described, the commonest of which are fever, malaise, diarrhoea, myalgia, arthralgia, sore throat, headaches, lymphadenopathy and a maculopapular rash (De Jong et al 1991). The com-

Table 7.2 Baseline investigations of a new HIV-seropositive individual

Investigation	Reason
Virology	
HIV antibody*	confirmation
HIV (p24) antigen	prognostic marker
CMV antibody	? cofactor; future disease
Hepatitis Screen (A,B,C)	1. if HBs Ab -ve consider immunization
	2. may develop chronic disease
	3. ? cofactor
Immunology	
T lymphocyte subsets	prognostic marker
$\beta2$ microglobulin/neopterin	prognostic marker
Microbiology	
Syphilis serology (VDRL/TPHA/FTA)	? occult/latent disease
Toxoplasma serology (dye test)	future disease
Biochemistry	
Urea, electrolytes and creatinine	assess disease state
Liver function tests	abnormal with infection or drugs/therapy
Calcium	malnourishment
Creatinine phosphokinase	may increase on zidovudine/with HIV
Amylase	may increase on ddI
Haematology	
Full blood count	HIV-related haematological
Differential	abnormalities
Film	(+ effect of treatment)

* HIV-1 antibody may take up to 3 months (and very rarely longer) to become positive from time of last risk; if in doubt repeat testing advised and check HIV antigen (may be present before antibody); CMV, cytomegalovirus

monest neurological manifestation is an aseptic meningoencephalitis (presenting with headache, fever, photophobia and confusion).

The time from infection with HIV-1 to clinical disease seems to vary between 1 and 4 weeks for the 'flu-like' illness and up to 6 weeks for neurological disease. The acute illness is self-limiting, though there is evidence that the duration of symptoms (> 14 days) predicts early progression to AIDS (Pedersen et al 1989).

During symptomatic primary HIV-1 infection, specific HIV antibodies are usually detectable in serum. However, HIV antigenaemia is an earlier feature of infection and there may be a window period when no antibody is detectable though the patient is in fact highly infectious. Repeat HIV antibody testing 6–12 weeks later may be needed to establish the diagnosis.

There is no evidence at present that anti-retroviral therapy given at the time of infection alters either the course of the seroconversion illness or the natural history of HIV. Occasionally sero-conversion may produce such a profound (but transient) fall in immunity that the patient may develop opportunistic infection. This should not be regarded as AIDS-defining, as once treated, immunity will return towards normal.

Asymptomatic HIV infection

The proportion of seropositives who will progress to AIDS is unknown. A San Francisco cohort study of gay men revealed that 11 years after sero-conversion, 19% of the population had no clinical symptoms or signs, and 3% had asymptomatic generalized lymphadenopathy (Rutherford et al 1990). However, it was also clear that the likelihood of developing AIDS was related to the duration of HIV-1 infection, with an estimated 11-year cumulative incidence of AIDS of 54%. Thus, although the majority of seropositives may ultimately develop AIDS, a large proportion will remain well for a long period of time.

Asymptomatic seropositives may see friends and partners progress to AIDS and die. Therefore, a large part of their management involves adequate counselling, support and education. They should be encouraged to self-report symptoms, and should feel that they have easy access to medical care when necessary. Typically, patients are reviewed 3-monthly, at which time full clinical examination is undertaken. In many clinics laboratory monitoring is performed (i.e. CD4 counts, HIV antigen and $\beta 2$ microglobulin) 6-monthly.

Persistent generalized lymphadenopathy (PGL), histologically a follicular hyperplasia, is often a worry for patients as they are aware that they have a sign of 'disease'. However, the prognosis in this subgroup is the same as that for clinically asymptomatic seropositives. Indications for investigation of HIV-related lymphadenopathy are: development of lymph nodes associated with symptoms (e.g. night sweats, weight loss); rapidly enlarging or painful nodes; and markedly asymmetrical nodes. Mediastinal adenopathy is unlikely to be due to

PGL and a further cause should be sought (e.g. lymphoma or mycobacterial disease).

Early symptomatic HIV infection

In practice, many 'asymptomatic' seropositives will have early symptoms or signs of HIV infection. These, however, may be non-specific or represent a worsening of a previous condition. Examples include folliculitis, molluscum contagiosum, seborrhoeic dermatitis, psoriasis and viral warts. The development of some conditions, though, indicates advancing disease and marked immunosuppression. These are often known as AIDS-related complex (ARC) and are summarized in

Table 7.3 Components of AIDS-related complex (ARC)

Persistent fever	persistent or recurring fever > 38°C for at least 2 weeks
Fatigue	persistent fatigue for at least 2 weeks
Diarrhoea	diarrhoea for at least 2 weeks
New rash	new skin rash that lasts for at least 2 weeks
Worse herpes	more frequent, more severe, longer duration
Bullous impetigo	by physical examination or by self-report
Oral hairy leukoplakia	by physical examination or self-report
Oral thrush	by physical examination (may be confirmed by KOH testing) or by self-report
Varicella zoster	shingles (uni- or multidermatomal)
Unintentional weight loss	unintentional weight loss of at least 10 lb (4.5 kg) unrelated to dieting
Night sweats	sweating at night for at least 2 weeks

Table 7.3. The presence of ARC is associated with an increased risk of AIDS; for example, on no antiretroviral therapy, 75% of patients with oral hairy leukoplakia will develop AIDS in 2–3 years.

Late symptomatic HIV infection

With advancing immunosuppression (CD4 count $< 200 \times 10^6/1$), patients become susceptible to a wide variety of infectious, neoplastic and infiltrative disorders. These correspond to Centers for Disease Control (CDC) stage IV disease and often represent an AIDS diagnosis (Table 7.1). Thera-

peutic intervention has improved post-AIDS median survival (currently 18 months), yet may also have altered the natural history of HIV: there is less early and survivable *Pneumocystis carinii* pneumonia (PCP) and more fatal lymphoma. The following section will deal with the management of common symptoms in the different organ systems and will conclude with a section on HIV-related tumours.

Respiratory disease

Pneumocystis carinii pneumonia

Respiratory disease is the commonest AIDS presentation. The typical picture is several days to weeks of breathlessness, dry cough, fevers and malaise with few respiratory signs. This is often due to PCP, which occurs in up to 70% of AIDS patients. Thus, any seropositive individual at risk of PCP (i.e. with laboratory evidence of immunosuppression: CD4 $< 200 \times 10^6/1$) (Graham et al 1991) who presents with a history of breathlessness should be assumed to have this until proven otherwise.

Certain clinical features may suggest other respiratory pathogens (e.g. purulent sputum, pleuritic chest pain and focal signs imply a bacterial pneumonia; pleural effusions are usually due to mycobacterial disease or Kaposi's sarcoma). However, dual pathogens are found in up to 30% of AIDS patients and bacterial infection (especially Gram-negative septicaemia) is now the commonest cause of HIV-related death.

The vigour with which the diagnosis is pursued will vary from centre to centre, though it is mandatory to perform a chest radiograph and either resting and exercise oxygen saturations (via a pulse oximeter) or arterial blood gases. In early disease these investigations may be normal, but typically the chest radiograph reveals bilateral alveolar and interstitial shadowing, predominantly lower zone, with absence of Kerley 'B' lines. Often the patient is either hypoxic at rest or markedly desaturates when exercised (e.g. oximetry 97% at rest, falls to 90% after 'step-ups' for 5–10 min. When doubt remains, thoracic computed tomography (CT) scans and radionuclear uptake methods (e.g. Technetium-99m DTPA) can provide further information.

For a definitive diagnosis, sputum, bronchoalveolar washings or lung parenchyma must be examined by histological, cytological or microbiological techniques. The methods employed are listed in Table 7.4. None of the procedures is without risk or discomfort to the patient, which may be important when considering the quality of an AIDS patient's life. Indeed the chance of PCP in a high risk individual is so great that simple scoring systems have been devised that attempt to dispense with the need for first-line invasive investigations (Smith et al 1992).

Table 7.4 Diagnostic investigations in HIV-related respiratory disease

Investigation	Method	Comment
Induced sputum production	hypertonic saline via ultrasonic nebulizer with postural drainage	unpleasant, time-consuming, poor yield without prior experience of technique
Fibreoptic bronchoscopy with bronchoalveolar lavage	180–240 ml buffered isotonic saline into right middle lobe or area of focal change	requires sedation, intra/post-procedure hypoxia well documented; may cause acute deterioration in sick patient; good diagnostic yield
Fibreoptic bronchoscopy with transbronchial biopsy	multiple biopsies of right lower lobe or area of focal change	high risk of complication in HIV, e.g. pneumothorax, bleeding; good diagnostic yield
Open lung biopsy		requires general anaesthetic; often ITU care postoperatively; useful if all else fails (+ patient can tolerate procedure)

ITU, intensive therapy unit

As mentioned earlier, PCP is the likeliest diagnosis, though similar presentations are found with viral (e.g. cytomegalovirus, herpes simplex virus) protozoal (*Toxoplasma*), fungal (*Candida*, *His-toplasma*, *Cryptococcus*), bacterial and mycobacterial infections – all of which occur with increased frequency in HIV disease. In practical terms, if someone is suspected of having PCP they should be started on therapy as soon as possible, with a diagnostic procedure planned for an appropriate time within the next few days (*Pneumocystis* can still be recovered after several weeks of treatment).

The standard therapy for PCP is either trimethoprim–sulphamethoxazole (cotrimoxazole) or pentamidine isethionate; although there is little to choose between the two in terms of efficacy (80% response rate) or duration of treatment (an initial 21 days). Cotrimoxazole is the usual first-choice drug as it can be given orally from the outset in mild disease or over the last part of the treatment course with more severe infection. Side-effects with both agents are common. Cotrimoxazole causes nausea, rash, fever and neutropenia in 40–80% of AIDS patients; whilst pentamidine will induce hypotension, hypoglycaemia and worsening renal function in up to 70% of AIDS patients. The response to either drug is slow and often clinical improvement is not obvious until day 5 of therapy.

If a patient continues to deteriorate after 5 days' treatment with trimethoprim–sulphamethoxazole (120 mg/kg per day), they may be switched to pentamidine (4 mg/kg per day), overlapping the two drugs by at least 48 h. In some patients cotrimoxazole is effective but causes marked adverse effects of uncontrolled nausea and vomiting. In this case, the second-line combination of trimethoprim (20 mg/kg per day) and dapsone (100 mg/day) may be more appropriate (surprisingly, 70% of patients who experience side-effects from cotrimoxazole tolerate this combination). Folinic acid (15 mg every 3 days) should be given when high-dose folate antagonists are used. Regular haematological and biochemical monitoring is necessary for all anti-PCP drugs.

Other drugs may have a role in 'salvage therapy' of PCP, where first-line treatments have failed. These include primaquine and clindamycin combination, trimetrexate, eflornithine (DFMO) and the promising new drug 566C80 (atovaquone). The results from the few studies that have been performed suggest that at best these drugs are effective in only about 50% of these cases, though it must be remembered that often they have been used where standard therapy has failed (Hughes 1991).

Prophylaxis against PCP relies heavily on either oral cotrimoxazole or nebulized pentamidine. There is benefit in both primary (no previous PCP, but CD4 $< 200 \times 10^6/1$ or CDC IV disease) and secondary prophylaxis (started immediately after the high-dose induction course). The San Francisco Community Prophylaxis Trial (Leoung et al 1990) established the standard pentamidine dose of 300 mg every 4 weeks via a jet nebulizer (Respirgard II). Recent work from the American AIDS Clinical Trials Group (ACTG 021) (Hardy et al 1992) demonstrated the superiority of cotrimoxazole (960 mg od) over pentamidine (300 mg/month via Respirgard II) in secondary prophylaxis (1-year estimated recurrence rate of 3.5% vs 18.5%). There was also a suggestion of cross-prophylaxis against *Toxoplasma* and bacterial infections in the cotrimoxazole group. However, there were a large number of adverse reactions to cotrimoxazole reported. Most clinicians now favour the use of cotrimoxazole as first-line prophylaxis and would use pentamidine in patients who are sulphonamide-intolerant. Other drugs – e.g. dapsone and Fansidar – have been explored as possible prophylactic agents. At present there is little efficacy data to recommend their routine use (CDC 1992A).

The first episode mortality rate of PCP has fallen from 20% to 7% whilst post-ventilation survival has risen from 14% to 55%. This is due to a number of factors including earlier detection of disease, aggressive PCP management and use of antiretroviral/prophylactic drugs. Some of the therapeutic strategies that seem to be important include the early use of systemic glucocorticoids: dose at least 60–80 mg prednisolone/day reducing after day 5 in moderate to severe PCP – i.e. PaO_2 < 70 mmHg (9.3 kPa); O_2 saturation $< 90\%$ on air; or alveolar–arterial gradient > 35 mmHg (4.7 kPa) (McGowan et al 1992); and appropriate selection of patients for either continuous positive pressure airway circuits (CPAP), where the patient is breathing spontaneously, and/or intubation with formal mechanical ventilation (Wachter et al 1992).

Mycobacterial disease

Since 1985 the number of cases of *Mycobacterium tuberculosis* (MTB) reported annually in the USA has risen by 16%. This is mainly due to coexistent HIV infection (Snider & Roper 1992). Globally the situation is similar with an estimated 4 million people co-infected with HIV and MTB. A large proportion of patients with MTB and HIV infection will have extrapulmonary disease (e.g. pleural, pericardial, lymphatic, central nervous system or genitourinary system involvement); whilst pulmonary MTB may itself be anatomically atypical (Elliot et al 1990). MTB can present at any stage of HIV disease and normally responds to standard quadruple or triple drug therapy. However long-term relapse (especially in the developing world) appears very common and so many physicians maintain patients on life-long isoniazid.

Multidrug-resistant MTB is seen increasingly frequently in the USA. Clinical features that suggest its presence include continued fever, worsening pulmonary infiltrates, sputum smear positivity and extrapulmonary MTB cultures whilst on standard treatment. It is extremely difficult to treat, has a high mortality, and has been implicated in several outbreaks of nosocomial MTB. It has arisen from non-compliance with treatment and poses a major threat to the HIV-infected population.

The opportunist pathogen *Mycobacterium avium intracellulare* complex is a much later finding in HIV disease, presenting as disseminated infection a mean of 7–15 months after AIDS diagnosis when CD4 counts are below $100 \times 10^6/1$. Its clinical features are often non-specific – e.g. fever, night sweats, malaise, anorexia, weight loss and anaemia. Occasionally it may present in a specific organ system – e.g. gut infiltration or within the lung parenchyma. The presence of *Mycobacterium avium intracellulare* complex reduces patient survival, probably via general malnutrition and cachexia. It can be diagnosed on the basis of culture from any normally sterile site (e.g. blood, bone marrow). Treatment remains a problem due to widespread drug resistance, though there is some optimism that rifabutin, amikacin and the new macrolides (e.g. clarithromycin) may be more effective (Scoular et al 1991). The current recommended regimen is combination therapy with clarithromycin, ethambutol and rifabutin. Rifabutin has also been used with moderate success as a primary prophylactic agent in patients with CD4 $< 200 \times 10^6/1$ and AIDS. An important point to consider, however, is that drug therapy may do little to help the patient long term yet may markedly reduce the quality of the life that remains.

Gastrointestinal disease

The three common presentations of disease are oral disease, difficulty swallowing and diarrhoea.

Oral disease

All patients with HIV infection should be encouraged to see their own (or a hospital-recommended) dentist on a regular basis as gingivitis and periodontitis are common. Most dentists recommend 6-monthly follow-up by a dental hygienist. An acute attack of gingivitis will usually respond rapidly to metronidazole and penicillin, though the antibiotics may cause oral thrush.

Patients with oral candidiasis may complain of loss of taste, a dry mouth or may have noticed the fungus' appearance. The presence of oral thrush should prompt enquiry regarding any difficulty or discomfort swallowing as the patient may also have oesophageal candidiasis. If there is no indication of this, then a short course of an azole antifungal (e.g. fluconazole or ketoconazole) will be effective. Cheaper alternatives (e.g. nystatin pastilles or amphotericin lozenges) are unfortunately not so successful. Oral *Candida* may recur; however, using an azole antifungal agent for prophylaxis tends to lead to resistant infection. Intermittent treatment courses should therefore be used.

Mouth ulcers may result from a variety of causes and should always be swabbed for microbiological, mycobacterial and virological culture. Painful ulcers are usually due to herpes simplex (HSV) and respond to acyclovir 400 mg qds for 5 days or until the ulcer has healed. Any ulcer that has not resolved or increases in size may need biopsy for histological diagnosis. Acyclovir-resistant herpes is now more commonly seen, and here topical trifluridine appears to be effective. Giant aphthous ulceration is also well recognized in HIV disease,

and is treated with thalidomide which can be prescribed on a named patient basis.

Oral hairy leukoplakia appears as a whitish lesion on the lateral border of the tongue. It represents heaped up hyperparakeratotic epithelium which is presumed to have proliferated in response to Epstein-Barr virus stimulation. It is often asymptomatic, though its prognostic significance has been mentioned earlier. Some cases may respond to either high-dose acyclovir (800 mgs qds) or topical retin-A.

Difficulty swallowing

Difficulty swallowing is a frequent symptom as it usually indicates an opportunistic infection. Commonly it is due to candidal oesophagitis, but may result from cytomegalovirus (CMV) or herpes simplex virus oesophagitis (both usually more painful), or obstruction from tumour (e.g. Kaposi's sarcoma). Endoscopy rather than barium swallow tends to be the investigation of choice as here there is little risk of perforation. Endoscopy also enables biopsies to be taken which should be sent to cytology/histopathology, microbiology and virology. Treatment is as necessary (e.g. for *Candida*, fluconazole 150–400 mg/day for 14 days; ganciclovir or foscarnet for CMV infection).

Diarrhoea

Diarrhoea occurs in 30–50% of North American and European patients with AIDS, and in nearly 90% of those from the developing world (often with marked cachexia – 'slim disease'. There is increasing evidence that protracted diarrhoea (i.e. > 3 liquid or semiformed stools most days per week for > 4 weeks) will usually have a specific pathogenic cause, though not always a specific treatment (Quinn et al 1992).

Diarrhoea may be profuse, watery and associated with crampy abdominal pains and dehydration as seen with *Cryptosporidium* or *Isospora belli* and microsporidial species. It may be dysenteric with fever, malaise, abdominal pain and blood and pus in the motion (e.g. CMV colitis, *Salmonella* dysentery), or it may be associated with malabsorption and weight loss (e.g. giardiasis).

Step-wise investigations are summarized in Table 7.5.

Table 7.5 Step-wise investigation of HIV-related diarrhoea

1. Stools and stool chart (1 divided sample on ≥ 3 consecutive days – best results with semiformed/liquid stool)	microscopy, culture for dysenteric pathogens ova, cysts, parasites mycobacterial culture *Clostridium difficile* toxin (drug-induced pseudomembranous colitis) viral culture (CMV, HSV, adenovirus)
2. Sigmoidoscopy & rectal biopsy	histology bacteriology mycobacteriology virology
3. Colonoscopy and biopsy	as for number 2
4. Duodenoscopy and duodenal brushings and duodenal juice aspiration	'HIV villous atrophy' ova, cysts, parasites biopsy macroscopic lesions
5. Electron microscopy of tissue samples	microsporidia species

CMV, cytomegalovirus; HSV, herpes simplex virus

CMV colitis occurs in about 13% of AIDS patients. The diagnosis should be based strictly on either histology or culture as treatment involves 2–3 weeks of ganciclovir or foscarnet, both of which are currently available only intravenously and both of which have serious side-effects (neutropenia and renal impairment, respectively). At present there is no consensus on maintenance therapy for isolated CMV gastrointestinal disease and our practice is not to give maintenance therapy unless gastrointestinal disease is recurrent.

CMV has been implicated in the pathogenesis of both HIV cholangiopathy (similar radiologically to sclerosing cholangitis) and HIV pancreatitis. So, too, have *Cryptosporidium* species which are isolated in the stool of up to 25% of AIDS patients. *Cryptosporidium* can cause profound malabsorption which may not respond at all to treatment. Therapeutic strategies include macrolide antibiotics (e.g. azithromycin) and azoles (e.g. fluconazole); though often symptomatic therapy (fluids and antidiarrhoeals) is all that can be offered.

Diarrhoea may be rarely due to gut wall infiltration by tumours such as Kaposi's sarcoma or lymphoma, which may be revealed at endoscopic examination.

General measures

Nutrition is an important part of general AIDS/HIV management. The mechanisms promoting malabsorption and cachexia are not clearly understood, though the precipitous weight loss in AIDS seems to be related to infection (low serum albumin, normal or raised metabolic rate) (Grunfeld & Feingold 1992). In early disease general 'healthy eating' guidelines are probably adequate, whilst in advanced HIV infection specialist dietetic help is needed to advise on enteral and parenteral feeding.

Neurological disease

Direct HIV infection

HIV may cause direct neurological disease, affecting the brain ('HIV encephalopathy'), the spinal cord (presenting as a vacuolar myelopathy with long tract signs and a sensory level) and the peripheral nervous system (e.g. symmetrical peripheral neuropathy, mononeuritis multiplex, autonomic neuropathy). HIV encephalopathy is characterized by abnormalities of cognition, motor function and behaviour. It is the AIDS-defining illness in less than 5% of cases yet is a common histological finding at post mortem. There is some evidence that antiretroviral therapy may slow down the progressive deterioration (Schmitt et al 1988), though in practice most patients with HIV encephalopathy require supportive care within weeks to months.

Opportunist CNS disease

Opportunistic infection is the commonest cause of neurological dysfunction. *Toxoplasma* encephalitis (the commonest AIDS-defining neurological disease) may present either as a space-occupying lesion with or without focal signs, as a seizure or as a depressed level of consciousness. In 95% of cases *Toxoplasma* encephalitis is a reactivation of past infection. The diagnosis is made by the history, examination and CT brain scan appearance which will show one or more areas of hypodense oedema, often with contrast ring-enhancement signifying abscess formation. Treatment is started for toxoplasmosis on a presumptive basis as *Toxoplasma* encephalitis is common and will respond to therapy, whereas the other likely causes of this picture have a uniformly poor outlook. Indications for brain biopsy include failure of therapy (after about 2 weeks), atypical CT findings and negative *Toxoplasma* serology with previous good quality of life (Barker & Holliman 1992).

Standard treatment is 4–8 weeks of sulphadiazine 6–8 gms/day with pyrimethamine 75 mg/day plus folinic acid supplements. Clindamycin is an effective substitute for sulphadiazine if there is sulphonamide intolerance. Lower dose maintenance therapy needs to be life-long. Recent work suggests that primary prophylaxis with dapsone and pyrimethamine may prevent *Toxoplasma* reactivation (and hence disease). This needs further confirmation but may be important for patients who are *Toxoplasma* IgG-positive.

Other causes of focal neurological dysfunction include progressive multifocal leukoencephalopathy (a degenerative disease due to a papova virus, also carrying a poor prognosis); and much more rarely tuberculoma, bacterial abscess (usually in drug addicts) and viral and fungal infections. Focal neurological abnormality may also be caused by primary central nervous system lymphoma. The diagnosis is made by brain biopsy. Response to radiotherapy is usually disappointing.

Diffuse central nervous system dysfunction may present as drowsiness, confusion or behaviourial changes. It is important to exclude metabolic (e.g. systemic infection, hyponatraemia) and hypoxic causes (undiagnosed chest infection). Drugs can also be a potent cause of confusion (e.g. opiates for pain relief). Infections may also produce this sort of picture and include cryptococcal meningitis (which may have minimal associated meningism). This responds in only 40–50% of cases to either amphotericin B or the less toxic fluconazole (200–400 mg/day) (Saag et al 1992). Bacterial and mycobacterial meningitis can present like this, as will CMV/HSV encephalitis in the immunosuppressed. Recent reports have stressed the danger of missing active neurosyphilis and thus it is important that routine 'work-up' includes MRI/CT brain scan; then lumbar puncture with CSF analysis to cytology (lymphoma, fungi), microbiology, mycobacteriology, serology laboratory, virology and biochemistry.

Retinal involvement is usually due to CMV disease and is a fairly late AIDS event. The patient may complain of 'floaters' or loss of vision and to save the eye treatment should be started as soon as possible. Post-induction maintenance therapy is important and should be given indefinitely. A recent trial compared the benefits of foscarnet and ganciclovir and appeared to show a survival advantage for the former (median 12.6 vs 8.5 months) (SOCA 1992). However, oral maintenance ganciclovir may soon be available, reducing the need for permanent indwelling lines – which would be a considerable advance as patients frequently develop septicaemia requiring multiple line changes.

Haematological disease

The haematological manifestations of HIV are protean and may result from HIV infection per se; opportunist disease (e.g. anaemia from disseminated *Mycobacterium avium intracellulare* complex, bone marrow infiltration by lymphoma); or the drug therapy used in treating these conditions (Costello 1990). Cytopenias may be due to either increased destruction or failure of production. Any form of cytopenia can be present, though typically HIV will cause more thrombocytopenia than will either drugs or opportunist infections; whilst drugs such as cotrimoxazole, zidovudine and ganciclovir produce neutropenia and anaemia. Zidovudine causes a macrocytosis irrespective of the haemoglobin level in 90% of patients. Vitamin B12 and folate levels are usually normal.

Promising results have been found with both granulocyte colony stimulating factor (G-CSF) and granulocyte – macrophage colony stimulating factor (GM-CSF) in reversing zidovudine-induced and HIV-related leucopenia (Mitsuyasu 1991). However, apart from the anticipated side-effects of flu-like symptoms, and high cost, there is a potential disadvantage with GM-CSF, in particular, in that it can stimulate macrophages which may lead to increased HIV replication within these retroviral reservoirs. Fortunately this has not been borne out in clinical practice. Recombinant erythropoietin has been shown to correct zidovudine-induced anaemia in patients with low endogenous erythropoietin (Fischl et al 1990a).

HIV-related neoplastic disease

Kaposi's sarcoma is the main non-infectious AIDS complication. It is more common in homosexual than heterosexual men, and is rare in women, particularly in women of Caucasian origin. It can behave as a benign solitary tumour or rapidly develop multicentrically to involve the gut, lungs and lymph nodes. It is commonly found on the skin and palate and resembles at first a bruise that then becomes a purplish nodule. Treatment can be expectant or, if required, local radiotherapy or cryotherapy is often effective for Kaposi's sarcoma involving the skin. Intralesional chemotherapy can also be used, though if Kaposi's sarcoma is extensive or involves the viscera, systemic chemotherapy is advocated. Median survival time with extensive disease is 8–10 months. Interferon-a exerts an antiproliferative action on Kaposi's sarcoma. It appears to be most successful if given with zidovudine to an individual with a relatively intact immune system (CD4 > $200 \times 10^6/1$) (Fischl et al 1991), and thus it should be considered early in patients with Kaposi's sarcoma.

Non-Hodgkin's lymphoma is an AIDS-defining condition which can be either primary central nervous system or systemic. The former appears to be associated with Epstein-Barr virus and carries a very poor prognosis (median survival under 2 months) whilst the latter responds to chemotherapy, though often relapses several months later (Levine 1992).

It seems that improving the treatment and prophylaxis of HIV-related infection leads to an increased recognition of HIV-related tumours. Examples include cervical carcinoma (Maiman et al 1990) and squamous cell carcinoma of the anus.

Antiretroviral therapy

In the long term, antiretroviral therapy is the only hope of eradicating established HIV infection. At present the licensed agents can only inhibit HIV reverse transcriptase (suppressing HIV replication by blocking the synthesis of viral DNA) and thus are not curative. These drugs need to be taken lifelong and so questions of short- and long-term toxicity and sustained effect become paramount. Zidovudine (azidothymidine, AZT) is the only agent of proven efficacy (prolonged survival, reduction in opportunistic infections and improved quality of life) for the treatment of AIDS (Fischl et al 1987, Vella et al 1992). In America, in addition, the dideoxynucleoside analogue didanosine (ddI) and dideoxycytidine (ddC) are licensed for use. Drug trials with these agents have been hampered by the length of time required for clinical end-points (e.g. death, development of AIDS), and thus ddI and ddC have been deemed efficacious on the basis of favourable changes in surrogate immune markers (e.g. CD4 count and HIV antigen) (Lambert et al 1990) which appear to predict short-term risk for clinical progression rather than survival (Jacobson et al 1991).

The value of treatment in patients who are less symptomatic (Fischl et al 1990b) or even asymptomatic (Volberding et al 1990) is not as yet clearly defined. Placebo-controlled studies to date have only demonstrated a reduction in rate of fall of CD4 count and a delayed progression to AIDS, but no improvement in survival. In a recent observational study, Graham showed zidovudine reduced mortality by slowing the progression to AIDS. However, this survival advantage had disappeared after the 2nd year of follow-up (Graham et al 1992). The results of the Veterans Affairs Cooperative Study suggest that 'early versus late' zidovudine use may be a trade-off between a longer pre-AIDS symptom-free period and a presumably improved quality and quantity of life once AIDS has developed (Hamilton et al 1992). Zidovudine is at present licensed for use at the onset of symptoms, or when the CD4 count is persistently < $200 \times 10^6/1$, or is rapidly declining from $500 \times 10^6/1$. We believe that in the latter case treatment should be discussed with the patient who should then make his/her own decision regarding therapy.

Zidovudine is a toxic drug. It can cause bone marrow suppression, nausea, vomiting, myositis, headache and insomnia. These effects are dose-related and can be severe enough to warrant stopping the drug. Fortunately, much smaller doses than first used seem equally efficacious (Volberding et al 1990, Nordic MRC 1992) and the standard prescribed regimen is now 400–600 mg/day in divided doses. Zidovudine used at this dosage level is associated with much less toxicity. Zidovudine also appears to be safe during pregnancy (Sperling et al 1992), though there are no data to show that it will influence vertical transmission of HIV from mother to infant.

Zidovudine appears to have a limited clinical duration of effect, which may correspond to in vitro resistance (Tudor-Williams et al 1992). This can be demonstrated after as little as 6 months of therapy (Larder et al 1989) and is present in all AIDS/ARC patients at 18 months. No cross-resistance has been found with other antiretrovirals, and dideoxynucleoside analogues may be of value in these situations. For example, the recent ACTG 116B/117 trial comparing zidovudine 600 mg/day with two doses of ddI (500 mg/day and 750 mg/day) in patients who had tolerated AZT for more than 16 weeks revealed a significant decrease in the number of opportunist infections in the 500-mg ddI group. This effect, however, was seen only in those entering the study with ARC or asymptomatic disease, and there was no difference in survival between any treatment arms.

Zidovudine sensitivity may return once the drug is stopped (St Clair et al 1991). This, plus the different toxicity profiles of zidovudine and the dideoxynucleoside analogues (ddI – pancreatitis and peripheral neuropathy; ddC – peripheral neuropathy), has led to trials of combination chemotherapy with some encouraging early results (Meng et al 1992). On the basis of this, the American Food and Drug Administration recently licensed ddC for use in combination with zidovudine.

At present there are no other licensed antiretroviral agents. Several clinical trials of non-nucleoside analogue reverse transcriptase inhibitors, e.g. TIBO derivatives (active almost solely against HIV-1 and responsible for profound single agent resistance), tat antagonists and retroviral protease inhibitors are underway. Soluble CD4 has generated interest, though doubts remain whether this fluid phase intervention can limit in vivo cell to cell spread. Cytokines and interferons are also under investigation, though whether they are useful as pure antiretroviral agents remains unclear.

Vaccines against HIV are now being tested for safety and immunogenicity in several clinical trials in both HIV-positive and -negative volunteers. Most vaccines are based on HIV envelope proteins, e.g. gp 160 (Dolin et al 1991), though some use whole killed virus. Results so far suggest that a cellular but not humoral immune response is generated and sustained over at least a 2-year period. The clinical significance of this remains unclear.

The aims of medical HIV care are to prevent person to person spread, slow down disease progression and stop opportunist events. A cure is unlikely to be found, though the judicious use of immunotherapy, antiretrovirals and prophylactic drugs tailored to the individual through laboratory markers will continue to improve the quality and quantity of life of people infected with HIV.

REFERENCES

Aledort L M, Hilgartner M W, Pike M C et al 1992 Variability in serial CD4 counts and relation to progression of HIV-1 infection to AIDS in haemophilic patients. Br Med J 304: 212–216
Barker K F, Holliman R E 1992 Laboratory techniques in the investigation of toxoplasmosis. Genitour Med 68: 55–59
Bor R, Miller R, Johnson M A 1991 A testing time for doctors: counselling patients before an HIV test. Br Med J 303: 905–907
Centers for Disease Control 1981 Pneumocystis pneumonia – Los Angeles. MMWR 30: 250–252
Centers for Disease Control 1992a Recommendations for prophylaxis against pneumocystis carinii pneumonia for adults and adolescents infected with human immunodeficiency virus. MMWR 41: 1–11
Centers for Disease Control 1992B Addendum to the proposed expansion of the AIDS surveillance case definition. October 22
Costello C (ed) 1990 Haematology in HIV disease. Clin Haematol 3: 1–218
De Jong M D, Hulsebosch H J, Lange J M A 1991 Clinical, virological and immunological features of primary HIV-1 infection. Genitour Med 67: 367–373
Dolin R, Graham B S, Greenberg S B et al 1991 The safety and immunogenicity of a human immunodeficiency virus type 1 (HIV-1) recombinant gp 160 candidate vaccine in humans. Ann Intern Med 114: 119–127
Elliot A M, Luo N, Tembo G et al 1990 Impact of HIV on

tuberculosis in Zambia: a cross sectional study. Br Med J 301: 412–415

Fischl M A, Richman D D, Grieco M H et al 1987 The efficacy of azidothymidine (AZT) in the treatment of patients with AIDS or AIDS related complex: a double-blind placebo-controlled trial. N Engl J Med 317: 185–191

Fischl M A, Galpin J E, Levine J D et al 1990a Recombinant human erythropoietin for patients with AIDS treated with zidovudine. N Engl J Med 322: 1488–1493

Fischl M A, Richman D D, Hansen N et al 1990b The safety and efficacy of zidovudine (AZT) in the treatment of subjects with mildly symptomatic human immunodeficiency virus type 1 (HIV) infection. Ann Intern Med 112: 727–737

Fischl M A, Uttamchandani R B, Resnick L et al 1991 A phase 1 study of recombinant human interferon-alpha or human lymphoblastoid interferon alpha and concomitant zidovudine in patients with AIDS-related Kaposi's sarcoma. J Acq Immune Defic Synd 4: 1–10

Graham N M H, Zeger S L, Park L P et al 1991 Effect of zidovudine and pneumocystis carinii pneumonia prophylaxis on progression of HIV-1 infection to AIDS. Lancet 338: 265–269

Graham N M H, Zeger S L, Park L P et al 1992. The effects on survival of early treatment of human immunodeficiency virus infection. N Engl J Med 326: 1037–1042

Grunfeld C, Feingold K R 1992 Metabolic disturbances and wasting in the acquired immunodeficiency syndrome. N Engl J Med 327: 329–337

Hamilton J D, Hartigan P M, Simberkoff M S et al 1992 A controlled trial of early versus late treatment with zidovudine in symptomatic human immunodeficiency infection: results of the veterans affairs cooperative study. N Engl J Med 326: 437–443

Hardy D, Holzman R, Feinberg J et al 1992 Trimethoprim-sulfamethoxazole (T–S) vs aerosolized pentamidine (AP) for secondary prophylaxis of pneumocystis carinii pneumonia (PCP) in AIDS patients: a prospective, randomised controlled clinical trial. AIDS Clinical Trials Group. Third European Conference on Clinical Aspects and Treatment of HIV infection, Paris

Hughes W T 1991 Prevention and treatment of pneumocystis carinii pneumonia. Annu Rev Med 42: 287–295

Jacobson M A, Bacchetti P, Kolokathis A et al 1991 Surrogate markers for survival in patients with AIDS or AIDS related complex treated with zidovudine. Br Med J 302: 73–78

Lambert J S, Seidlin M, Reichman R C et al 1990 2' 3'-dideoxyinosine (ddI) in patients with the acquired immunodeficiency syndrome or AIDS-related complex: a phase 1 trial. N Engl J Med 322: 1333–1340

Larder B A, Darby G, Richman D D 1989 HIV with reduced sensitivity to zidovudine (AZT) isolated during prolonged therapy. Science 243: 1731–1734

Leoung G S, Feigl D W Jr, Montgomery A B et al 1990 Aerosolized pentamidine for prophylaxis against pneumocystis carinii pneumonia – the San Francisco community prophylaxis trial. N Engl J Med 323: 769–775

Levine A M 1992 AIDS-associated malignant lymphoma. Med Clin N Am 76: 253–268

McGowan J E Jr, Chesney P J, Crossley K B et al 1992 Guidelines for the use of systemic glucocorticosteroids in the management of selected infections. J Infect Dis 165: 1–13

Maiman M, Fruchter R G, Serur E et al 1990 Human

immunodeficiency virus infection and cervical neoplasia. Gynecol Oncol 38: 377–382

Mitsuyasu R T 1991 Use of recombinant interferons and hematopoietic growth factors in patients infected with human immunodeficiency virus. Rev Infect Dis 13: 979–984

Meng T C, Fischl M A, Boota A M et al 1992 Combination therapy with zidovudine and dideoxycytidine in patients with advanced human immunodeficiency virus infection. A phase I/II study. Ann Intern Med 116: 13–20

Moss A R, Bacchetti P 1989 Natural history of HIV infection. AIDS 3: 55–61

Nordic Medical Research Councils' HIV Therapy Group 1992 Double blind dose–response study of zidovudine in AIDS and advanced HIV infection. Br MedJ 304: 13–17

Pedersen C, Lindhart B O, Jensen B L et al 1989 Clinical course of primary HIV infection: consequences for subsequent course of infection. Br MedJ 299: 154–157

Quinn T C, Strober W, Janoff E N et al 1992 Gastrointestinal infections in AIDS. Ann Intern Med 116: 63–77

Royce R A, Luckmann R S, Fusaro R E et al 1991 The natural history of HIV infection: staging classifications of disease. AIDS 5: 355–364

Rutherford G W, Lifson A R, Hessol N A et al 1990 Course of HIV-1 infection in a cohort of homosexual and bisexual men: an 11 year follow up study. Br MedJ 301: 1183–1188

Saag M S, Powderly W G, Cloud G A et al 1992 Comparison of amphotericin B with fluconazole in the treatment of acute AIDS-associated cryptococcal meningitis. N Engl J Med 326: 83–89

St Clair M H, Martin J L, Tudor-Williams G et al 1991 Resistance to ddI and sensitivity to AZT induced by a mutation in HIV-1 reverse transcriptase. Science 253: 1557–1559

Schmitt F, Bigley J, McKinnis R 1988 Neuropsychological outcome of zidovudine treatment of patients with AIDS and AIDS related complex. N Engl J Med 299: 819–821

Scoular A, French P, Miller R F, 1991 Mycobacterium avium-intracellulare infection in the acquired immunodeficiency syndrome. Br J Hosp Med 46: 295–300

Smith D, Forbes A, Gazzard B 1992 A simple scoring system to diagnose pneumocystis carinii pneumonia in high-risk individuals. AIDS 6: 337–338

Snider D E Jr, Roper W L 1992 The new tuberculosis. N Engl J Med 326: 703–705

Sperling R S, Stratton P, O'Sullivan M J et al 1992 A survey of zidovudine use in pregnant women with human immunodeficiency virus infection. N Engl J Med 326: 857–861

Studies of ocular complications of AIDS (SOCA) Research Group, in collaboration with the AIDS Clinical Trials Group 1992 Mortality in patients with the acquired immunodeficiency syndrome treated with either foscarnet or ganciclovir for cytomegalovirus retinitis. N Engl J Med 326: 213–220

Tudor-Williams G, St Clair M H, McKinney R E et al 1992 HIV-1 sensitivity to zidovudine and clinical outcome in children. Lancet 339: 15–19

Vella S, Giuliano M, Pezzotti P et al 1992 Survival of zidovudine-treated patients with AIDS compared with that of contemporary untreated patients. JAMA 267: 1232–1236

Volberding P A, Lagakos S W, Koch M A et al 1990 Zidovudine in asymptomatic human immunodeficiency virus infection: a controlled trial in persons with fewer than 500 CD4-

positive cells per cubic millimeter. N Engl J Med 322: 941–949

Wachter R M, Luce J M, Hopewell P C 1992 Critical care of patients with AIDS. JAMA 267: 541–547

World Health Organization 1991 Current and future dimensions of the HIV/AIDS pandemic – a capsule summary. WHO, Geneva

8. Clinical management of HIV disease in developing countries

Anton Pozniak

INTRODUCTION

The human immunodeficiency virus (HIV) has spread more extensively in sub-Saharan Africa than in any other region of the world to date; 60% of the 10 million HIV infections world-wide have occurred in this continent with at least one in 40 adults infected (N'Galy & Ryder 1988, Chin 1990). The significance of this epidemic is disturbing, as the region has less than 10% of the world's population (Berkley 1992). Many reasons why the HIV epidemic has become so severe in sub-Saharan Africa are set by the social realities of Africa: the migrant labour system, rapid urbanization, constant war, high levels of military mobilization, landlessness, poverty and, until the advent of HIV, unchecked population growth. Nevertheless, 70 million HIV infections are predicted for Africa during the next 25 years, leading to a mean decrease of 12 years in life expectancy and 4.5 million deaths annually (Way & Stanecki 1991, Chin 1992).

HIV infections and deaths are increasing not only in Africa but also in other developing countries such as Latin America, the Caribbean and especially Asia. This mainly heterosexual epidemic is having profound effects on family life and is bringing into sharp focus the problems of women with, or at risk of, HIV. Three million women world-wide have already been infected with HIV and half a million have developed AIDS; an estimated two million women will die of AIDS during the 1990s (Preble 1990).

Most of what is known about HIV disease in women has been derived from studies of prostitutes or pregnant women, or those which have focused primarily on perinatal issues, and women are seen as 'only whores and mothers' (Carovano 1991). Women in Africa have been portrayed as dangerous vectors of AIDS and many epidemiological investigations have emphasized the study of female prostitutes to the exclusion of other women. The data are often interpreted as meaning that without prostitutes there would be no epidemic (Padian 1987), but what may really be happening is that these women infected by their clients are experiencing the brunt of the epidemic (Bassett & Mhloyi 1991). The extent to which the propagation of the epidemic depends on prostitution is unknown. The other image of a woman in the AIDS epidemic is a pregnant one, who might infect her child. This image reinforces the notion that mothers are solely responsible for a child's serostatus. All women, whether pregnant or not, are at risk of HIV infection (Panos Institute 1990) and this chapter will discuss the broad issues of management of HIV disease in women in developing countries, especially concentrating on what is known in Africa.

SEXUAL BEHAVIOUR

Sub-Saharan African societies have important historical, cultural and economic differences that can affect sexual behaviour, both in the cities and in isolated villages, and these societies should not be unthinkingly combined (Larson 1989). There is a great diversity in the form and nature of marital and extramarital relationships throughout this region, yet cross-cultural studies are increasingly finding uniformities that display some coherence between cultural, sexual and economic factors (Guyer 1981). People with common traditions living in an area such as Central Africa can share certain values, symbols and rituals of overriding importance (Christakis & Fox 1992). In many African societies, for example, the person is seen as an extension of the family, and an intermediary between ancestors and future generations. Although there has been some division into urban and rural life within Africa, it has not removed Africans completely, either physically or socially, from traditional village existence, and many urban residents tend to live in village-like enclaves with persons of the same tribe and rural origin. Sexual behaviour of women depends on the understanding of traditions, culture and economic status. For example, in many parts of sub-Saharan Africa women receive their sex education between the ages of 12 and 16 years from maternal aunts or grandmothers, and girls are sometimes sent to villages from urban townships in order to learn about sexual matters from rural aunts. They are told about their future duties as wives (Gelfand 1979, Larson 1989), and how to make relationships with the husband's relatives. In some regions polygamy is taken for granted, and both sexes grow up in an environment where it is accepted. Sex education for girls is preparative, and continues until they marry.

Much more emphasis is placed on a girl's purity than on a boy's, and in some societies adolescent girls can undergo routine inspection for virginity between once a month and twice a year until the girl marries (Gelfand 1979). Virginity at first marriage is expected of girls in Eastern and Central Africa, and where premarital sexual intercourse does occur, the woman's kin are concerned that pregnancy, not loss of virginity, will spoil a marriage (Molnos 1973, Bongaarts et al 1984). Consequently, the level of premarital births is usually below 5% of the total number of annual births. Male chastity is not praised, and male premarital experience is often limited to rare contacts with prostitutes (Page & Lesthaeghe 1981). Men tend to marry later than women because of dowry problems, polygamy levels, migration and man shortage. Punishment for adultery is strict, but a long period of sexual abstinence postpartum is a major reason for many monogamous marriages to seek sex elsewhere. Urbanization has reduced sexual control and so has led the way from traditional marriages to more cohabitation and changes in sexual practices, and bar girls and prostitutes have become alternative male sexual outlets (Page & Lesthaeghe 1981). Within cities sexual permissiveness for women has changed, but what has emerged is a more sophisticated sexual structure allowing mistresses, love affairs and concubines.

Many societies in Africa are patrilineal and marriages are accompanied by payments of a bride price in compensation to the wife's family for loss of her labour, reproductive capacity, and as a token of respect from one family to another (Larson 1989). This payment can be substantial and may take many years to complete. Male commitment to marriage is primarily to financially support his wife and children that become part of the male lineage. Wealthy men can have more than one wife, but polygamy has now become too expensive (Bassett & Mhloyi 1991).

Male migration has left women as heads of household in the rural areas, and separation has become a feature of life in many parts of Africa (Riddell 1982). Sexual relationships outside marriage have also changed, with husbands having other partners in towns. These liaisons can lead to loss of cash income from the towns back to the rural areas, and sometimes rural income might be used to supplement urban expenses. Men who can not afford to maintain urban wives as well as their rural wives might opt for more casual arrangements. Multiple relationships that arise in urban settings are not rare and exchange of sex for money or for other goods and services is not always considered to be prostitution (Day 1989). Reward of sexual services may range from occasional cash payments to stable partners through to supplementation of incomes with gifts. Women who work as seasonal labourers can support themselves off-season by selling sex, and others sell or are forced to have sex to meet a specific obligation, such as school fees or job security. These behaviour patterns may not only be found in cities but also in some rural areas where there are business centres, in army camps and similar locations which provide the setting for exchanges to occur. It is important to emphasize that there are strong social sanctions that exist against women who engage in extramarital sex, and for the vast majority of women, sexual relationships occur in the context of marriage (Lindan et al 1991); by the age of 20–

24 years, 75% of women in Zimbabwe have been married (UNICEF 1985).

In many parts of the developing world, women are born into inequity characterized by negligence and ecological handicap, lack of educational opportunity, low societal status, early marriages and excess fertility (Ramalingaswami 1992). Many factors that predispose African women to illness, such as poverty, malnutrition, uncontrolled fertility and the complications of childbirth, also increase the risk of their acquiring HIV infection (Ulin 1992). Women have little bargaining power to negotiate safe sex with their partners, and few of them have control over the sexual behaviour of their men (Ankrah 1991). Economic dependency of women on men is one of the most important factors for female prostitution.

Men who have travelled out of rural communities to urban centres in search of employment may acquire the HIV virus in the cities and carry it back to infect rural wives (Latif et al 1989, Jochelson et al 1991). Women are also leaving rural areas and migrating to the city but without any economic and personal autonomy (Ulin 1992). Traditional attitudes towards marriage and sexuality have changed, and in the larger cities of Africa new forms of sexual relationships including prostitution and small circles of interchanging lovers occur. Land expropriation, rural impoverishment and forceful introduction of male migrant labour have resulted in patterns of sexual relations characterized by multiple partners (Ankrah 1991). Traditional patriarchal values reinterpreted in European law have resulted in further segregation of women and the limited right to female ownership has been withdrawn. Sexual relationships with men, either within marriage or outside, have become inextricably linked to economics and social survival. In townships in South Africa, although the level of AIDS knowledge amongst mothers was high, sexual behaviour was characterized by high pregnancy rates and a high proportion of women having children by more than one consort (Abdool-Karim et al 1991).

SPREAD OF HIV IN CENTRAL AFRICAN COUNTRIES

Since the mid-1970s HIV has followed the routes of trade and population movements, and conditions in war-torn areas have contributed to its spread. There appears to be an urban/rural gradient in terms of the percentage of people infected, the seroprevalence rates in urban and rural areas ranging from 5 to 12% in some rural settings (Dolmans et al 1989) to 8 to 30% in urban areas (Melbye et al 1986). This trend will probably not be sustained because of frequent movement between town and rural areas, migrant labour and a general trend for urban migration, which in Africa is the highest in the world (United Nations 1987).

Since the early 1980s HIV has spread rapidly in groups such as female prostitutes, but much more slowly and at various rates in the general population (Nkowane 1990). The reasons for this particular epidemiological pattern are not clear, but demographic factors as well as the presence of sexually transmitted disease may have influenced the dynamics of the epidemic. The annual HIV seroconversion rate was 1% per year over 2 years in one cohort in Zaire (Mann et al 1986a), and in another it remained stable over 2 years at 0.8% (Piot & Carael 1988). HIV seroprevalence studies have been done in many parts of Africa, usually as cluster studies in blood donors or in high risk groups such as prostitutes, in whom there is up to 88% seropositivity (Van de Perre et al 1985, Quinn et al 1986, Piot et al 1987). There has been an alarming rate of rise in HIV seroprevalence among a cohort of Nairobi prostitutes (Piot et al 1987) and a rapid dissemination of HIV infection in this particular risk group in Africa (Kreiss et al 1986, Simonsen et al 1990).

To define the seroprevalence rates in the general population is more difficult, and so data are collected from other groups considered to be at risk from sexual transmission (Odehouri et al 1989). In pregnant women from Nairobi between 1989 and 1991 the annual incidence rate of HIV infection was 4% (Temmerman et al 1992). HIV seroprevalence among women less than 25 years of age increased from 5.6% in 1989 to 13.2% in 1991, and increased in those over 25 years of age from 6.8% in 1989 to 12.7% in 1991. This pattern is similar to that in other African countries such as Uganda, Rwanda, Zambia, Malawi (Miotti et al 1990), Cameroon and Zimbabwe (Mahomed et al 1991), although slower rates of spread have been reported from Zaire, Mali and some regions in the Congo (Lallemant et al 1992).

The prevalence of HIV-1 infection is very high even among women (in particular teenagers) who did not report at-risk sexual behaviour. The relatively conservative sexual behaviour of women outside of high risk groups indicated that any change in their sexual behaviour would have little impact on the risk of HIV-1 infection. In a study from Rwanda (Allen et al 1991), male partners who consumed alcohol or who had a high income were more likely to transmit HIV-1 infection to their female partners. These data have led some to believe that it is more important to direct education programmes towards changing male sexual behaviour than to target women outside of core groups.

MAJOR RISK FACTORS FOR HIV ACQUISITION

Sexually transmitted disease (STD) in the form of genital ulceration has the strongest association with transmission of HIV (Nsubuga et al 1990, Jessamine et al 1990). Other risk factors for transmission of HIV have been reported and include non-ulcerative sexually transmitted diseases (Kreiss et al 1986, Manoka et al 1990), number of sexual partners (Clumeck et al 1985), a history of prostitution or contact with a prostitute (Kreiss et al 1986, Quinn et al 1986, Mann et al 1988b) and the presence of an intact foreskin (Cameron et al 1989). How many of these factors have their association because they are also associated with genital ulcer disease is not known. Evidence also suggests that sexual transmission of HIV is more likely among couples if the index case acquired HIV sexually rather than from transfusion of blood products (Holmes & Kreiss 1988).

Sexual transmission of HIV through vaginal-penile intercourse is a major route of acquisition of HIV-1 amongst prostitutes in Nairobi (Plummer et al 1991). The incidence of HIV-1 infection in these women was 67% over 30 months of follow-up. *Chlamydia trachomatis* infection and genital ulcers appeared to facilitate HIV-1 transmission. In this study gonorrhoea rates and number of sex partners were unrelated to HIV acquisition. Oral contraceptive use appeared to facilitate transmission but this association was not conclusive. It is possible that an increase in ectopy or risk of *Chlamydia* associated with pill use may enhance HIV transmission. Condoms would give some protection to these women, as barrier methods extend the protection against HIV-1 infection, even with incomplete condom use, and they also protect against genital ulceration and *Chlamydia trachomatis* infection. Convincing men to use them is difficult (Goldberg et al 1989). Only 35% of men in a national survey (Mbivzo & Adamchak 1989), and only 7% of child-bearing women in Rwanda (Lindan et al 1991) said they had ever used them. Transmission occurs even though intercourse does not continue during menstruation, and there is a lack of association with insertion of objects into the vagina, or with potential non-sexual routes such as injections, scarification and blood transfusion (Quinn et al 1986).

As heterosexual transmission of HIV may be enhanced in the presence of other sexually transmitted disease, female prostitutes are at increased risk of acquiring and transmitting HIV infection. In a survey conducted in 1986 in Kinshasa, Zaire, 27% of female prostitutes were HIV antibody-positive (Mann et al 1988a), rising to 35% in 1988 (Nzila et al 1991). Among men in Kinshasa, of 7,000 male employees in two worksites, 28% admitted having had sex with a prostitute in the last year (Ryder et al 1990). Thirty-five percent of this group were HIV-positive, and 16% had syphilis, 23% gonorrhoea, 13% *Chlamydia*, 22% *Trichomonas* and 10% *Candida*. Not only is there a high prevalence of HIV infection among prostitutes in African cities, but there is also a high burden of many other STDs amongst prostitutes. In Nairobi, the HIV seroprevalence rose from 30 to 90% in prostitutes between 1985 and 1987 (Piot et al 1987). The reason for the differences between Kinshasa and Nairobi is not clear, but the Kinshasa population were less stable, with 23% of the Kinshasa prostitute population being new recruits. There was also a lower number of partners amongst Kinshasa prostitutes, lower prevalence of HIV infection amongst clients and a lower prevalence of genital ulcerative disease. More men in Kinshasa were circumcised (95%), compared with Kenya (about 75%).

Blood transfusion has probably accounted for 5–10% of all AIDS cases in Africa (Mann et al 1986a, Piot & Carael 1988). The proportion of blood donors who are HIV-positive is greater in Africa than in the developed world, and the use of unscreened blood led to many recipients, especially children, being infected (Kayembe et al 1986, Mann et al 1986b). However, these problems are being solved; Zimbabwe was the third country in the world to screen their blood and blood products for HIV, and many other African countries have developed comprehensive blood screening programmes. Nevertheless, in spite of a well-developed blood transfusion service, the risk of HIV-1 infection from blood transfusion in Africa is 5.4–10.6/1000 units (Savarit et al 1992).

Intravenous drug use is not common in Africa (Conlon 1988), and even when it occurs it contributes little to HIV seropositivity rates compared to heterosexual spread. No association has been found between frequency of needle exposure, for whatever reason, and HIV seropositivity in groups such as prostitutes (Kreiss et al 1986; Le Page et al 1986).

In Uganda, women were found to have a higher seroprevalence compared to men at 1.4 to 1.0 (Berkley et al 1990). Possible reasons for this are that men are more likely to be admitted to hospital, and therefore tested; that there is a differential rate of progression to HIV illness in infected men and women with a faster progression in men; that there is an increased efficiency in transmission from men to women, compared to women to men (Padian 1987, Friedland & Klein 1987); that women are infected at a younger age than men; that there are possible gender differences in infectiousness and susceptibility to HIV infection; and that women may survive longer than men. The medium maternal age at first childbirth is 18 years in Uganda, during the peak of risk of HIV sero-prevalence infection. The Ugandan woman's perceived mean ideal total number of children is seven, which has implications for vertical transmission. Clearly, young women should be considered a high risk group requiring immediate and intensive education.

FERTILITY AND TRANSMISSION RATES

African women have traditionally some of the highest fertility rates in the world, with an average total lifetime fertility in excess of six children (Ryder et al 1991). HIV seroprevalence of women of child-bearing age in sub-Saharan Africa is estimated at approximately 2500 per 100 000 women compared with South America, 200 per 100 000; North America, 140 per 100 000; and Europe, 70 per 100 000 (Chin 1990). Over the next decade 80% of all children with HIV infection acquired during the perinatal period will be born in Africa (Chin 1990).

Maternal-fetal HIV transmission appears to occur at a rate of 20–40% in Africa. Little information has been reported on fertility rates in women who are infected with HIV-1 (Schrijvers et al 1991). In a study in Zaire (Ryder et al 1991), less than 25% of HIV-1-positive women used any form of birth control during the 3-year follow-up period; however, at the end of this period, 33% of sexual partners of women with AIDS were using condoms. Fertility rates were consistently lower in seropositive women compared with seronegative women, and among HIV-positive women, those most advanced in their immunosuppression had the lowest fertility rate. It has not been determined whether these rates were due to lower rates of sexual activity or were due to the primary effects of HIV infection. The knowledge of HIV-1-seropositive status has been shown to have a lack of influence on child-bearing behaviour in HIV-1-seropositive intravenous drug-using women in Europe and North America, as well as in heterosexual African women. More than 97% of all HIV-seropositive women in the Zaire study were unwilling to inform their sexual partners because of fear of divorce; this consequently led to a low use of condoms.

BREAST-FEEDING

Breast-feeding is a significant factor in maternal-child transmission of HIV, and advice in industrialized countries is to encourage bottle feeding by HIV-positive mothers. Breast-feeding is usually universal and prolonged in Africa (WHO 1982), and access to artificial feeding bottles is limited.

Poverty makes any change to artificial feeding unlikely as well as undesirable in rural areas (Nicoll et al 1990). In urban centres, artificial feeds are often available and the possibility exists of their unscrupulous commercial promotion. Although there could be a change towards artifical feeding once doubts are raised over the safety of breast-feeding, because of competing causes for perinatal mortality any population change to artificial feeding in urban areas would result in infant and child wastage (Nicoll et al 1990). Consequently, in the developing world, promotion of breast-feeding will need to be strengthened (Oxtoby 1988).

HIV INCIDENCE AND MORTALITY IN WOMEN

At present half a million women die every year throughout the world from causes related to pregnancy and childbirth, and over 99% of these deaths take place in developing countries (Ramalingaswami 1990). The dynamics of the HIV epidemic are such that AIDS will emerge as a leading cause of death in women between 20 and 40 years of age in the 1990s (De Cock et al 1990). Rising HIV infection rates in women of reproductive age with their high birth rates lead to an increase in the incidence of perinatal transmission, and so infant and child mortality rates will rise by 10 and 15%, respectively, by the beginning of the 21st century (Chin 1992). Even seronegative children will have a poorer chance of survival as their seropositive mothers become ill and household management and child care deteriorate.

The 2 year mortality from one study of 260 HIV-positive women from Rwanda was 7%, which was 20 times the mortality of the HIV-negative cohort (Lindan et al 1992). HIV disease accounted for 90% of all deaths among child-bearing urban Rwandan women. In the same study, however, it was shown that mortality among patients with AIDS was low compared with that reported from other studies in Africa, although these latter studies were based on hospitalized patients presenting late in the course of disease, and not on outpatients. Baseline predictors of mortality (in order of descending risk) in women with HIV infection were:

1. Low body mass index ($< 21 \text{ kg} / \text{m}^2$)

2. Low income
3. Erythrocyte sedimentation rate $> 60 \text{ mm} / \text{h}$
4. Chronic diarrhoea
5. History of herpes zoster in the previous 5 years
6. Oral *Candida*

Women of low socio-economic status, who may lack adequate nutrition, had a two- to threefold mortality. An elevated erythrocyte sedimentation rate was related to poor outcome, more so than the absolute lymphocyte count, and anaemia and leucopenia were also associated with an increased risk of death. Survival was reduced among women over 30 years of age, and in those who had had gonorrhoea or syphilis or more than one lifetime sexual partner. The majority of women died from wasting syndrome; extrapulmonary tuberculosis, cryptococcal meningitis and Kaposi's sarcoma were also causes of death. In Zambia, HIV-infected patients attending a sexually transmitted disease clinic had a mortality of 4–6% in 18 months (Hira et al 1990), which was similar to the Rwandan figure.

TRADITIONAL MEDICINE AND HEALERS

There is an incomplete understanding of health-seeking behaviour in African nations because research has focused almost exclusively on 'traditional' and 'orthodox' medicine. Traditional and orthodox medicine systems may be used simultaneously by patients or might be used in sequence (Gelfand et al 1985, Ankrah 1991). This dual model does not consider self-treatment, traditional family and community medical knowledge, and various popular therapeutic systems (Cavender 1991). Relatives and carers play a consulting role for the sick, and they help define an illness and select the appropriate therapy. In Zimbabwe, for example, the Shona consider illness as having both normal and abnormal causes. Minor ailments are regarded as normal since they occur from time to time in the life of the individuals and disappear completely. Illnesses that linger too long or fail to respond to treatment become an abnormal illness, and are supernaturally based. They can be identified and treated only by traditional healers. In one study in Uganda, patients felt they could be cured only by traditional healers, not by orthodox medicine, and in Zambia it is believed by some that a woman must have sex with a relative almost immediately after her husband's death as part of a cleansing system for widows.

Medicinal blood-letting, ritual and medicinal scarification, group circumcision, genital tattooing and shaving of body hair are customs that may be potential modes of HIV transmission (Hrdy 1987), but it is not likely that traditional medicine contributes greatly as fresh razor blades are used by the traditional healers, not hollow instruments such as needles (Pela & Platt 1989). Traditional vaginal agents such as herbs or stones used for tightening or treatment of discharge may play some part in transmission of HIV due to their irritative and erosive effect on mucosal surfaces (Dallabetta et al 1990).

Traditional health care systems are important. In Zimbabwe in 1982, 68% of deliveries nationally were by traditional birth attendants and in 1988 in a study of 76 pregnant women, 28 were delivered by traditional birth attendants. The reason for pregnant women using traditional medicine was thought to be that the spiritual aspects of health were not catered for by orthodox health systems. In South Africa many people went to traditional healers for the treatment of their STDs. In Zimbabwe traditional healers including traditional midwives have formed an association called Zinatha. Its representatives are on the AIDS Control Programme Education Committee. Guidelines for healers' instruments have been prepared and patients are encouraged to take their own razor blade, as cutting the skin is a traditional healing practice.

CLINICAL MANIFESTATIONS

The disease pattern in HIV-positive patients in the developing world has its own particular characteristics (Quinn et al 1986). In one study of 299 seropositive clinically ill adults, 61% had diarrhoea, fever and weight loss; 28% had CDC $1VC_2$, the majority of these being tuberculosis (Brown 1990); and other studies show similar findings (Reeve 1989). There is a lack of data regarding clinical problems of women in the developing world. Most studies have not highlighted any gender differences.

Gynaecological problems

Gynaecological problems such as cervicitis, salpingitis, vaginitis, genital ulcers, genital warts and cervical dysplasia may be more frequent and severe and/or less responsive to treatment among women with HIV infection compared to women without HIV infection. There are few specific data on cervical changes in women living in the developing world, though from the developed world, data suggest that invasive cervical carcinoma appears to be more common among women with HIV infection (Carpenter et al 1991, Wofsy et al 1992). One study from Tanzania (ter Meulen et al 1992) observed no association between the prevalence of HIV and the frequency of cytological abnormalities or cancer. Refractory vaginal candidiasis is frequently seen among HIV-infected women (Rhoads et al 1987, Imam et al 1990, Carpenter et al 1991), but studies in the developing world have not been as extensive as those in the developed world. Oral antifungal agents are expensive and topical therapy with nystatin pessaries or local gentian violet is usually prescribed.

Gastrointestinal disease

In Zaire and Uganda chronic diarrhoea and severe weight loss is common, with an overall frequency of 30–80% (Serwadda et al 1985; Antony et al 1988). This syndrome is known locally as 'Slim' (Serwadda et al 1985). The diarrhoea may be intermittent with asymptomatic periods followed by diarrhoeal episodes. Infective causes are found in 30–80% depending on the extent of the investigations, but obviously in Africa there are limited resources for sophisticated investigation. *Cryptosporidium* was found in 10–21% and *Isospora* in 7% in studies from Zaire and Uganda (Henry et al 1986; Quinn et al 1986, Sewankambo et al 1987) and in other developing countries the figures have been as high as 40% and 15%, respectively (Pape et al 1989). There are some data to suggest that some cases of slim are due to disseminated tuberculosis.

Treatment in Africa is usually symptomatic and supportive as extensive investigation beyond microscopy and culture is not widely available. Helminth infestation is found to a comparable degree in both HIV-positive and HIV-negative persons although one study has shown that a large proportion of HIV-positive children with chronic diarrhoea had intestinal parasites which might have been responsible for their symptoms (Cegielski et al 1990).

Oral *Candida* is a sensitive clinical marker of immunosuppression (Kaslow et al 1987) and is common in African HIV patients (Tavitian et al 1986b). Extension into the oesophagus causing dysphagia often occurs and is usually diagnosed clinically. Topical therapy for oral disease helps but is sometimes unsatisfactory and oral long-term systemic agents are then given. Ketoconazole is not available in all countries and its cost, reports of resistant strains, and concern over its toxicity limit its use (Tavitian et al 1986a). Even fewer countries can afford the newer azole compounds such as fluconazole but gentian violet appears to be a cheap and effective anticandidal drug. In one study it was more useful than topical nystatin and short-course ketoconazole (Nyst et al 1990). Its use as first-line treatment in Africa for oral thrush will continue. Vaginal pessaries can be cut into pieces and sucked as a cheap alternative to lozenges.

Lung disease

Acute pneumococcal pneumonia is a common illness in Africa (Slack et al 1976) and appears to be on the increase because of its association with HIV. High rates of pneumococcal bacteraemia have been reported in patients with HIV (Gilks et al 1990a). Epidemiological data strongly suggest that acute bacterial pneumonia is an important cause of death in some high risk groups, even though acute bacterial pneumonia is not part of AIDS surveillance.

In, one cross-sectional survey of adults acutely admitted to hospital in Nairobi, pneumococcal and *Salmonella typhimurium* bacteraemia accounted for almost one-quarter of HIV-related acute medical admissions and the mortality from these episodes of bacteraemia was higher in the HIV-positive patients (Gilks et al 1990b). The *S. typhimurium* bacteraemia was often resistant to therapy with resulting prolonged bacteraemia and recurrence.

It is debatable whether *Pneumocystis carinii* pneumonia (PCP) is an important opportunistic infection in Africa, although it has been well documented in Africans with AIDS living in Europe (Clumeck et al 1984, Biggar et al 1984). Before AIDS, PCP was occasionally found in Africa in immunosuppressed patients in Nigeria (Abioye 1967), the Congo (Thijs & Janssen 1963) and the Republic of South Africa (Pepler 1958). Although thought to be uncommon (Serwadda et al 1989), PCP has occurred in HIV-positive patients with pneumonia in several African countries (Batungwanayo et al 1990; Nelson et al 1990); 22% of patients with HIV and clinical or radiological pneumonia were found to have PCP in one study from Zimbabwe (McLeod et al 1989), the clinical picture being similar to that seen in patients in the developed world. In that study the numbers studied were small and highly selected, and many of the diagnoses were made on cytology and may have overemphasized the importance of PCP.

In Zambia, 4/27 AIDS patients with clinical pneumonia of unknown aetiology were found to have probable trophozoites of *Pneumocystis*, although no cysts were present in their sputum and no definite diagnosis of PCP was made (Elvin et al 1989). The reason for the global variation in prevalence of PCP may be due to lack of diagnostic skills, facilities and technique (such as induced sputum or 'Diff-quick' staining). Genetic or environmental differences remain speculative. It may well be, and there are some supportive data, that other infections, especially TB, infect HIV patients earlier in their immune suppression and that patients die from these initial or subsequent infections before their CD4 count drops below 200 cells/mm^3 placing them at high risk of developing PCP (Elvin et al 1989).

Primary prophylaxis is not indicated for patients from countries in which PCP is rarely found. It would be difficult to initiate even if PCP were a problem, due to lack of CD4 monitoring. Treatment for PCP in Africa is usually with high-dose oral cotrimoxazole due to the lack of availability and the cost of intravenous preparations. Prophylaxis with cotrimoxazole or dapsone is encouraged after a first episode of PCP, but pentamidine, whether nebulized or parenteral, is expensive and not often used.

Tuberculosis

Between 25 and 81% of hospitalized patients with tuberculosis in Africa are HIV-positive (Colebunders et al 1989, Elliott et al 1990, Batungwanayo et al 1992). Differences in these rates may be due to selection of rural or urban populations, the amount of suspected or proved TB reported (Pape & Johnson 1988, Harries 1990), and difference in national HIV sero-prevalence. There is a lack of information existing about the relationship between TB and HIV infection in women, but in Zaire, HIV-positive women have a 26-fold increased risk of developing tuberculosis compared with seronegative women after a medium follow-up of 32 months (Braun et al 1991). HIV co-infection has led to a decreased usefulness of several important methods of tuberculosis diagnosis. The chest X-ray can be abnormal with atypical or non-specific changes (Barnes et al 1991). Persons with HIV and TB may have false-negative tuberculin tests due to anergy, and HIV-infected patients with active TB are less likely to be sputum smear-positive than HIV-negative patients (Louie et al 1986, Colebunders et al 1989, Elliott et al 1990). Sputum cultures are rarely performed in the developing world and so surveillance of the epidemic and of the emergence of any drug-resistance can be problematic. Drug reactions to thiacetazone, a commonly used drug in the developing world, are frequent and can be fatal in HIV-positive patients (Nunn et al 1991, Pozniak et al 1992a), but alternative therapies are more costly. In countries such as Uganda, where there is a 2% annual risk of infection of tuberculosis and a 20% HIV prevalence, the incidence of active TB may rise 12-fold by the year 2000 to 4218 per 100 000 (Schulzer et al 1992). As tuberculosis will infect both HIV-positive and HIV-negative women, this will have a profound impact on family life and economy and will add to the developing world's problems (Anderson et al 1988, Murray 1990). With the spread of HIV into Asia, where 25% of the world's total TB cases occur (Nsengiyumva 1982), the cursed duet of TB and HIV will have a disastrous impact on the tuberculosis control programme (GPA/WHO 1990). The use of primary prophylaxis is being investigated but may be impractical.

BCG continues to be given at birth, bearing in mind the WHO guidelines as regards HIV status.

Tumours

The new aggressive form of Kaposi's sarcoma was first recognized in Zambia (Bayley et al 1985) and it accounts for about 90% of all the Kaposi's sarcoma seen in Africa. It is uncommon in women and the reason for this is unknown. Treatment with radiotherapy and cytotoxic drugs can be given only at large centres. Patients often present late, commonly with lung involvement (Pozniak et al 1992b), and although treatment may relieve symptoms it has little effect on survival.

Skin disease

The incidence of herpes zoster in HIV-positive patients is seven times greater than that of the general population (Friedman-Kien et al 1986), and the incidence of HIV seropositivity in members of high risk groups who present with zoster is 92% (Colebunders et al 1988b, Van De Perre et al 1988). The positive predictive value of a history of shingles for HIV positivity is 90% and the progression by such HIV-positive individuals to AIDS is at the rate of about 1% per month after presentation (Melbye et al 1987). Zoster often occurs as the first manifestation of progressive HIV infection, preceding *Candida* and oral leukoplakia by an average of 1.5 years (Colebunders et al 1988a). The clinical presentation may be typical with radicular pain or dermatomal eruption, but involvement of two or more dermatomes and dissemination are common, morbidity and mortality are increased and clinical relapse frequent. Spontaneous healing occurs, but the rate of post-herpetic neuralgia is undefined in Africa. Treatment with acyclovir, especially high-dose intravenous therapy (Hoppenjans et al 1990), is too costly and impracticable for Africa. Lesions are often treated with local gentian violet and analgesia given for the acute stage.

One of the most specific skin diseases in Africans is an itchy widespread nodular prurigo (Liautaud et al 1989) which occurred in 21% of HIV-infected patients in Zaire (Piot et al 1984). It has been suggested that the skin lesions are a peculiar reaction pattern to insect bites in immunosuppressed persons (Sundharam 1990), but its actual aetiology is not known and treatment is symptomatic.

Neurological disease

HIV and neurological morbidity and mortality is little documented in the developing world. Early case reports of Africans treated in Europe described cerebral toxoplasmosis or cryptococcal meningitis (Van De Perre et al 1984; Clumeck et al 1984). In one study from Tanzania, 10.5% of 200 patients with HIV had an obvious focal neurological disorder such as cranial nerve palsies, hemiparesis or paraparesis; 72% of the rest had less obvious neurological disorders including dementia (54%), retinopathy (23%), areflexia (21%), pyramidal tract signs (19%) and tremor and coordination impairment (Howlett et al 1989). Guillain-Barré syndrome (Thornton et al 1989), facial palsy (Belec et al 1989), painful peripheral neuropathy and psychiatric syndromes appear to be increasing in Africa and many patients with severe immunosuppression appear demented.

Meningeal infection with *Cryptococcus* is common in some parts of Africa and in one study occurred in 8% of HIV-positive patients admitted with a fever (Bogaerts et al 1990). There was a sevenfold increase in cryptococcal meningitis in 1978–84 compared with 1973–77 in Rwanda (Vandepitte et al 1983), due to the interaction with HIV. Unfortunately for clinicians working in low technology areas the diagnosis can be difficult as signs and symptoms of meningitis may be lacking and cerebrospinal fluid (CSF) changes less marked in HIV-positive patients (Masci 1987). Cryptococcal antigens in the blood and CSF are useful investigations but expensive and technology-dependent; however, India ink staining of CSF is simple, needing only a microscope. Treatment requires intravenous amphotericin and/or oral fluconazole. Some African countries cannot treat cryptococcal infection as it is too costly and there can be difficulty in drug availability.

Toxoplasmosis is thought to be commoner in patients from Africa than in those from Europe or the USA (Biggar 1986), but the true incidence of CNS toxoplasmosis causing focal abscess or diffuse meningoencephalitis is not known; studies

in West Africa show that it is common at post-mortem in patients with neurological disease (Lucas et al 1992). Clinicians face a diagnostic dilemma, as neurological disease can be confused by the common occurrence of pyogenic abscess, tuberculous meningitis and meningovascular syphilis, which produce similar clinical syndromes to toxoplasmosis.

Sexually transmitted diseases – genital ulceration

Sexually transmitted diseases are a major health problem in parts of Africa and are many times more common than in Europe. Genital disease is a major risk factor for HIV transmission (Simonsen et al 1988, Greenblatt et al 1988) and one suggestion to curb HIV is to control STD, especially ulcerative disease (Pepin et al 1989, Kirby et al 1991, Plummer et al 1991). In light of this, some countries such as Zimbabwe, which reported one million STDs in 1989 (Annual Report 1989), now have national STD programmes linked to the HIV prevention strategy. Prompt treatment and follow-up can be supervised at a clinic or outstation level using algorithms and attendances reinforced with positive sexual and reproductive health messages.

Against the background of high rates of STD, HIV transmission occurs, and in most cases it is the male partner who introduces HIV infection to the family unit. In one study, 40% of HIV-negative men have reported a STD in the previous year, and 67% have paid money for sex. These men could not be characterized as being low risk (Bassett et al 1990).

Chancroid ulceration more often persists in the HIV-positive person in spite of standard antibiotic treatment (Cameron et al 1988), and this lack of responsiveness has been used as a predictor for HIV status. Chancroid is the primary cause of genital ulcer (85%) in STD clinic attendants and prostitutes in Nairobi (Nsanze et al 1981). Two cross-sectional studies have shown a correlation between genital ulcer or a history of genital ulcer and HIV seropositivity (Greenblatt et al 1988; Simonsen et al 1988). In a prospective study in 293 HIV-negative men who had sexual contact with prostitutes, genital ulcer disease was associated with a sevenfold increased risk of subsequent

HIV seroconversion when compared with those that developed a urethral discharge (Cameron et al 1988). In Nairobi, prostitutes' HIV seroconversion was associated with antecedent occurrence of genital ulcer, even when sexual activity and condom use were taken into account (Plummer et at 1988). Transmission of HIV to wives of HIV-positive men is much more likely if the man has a history of genital ulcer (Latif et al 1989).

Although a positive Treponema pallidum haemagluttination test result is associated with HIV positivity in Nairobi prostitutes (Kreiss et al 1986), the same was not found in Kinshasa (Mann et al 1988a; Kivuvu et al 1990) or in Nairobi male STD attenders (Simonsen et al 1988), and the association between syphilis and HIV is not unequivocally established. In pregnant women in Nairobi a parallel rise in syphilis seroreactivity was noted in an HIV-infected cohort (Temmerman et al 1992), which would be compatible with an increased susceptibility to HIV-1 among individuals with syphilis, or increased susceptibility to syphilis acquisition among HIV-1-seropositive individuals, although both could be markers of common exposure.

Lack of male circumcision is associated with HIV infection (Greenblatt et al 1988; Simonsen et al 1988; Bongaarts et al 1989; Cameron et al 1989). An increase in balanitis (Parker et al 1983), a large surface area for contact with HIV, increased trauma and viral inoculum trapping have all been suggested to explain this fact (Moss & Kreiss 1990). The rates of circumcision vary in Africa but there is an inverse correlation with HIV sero-prevalence (Cameron et al 1988).

TREATMENT AND COST ISSUES

Antiviral therapy is little used in the developing world. There are some units in Bangkok and in Zaire where azidothymidine (AZT, zidovudine) is given to selected patients, and in Bangkok there is limited availability of 2',3'–dideoxyinosine (ddI, didanosine). These drugs, either separately or in combination, are far too expensive for most health care budgets to afford, and the laboratory monitoring required for initiation and follow-up of therapy is just not available to most people living in these areas. The annual cost of AZT is estimated

at $1200 US per annum and $2000 US per annum for ddI (Panos Dossier 1992). Government health allocations and expenditure for AIDS care ranges from 0.5% in Botswana to 21.4% in Rwanda (Berkley 1992). Total treatment cost per patient with AIDS in Africa has been estimated to be about $150 US in the public system and $1700 US in the private system. In contrast, per capita expenditure for health care averages $15 US (Panos Dossier 1992). Supplies of drugs, such as essential antibiotics etc., can be erratic, and a change to what may appear rational prescribing in the developed world may be irrational in the developing world because of cost and availability. Patients in the developing world rarely have opportunities to be involved in research of novel compounds, but vaccine trials are about to start in Africa and debate over the ethics of such trials continues.

Many countries have been tackling the HIV epidemic from the 'grass-roots'. In Uganda, Taso provides a counselling, education and prevention service. There is a home-based care programme for people with HIV infection centred around Chikankata in Zambia. In Zimbabwe there is a family AIDS counselling trust and other organizations concerned with home care (Report 1990). Almost all Southern African countries have developed a non-governmental organization network for AIDS support. There has been a move for more direct local leadership in combating HIV infection with the use of elders, and targeted AIDS education campaigns can be run locally with distribution of condoms and education in schools.

PREVENTION AND WOMEN'S HEALTH

Health programmes in the developing world have become over-burdened, but HIV is not just a medical or health problem. Compounding the problem are poverty and a deteriorating social situation and economic structure (Figure 8.1). Men and women must share the burden of HIV and responsibility for its prevention, and need to find ways to negotiate about safer sexual behaviour. Knowledge alone of how HIV is transmitted, however, does not necessarily change behaviour. It is important that women are active participants in the development of HIV prevention strategy. In

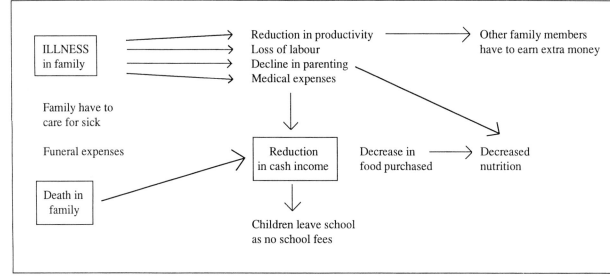

Figure 8.1   Impact of HIV/AIDS on the developing world family economy

order to accomplish this there should be a better understanding of how women perceive and respond to the HIV pandemic, and they should be supported so they can be as equals with their male partners and plan good sexual and reproductive health. This strategy may lead to changes in the way that women are perceived and act in a particular society. In order to cope with these changes there must be strengthening of women's established networks in and beyond their community. Education focused around local communities which are supported nationally and internationally should not only be health-orientated, but should also enable people to cope with changes in household structure, labour shortage and economic problems. In order to preserve life in the developing world, women must be allowed to play an active role.

REFERENCES

Abdool-Karim Q, Abdool-Karim S S, Nknomokazi J 1991 Sexual behaviour and knowledge of AIDS among urban black mothers. Implications for AIDS Intervention programmes. S Afr Med J 80(7):340–343

Abioye A A 1967 Interstitial plasma cell pneumonia (Pneumocystis carinii) in Ibadan. W Afr Med J 16:130

Allen S, Lindan C, Seriufilira A, Van de Perre P, Rundle A C, Nsengumuremyi F, Carael M, Schwalbe J, Hulley S 1991 Human immunodeficiency virus infection in urban Rwanda. Demographic and behavioural correlates in a representative sample of childbearing women. JAMA 266(12):1657–1663

Anderson R M, May R M, McLean A R 1988 Possible demographic consequences of AIDS in developing countries. Nature (London) 332:228–233

Ankrah E M 1991 AIDS and the Social Side of Health Soc Sci Med 32(9):967–980

Annual report 1989 Secretary for Health 1989. Government Printers, Harare, Zimbabwe

Antony M A, Brandt L J, Klein R S et al 1988 Infectious diarrhoea in patients with AIDS. Digest Dis Sci 33:1141–1146

Barnes P, Bloch A, Davidson P, Snider D 1991 Tuberculosis in patients with human immunodeficiency virus infection. N Eng J Med 324:1644–1650

Bassett M T et al 1990 HIV infection in urban men in Zimbabwe. Sixth International Conference on AIDS, San Francisco. Abstr No Th C 581

Bassett M T, Mhloyi M 1991 Women and AIDS in Zimbabwe: the making of an epidemic. Int J Health Serv 21:143–156

Batungwanayo J, Taelman H, Bogaerts J et al 1990 Pneumopathies et infection a VIH a Kigali, Rwanda, interet du lavage bronchoalveolaire (LBA) et de la biopsie transbronchique (BTB) pour le diagnostic etiologique. Fifth International Conference on AIDS in Zaire, Africa. Abstr FOD3

Batungwanayo J, Taelman H, Dhote R, Bogaerts J, Allen S, van de Perre P 1992 Pulmonary tuberculosis in Kagali, Rwanda – impact of human immunodeficiency virus infection on clinical and radiographic presentation. Am Rev Res Dis 146:53–56

Bayley A C, Downing R C, Cheingsong-Popov R, Tedder R, Dalgleish A C, Weiss R A 1985 HTLV-III distinguishes atypical Kaposi's sarcoma in Africa. Lancet 1:359–361

Belec L, Ghjerardi R, Georges A J et al 1989 Peripheral facial paralysis and HIV infection: report of our African cases and review of the literature. J Neurol 236:411–414

Berkley S 1992 HIV in Africa: what is the future? Ann Intern Med 16:339–341

Berkley S, Naamara W, Okware S, Downing R, Konde-Lule J, Wawer M, Musagaara M, Musgrave S 1990 AIDS and

HIV infection in Uganda – are more women infected than men? AIDS 4(12):1237–1242

Biggar R J 1986 The AIDS problem in Africa. Lancet 1: 79–82

Biggar R J, Bouvet E, Ebbesen P et al 1984 Epidemiology of AIDS in Europe. Eur J Cancer Clin Oncol 20:165–167

Bogaerts J, Taelman H, Abdel Aziz M et al 1990 Cryptococcose et sida au Rwanda, etude epidemiologique. Fifth International Conference on AIDS in Africa, Zaire. Abstr FOD2

Bongaarts J, Frank O, Lesthaeghe R 1984 The proximate determinants of fertility in sub-Saharan Africa. Pop Devel Rev 3:511–537

Bongaarts J, Reining P, Way P et al 1989 The relationship between male circumcision and HIV infection in African populations. AIDS 3(6):373–377

Braun M M, Badi N, Ryder R W et al 1991 A retrospective cohort study of the risk of tuberculosis among women of childbearing age with HIV infection in Zaire. Am Rev Resp Dis 143(3):501–504

Brown R C 1990 Seroprevalence and clinical manifestations of HIV-1 infection in Kananga, Zaire. AIDS 4(12):1267–1269

Cameron D W, Plummer F A, D'Costa L J et al 1988 Prediction of HIV infection by treatment failure for chancroid, a genital ulcer disease. Fourth International Conference on AIDS, Stockholm, Sweden. Abstr 7637

Cameron D W, Simonsen J N, D'Costa L J et al 1989 Female to male transmission of human immunodeficiency virus type 1: risk factors for seroconversion in men. Lancet 19(2):403–407

Carovano K 1991 More than mothers and whores: redefining the AIDS prevention needs of women. Int J Health Serv 21(1):131–142

Carpenter C J, Mayer K H, Stein M D, Liebman B D, Fisher A, Fiore T C 1991 Human immunodeficiency virus infection in North American women: experience with 200 cases and a review of the literature. Medicine 70: 307–325

Cavender A P 1991 Traditional medicine and an inclusive model of health seeking behaviour in Zimbabwe. Central Afr J Med 37(11): 362–369

Cegielski P, Msengi Abel, Dukes C et al 1990 Intestinal parasites associated with HIV infection in children with chronic diarrhoea in Dar we Salaam. Fifth International Conference on AIDS in Zaire, Africa. Abstr W P E 4

Chin J 1990 Current and future dimensions of the HIV/AIDS pandemic in women and children. Lancet 336(8790): 221–224

Chin J 1992 Present and future dimensions of the HIV/AIDS pandemic. In: Giraldo G (ed) Science challenging AIDS. Karger, Basel, p 33–50

Christakis N A, Fox F C 1992 Informed consent in Africa. N Engl J Med 327: 1101–1102

Clumeck N, Jonnet J, Taelman H et al 1984 Acquired immunodeficiency syndrome in African patients. N Engl J Med 310: 492–497

Clumeck N, Robert-Guroff M, Van de Perre P et al 1985 Seroepidemiological studies of HTLV-III antibody prevalence among selected groups of heterosexual Africans. JAMA 254: 2599–2602

Colebunders R L, Izaley L, Musampu M et al 1988a BCG vaccine abscesses are unrelated to HIV infection. JAMA 15; 259(3): 352

Colebunders R, Mann J M, Francis II et al 1988b Herpes zoster in African patients: a clinical predictor of human

immunodeficiency virus infections. J Infect Dis 157(2): 314–318

Colebunders R L, Ryder R W, Nzilambi N et al 1989 HIV infection in patients with tuberculosis in Kinshasa, Zaire. Am Rev Resp Dis 139(5): 1082–1085

Conlon C P 1988 Clinical aspects of HIV infection in developing countries. Br Med Bull 44: 101–114

Dallabetta G, Miotti P, Chphangwi J, Kiomba G, Saah A 1990 Vaginal agents as risk factor for acquisition of HIV-1. Fifth International Conference on AIDS in Zaire, Africa. Abstr FOA2

Day S 1989 Prostitute women and AIDS: anthropology. AIDS 2(6): 421–428

De Cock K M, Barrere B, Daiby L et al 1990 AIDS – the leading cause of adult death in the West African City of Abidjan, Ivory Coast, Science 17; 249(4970): 793–796

Dolmans W M V, van Loon A M, van den Akker R et al 1989 Prevalence of HIV-1 antibody among groups of patients and healthy subjects from a rural and urban population in Mwanza region, Tanzania. AIDS 3(5): 297–299

Elliott A M, Luo N, Tembo C et al 1990 Impact of HIV on tuberculosis in Zambia: a cross sectional study. Br Med J 301: 412–415

Elvin K M, Lumbwe C M, Kuo N P, Bjorkman K A, Kallenius G, Linder E 1989 Pneumocystis carinii is not a major cause of pneumonia in HIV infected patients in Lusaka, Zambia. Trans R Soc Trop Med Hygiene 83: 553–555

Friedland G H, Klein R S 1987 Transmission of the human immunodeficiency virus. N Engl J Med 317: 1125–1134

Friedman-Kien A E, Lafleur F L, Gendler E et al 1986 Herpes zoster: a possible early clinical sign for development of acquired immunodeficiency syndrome in high risk individuals. J Am Acad Dermatol 14: 1023–1028

Gelfand M 1979 Growing up in Shona society. Mambo Press, Harare, Zimbabwe, p 19

Gelfand M, Mavi S, Drummond R, Ndemera B 1985 The traditional medical practitioner in Zimbabwe. Mambo Press, Gweru

Gilks C F, Brindle R J, Otieno L S et al 1990a Life-threatening bacteraemia in HIV-1 seropositive adults admitted to hospital in Nairobi, Kenya. Lancet 1; 36(8714): 545–549

Gilks C F, Brindler R J, Otieno L S et al 1990b Extrapulmonary and disseminated tuberculosis in HIV-1 seropositive patients presenting to the acute medical services in Nairobi. AIDS 4: 981–986

Goldberg H I, Lee N C, Oberle M W, Peterson H B 1989 Knowledge about condoms and their use in less developed countries during a period of rising AIDS prevalence. Bull WHO 67(1): 85–91

GPA/WHO 1990 Current and future dimensions of the HIV/AIDS pandemic: a capsule summary. WHO 9

Greenblatt R M Lukehart S A, Plummer F A et al 1988 Genital ulceration as a risk factor for human immunodeficiency virus infection AIDS 2(1): 47–50

Guyer J I 1981 Household and community in African studies. Afr Studies Rev 24: 87–137

Harries A D 1990 Tuberculosis and human immunodeficiency virus infection in developing countries. Lancet 17; 335(8686): 387–390

Henry M C, De Clercq D, Lokombe B et al 1986 Parasitological observations of chronic diarrhoea in suspected AIDS adult patients in Kinshasa (Zaire). Trans R Soc Trop Med Hygiene 80:309–310

Hira S K, Ngandu N, Wadhawan D, Nkowne B, Baboo K S,

Macuacua R et al 1990 Clinical and epidemiological features of HIV infection at a referral clinic in Zambia. J Acq Immune Defic Synd 3(1): 87–91

Holmes K K, Kreiss J 1988 Heterosexual transmission of human immunodeficiency virus: overview of a neglected aspect of the AIDS epidemic. J Acq Immune Defic Synd 1: 602–610

Hoppenjans W B, Bibler M R, Orme R L, Solinger A M 1990 Prolonged cutaneous herpes zoster in acquired immunodeficiency syndrome. Arch Dermatol 126(8): 1048–1050

Howlett W P, Nkya W M, Mmuni K A, Missalek W R 1989 Neurological disorders in AIDS and HIV disease in the northern zone of Tanzania. AIDS 3(5): 289–296

Hrdy D B 1987 Cultural practices contributing to the transmission of human immunodeficiency virus in Africa. Rev Infect Dis 9: 1109–1119

Imam N, Carpenter C C, Mayer K H, Fisher A, Stein M, Danforth S B 1990 Hierarchial pattern of mucosal candida infections in HIV seropositive women. Am J Med 89(2): 142–146

Jessamine P G, Plummer F A, Ndinya-Achola J O, Wainberg M A, Wamola I, D'Costa L J, Cameron D W, Simonsen J N, Plourde P, Ronald A R 1990 Human immunodeficiency virus, genital ulcers and the male foreskin: synergism in HIV-1 transmission. Scand J Infect Dis Suppl 69: 181–186

Jochelson K, Mothibeli M, Leger J-P 1991 Human immunodeficiency virus and migrant labour in South Africa. Int J Health Serv 21(1): 157–173

Kaslow R A, Phair J P, Friedman H B et al 1987 Infection with human immunodeficiency virus: clinical manifestations and their relationship to immune deficiency. Ann Intern Med 107: 373–380

Kayembe K, Mann J M, Francis H et al 1986 Prevalence des anticorps anti-HIV chez les patients non atteints de SIDA ou de syndrome associe au SIDA a Kinshasa, Zaire. Ann Soc Belg Med Trop 66: 343–347

Kirby P K, Munyao T, Kreiss J, Holmes K K 1991 The challenge of limiting the spread of human immunodeficiency virus by controlling other sexually transmitted diseases. Arch Dermatol 127(2): 237–242

Kivuvu M, Malele B, Nzila N et al 1990 Syphilis among HIV + and HIV − prostitutes in Kinshasa: prevalence and serologic response to treatment. Fifth International Conference on AIDS in Zaire, Africa. Abstr T P C 7

Kreiss J K, Koech D, Plummer F A et al 1986 AIDS virus infection in Nairobi prostitutes: spread of the epidemic to East Africa. N Engl J Med 314:414–118

Lallemant M, Lallemant-Le Coeur S, Cheynier D, Nzingoula S, Jourdain G, Sinet M, Dazza M C, Larouze B 1992 Characteristics associated with HIV-1 infection in pregnant women in Brazzaville, Congo. J Acq Immune Defic Synd 5(3): 279–285

Larson A 1989 Social context of human immunodeficiency virus transmission in Africa: historical and cultural bases of East and Central African sexual relations. Rev Infec Dis 2(5): 716–731

Latif A S, Katzenstein D A, Bassett M T et al 1989 Genital ulcers and transmission of HIV among couples in Zimbabwe. AIDS 3: 519–523

Le Page P, Van de Perre P, Nsengumuremyi F et al 1986 Bacteraemia as predictor of HIV infection in African children. Acta Paediatr Scand 78: 763–766

Liautaud B, Pape J W, DeHovitz J A et al 1989 Pruritic skin lesions. A common initial presentation of acquired

immunodeficiency syndrome. Arch Dermatol 125(5): 629–632

Lindan C, Allen S, Carael M, Nsengumuremyi F, Van de Perre P, Serufilira A, Tice J, Black D, Coates T, Hulley S 1991 Knowledge, attitudes and perceived risk of AIDS among urban Rwandan women: relationship to HIV infection and behaviour change. AIDS 5(8): 993–1002

Lindan C P, Allen S, Serufilira A, Lifson A, Van de Perre P, Chen-Rundle A, Batungwanayo J, Nsengumuremyi F, Bogaerts J, Hulley S 1992 Predictors of mortality among HIV infected women in Kigali, Rwanda. Ann Intern Med 116: 320–328

Louie E, Rice L B, Holzman R S 1986 Tuberculosis and the human immunodeficiency syndrome. Chest 90: 542–545

Lucas S, Hounnou A, Beaumel A, Diomande M, Peacock C, Kadio A, Honde M, De Cock K 1992 The pathology of adult HIV infection in Abidjan, Cote d'Ivoire. VII International Conference on AIDS/III STD World Congress, Amsterdam, Abstr POB 375

McLeod D T, Neill P, Robertson V J et al 1989 Pulmonary diseases in patients infected with the human immunodeficiency virus in Zimbabwe, Central Africa. Trans R Soc Trop Med Hygiene 83: 694–697

Mann J M, Francis H, Quinn T, Asila P K, Bosenge N, Nzilambi N, Bila J K, Tamfum M, Ruti K, Piot P et al 1986a Surveillance for AIDS in a Central African City. Kinshasa, Zaire. JAMA 255(23):3255–3259

Mann J M, Francis H, Davachi F et al 1986b Risk factors for human immunodeficiency virus seropositivity among children 1–24 months old in Kinshasa, Zaire. Lancet 2: 654–656

Mann J M, Nzila N, Piot P et al 1988a HIV infection and associated risk factors in female prostitutes in Kinshasa, Zaire. AIDS 2:249–254

Mann J M, Chin J, Piot P, Quinn T 1988b The international epidemiology of AIDS. Sci Am 60–69

Mahomed K, Kasule J, Makuyana D, Moyo S, Mbidzo M, Tswana S 1991 Seroprevalence of HIV infection amongst antenatal women in greater Harare, Zimbabwe. Centr Afr J Med 37:322–325

Manoka A, Nzila N, Tuliza M et al 1990 Non ulcerative sexually transmitted diseases (STD) as risk factors for HIV infection. Fifth International Conference on AIDS in Zaire, Africa, Abstr F O A 1

Masci J R 1987 Clinical aspects of cryptococcosis in AIDS. In: Wormser G P, Stahl R E, Bottone E J (eds) AIDS and other manifestations of HIV infection. Noyes Publications, New Jersey. p 683–697

Mbivzo M, Adamchak D J 1989 Condom use and acceptance: a survey of male Zimbabweans. Centr Afr J Med 35:519–558

Melbye M, Njelesani E K, Bayley A, Mukelabai K, Manuwele J K, Bowa F J, Clayden S A, Levin A, Dalttner W A, Weiss R A et al 1986 Evidence for heterosexual transmission and clinical manifestations of human immunodeficiency virus infection and related conditions in Lusaka, Zambia. Lancet 2(8516): 1113–1115

Melbye M, Goedert J J, Grossman R J, Eyster M E, Biggar R J 1987 Risk of AIDS after Herpes zoster. Lancet 1: 728–731

Miotti P G, Dallabetta G, Ndovi E, Liomba G, Saah A J, Chiphangwi J 1990 HIV-1 and pregnant women: associated factors, prevalence, estimate of incidence and role in fetal wastage in Central Africa. AIDS 4(8):733–736

Molnos I 1973 A cultural source material for population

planning in East Africa. Beliefs and practices. Institute of African Studies, University of Nairobi. East African Publishing House, Nairobi, vol 3

Moss G B, Kreiss K 1990 The interrelationship between human immunodeficiency virus infections and other sexually transmitted diseases. Med Clin N Am 74(6):1647–1657

Murray C J L 1990 World tuberculosis burden. Lancet 28; 335(8696):1043–1044

Nelson A, Okonda L, Tuur S et al 1990 Pulmonary pathology of HIV infection in Zairians. Fifth International Conference on AIDS in Zaire, Africa. Abstr F P B 29

N'Galy B, Ryder R W 1988 Epidemiology of HIV Infection in Africa. J Acq Immune Defic Synd 1(6):551–558

Nicoll A, Killewo J Z, Mgone C 1990 HIV and infant feeding practices: epidemiological implications for sub-Saharan African countries. AIDS 4(7):661–665

Nkowane B M 1990 Prevalence and incidence of HIV in Africa: a review of data published in AIDS 1990. AIDS 5(Suppl 1): S7–15

Nsanze H, Fast M V, C'Cost L J et al 1981 Genital ulcers in Kenya: clinical and laboratory study. Br J Vener Dis 57:378–381

Nsengiyumva J M 1982 Tuberculose In: Meheus A, Butera S, Eylenbosch W, Gatera G, Kivits M, Musafili I(eds) Sante et maladies au Rwanda. Administration de la cooperation au development, Bruxelles p 238–259

Nsubuga P, Mugerwa R, Nsibambi J et al 1990 The association of genital ulcer disease and HIV infection at dermatology-STD clinic in Uganda. J Acq Immune Defic Synd 3(10):1002–1005

Nunn P, Kibuga D, Gathua S et al 1991 Cutaneous hypersensitivity reactions due to thiacetazone in HIV-1 seropositive patients treated for tuberculosis. Lancet 16; 37:(8742) 627–630

Nyst M, Lusakumunu K, Kapita B, Musongela L, Perriens J 1990. Comparative study of gentian violet, ketoconazole and nystatine to treat oral and oesophagial candidiasis in AIDS patients. Fifth International Conference on AIDS in Zaire, Africa. Abstr T P B 5

Nzila N, Laga M, Thiam M A et al 1991 HIV and other sexually transmitted diseases among female prostitutes in Kinshasa. AIDS 5(6):715–721

Odehouri K, De Cock K M, Krebs J W, Moreau J, Rayfield M, McCormick J B, Schoochetman G, Bretton R, Bretton G, Quattara D et al, 1989 HIV-1 and HIV-2 infection associated with AIDS in Abidjan, Cote d'Ivoire. AIDS 3(8):509–512

Oxtoby M J 1988 Human immunodeficiency virus and other viruses in human milk: placing the issues in broader perspective. Paediatr Infect Dis J 7:825–835

Padian N S 1987 Heterosexual transmission of acquired immunodeficiency syndrome: international perspectives and national projections. Rev Infect Dis 9:947–960

Page H J, Lesthaeghe R(eds) 1981 Child spacing in tropical Africa: traditions and change. Academic Press, London

Panos Dossier 1992 The hidden cost of AIDS. The challenge of HIV to development. The Panos Institute London. The Bath Press, Great Britain

Panos Institute 1990 Women and children at last? World AIDS 1(7):4–5

Pape J W, Johnson W D 1988 Epidemiology in the Caribbean. Bailliere's Clin Trop Med Comm Dis 3:31–42

Pape J W, Verdier R I, Johnson W D 1989 Treatment and prophylaxis of isospira belli infection in patients with the

acquired immunodeficiency syndrome. N Engl J Med 320(16):1044–1047

Parker S W, Stewart A G, Wren M N et al 1983 Circumcision and sexually transmissible disease. Med J Austr 2:288–290

Pela A O, Platt J J 1989 AIDS in Africa: emerging trends. Soc Sci Med 28(1):1–8

Pepin J, Plummer F A, Brunham R C, Piot P, Cameron D W, Ronald A R 1989 The interaction of HIV infection and other sexually transmitted diseases: an opportunity for intervention. AIDS 3(1):3–9

Pepler W J 1958 Pneumocystis Pneumonia. S Afr Med J 32:1003

Piot P, Carael M 1988 Epidemiological and sociological aspects of HIV infection in developing countries. Br Med Bull 44:68–88

Piot P, Quinn T C, Taelman H et al 1984 Acquired immunodeficiency syndrome in heterosexual population in Zaire. Lancet 2:65–69

Piot P, Plummer F A, Rey M A et al 1987 Retrospective epidemiology of HIV infection in Nairobi populations. J Infect Dis 155:1108–1112

Plummer F A, Cameron D W, Simonsen N et al 1988 Cofactors in male to female transmission of HIV. In: Programme and Abstracts of the Fourth International Conference on AIDS, Stockholm, Sweden. Abstr 4554

Plummer F A, Simonsen J N, Cameron D W et al 1991 Cofactors in male–female sexual transmission of human immunodeficiency virus type 1. J Infect Dis 163(2): 233–239

Pozniak A L, MacLeod G, Mahari M, Legg W, Weinberg J 1992a The influence of HIV status on single and multiple drug reactions to antituberculous therapy in Africa. AIDS 6:809–814

Pozniak A L, Latif A S, Neill P, Houston S, Chen K, Robertson V 1992b Pulmonary Kaposis's sarcoma in Africa. Thorax 47(9): 730–733

Preble E A 1990 Impact of HIV/AIDS on African children. Soc Sci Med 31(6): 671–680

Quinn T C, Mann J M, Curran J W, Piot P 1986 AIDS in Africa: an epidemiologic paradigm. Science 234(4779): 955–963

Ramalingaswami V 1990 Into inequity born: the state of health of the women in South Asia. Sci Public Affairs 6: 67–76

Ramalingaswami V 1992 The implications of AIDS in developing countries. In: Giraldo G (ed) Science Challenging AIDS. Karger, Basel, p 24–32

Reeve P A 1989 HIV infection in patients admitted to a general hospital in Malawi. Br Med J 298: 1567–1568

Report of the Southern African non-governmental organizations' conference on AIDS 1990 Harare, Zimbabwe

Rhoads J L, Wright C, Redfield R R, Burke D S 1987 Chronic vaginal candidiasis in women with human immunodeficiency virus. JAMA 257: 3105–3107

Riddell R 1982 Report of the commission of inquiry into incomes, price and conditions of service. Government of Zimbabwe, Harare

Ryder R W, Ndilu M, Hassig S E et al 1990 Heterosexual transmission of HIV-1 among employees and their spouses at two large businesses in Zaire. AIDS 4: 725–732

Ryder R W, Batter V L, Nsuami M, Badi N, Mundele L, Matela B, Utshudi M, Heyward W L 1991 Fertility rates in 238 HIV-1 seropositive women in Zaire followed for three years post-partum. AIDS 5(12): 1521–1527

Savarit D, De Cock K M, Schutz R, Konate S, Lackritz E,

Bondurand A 1992 Risk of HIV infection from transfusion with blood negative for HIV antibody in a west African city. Br Med J 305: 498–500

Schrijvers D, Delaporte E, Peeters M, Dupont A, Meheus A 1991 Seroprevalence of retroviral infection in women with different fertility statuses in Gabon, western equatorial Africa. J Acq Immune Defic Synd 4(5): 468–470

Schulzer M, Fitzgerald J M, Enarson D A, Grzybowski S 1992 An estimate of the future size of the tuberculosis problem in sub-Saharan Africa resulting from HIV infection. Tubercle Lung Dis 73: 52–58

Serwadda D, Mugerwa R D, Sewankambo N K et al 1985 Slim disease: a new disease in Uganda and its association with HTLV-III infection. Lancet 2: 849–852

Serwadda D, Goodgame R, Lucas S, Kocjan G 1989 Absence of pneumocystosis in Ugandan AIDS patients. AIDS 3(3): 47–48

Sewankambo N, Mugerwa R D, Goodgame R et al 1987 Enteropathic AIDS in Uganda. An endoscopic, histological and microbiological study. AIDS 1: 9–13

Simonsen J N, Cameron D W, Gakinya M N et al 1988 Human immunodeficiency virus infection among men with sexually transmitted diseases. Experience from a center in Africa. N Engl J Med 319(5): 274–8

Simonsen J N, Plummer F A, Ngugi E N et al 1990 HIV infection among lower socioeconomic strata prostitutes in Nairobi. AIDS 4(2): 139–144

Slack R C B, Stewart J D, Lewis C L H et al 1976 Acute pneumonia in adults in Nairobi. E Afr Med J 5(3): 480–483

Sundharam J A 1990 Pruritic skin eruption in the acquired immunodeficiency syndrome: arthropod bites? Arch Dermatol 126(4): 539

Tavitian A, Raufman J P, Rosenthal L E et al 1986a Ketoconazole resistant candida oesophagitis in patients with acquired immune deficiency syndrome. Gastroenterology 90: 443–445

Tavitian A, Raufman J P, Rosenthal L E 1986b Oral candidiasis as a marker for oesophageal candidiasis in the acquired immunodeficiency syndrome. Ann Intern Med 104: 54–55

Temmerman M, Mohamed Ali F, Ndinya-Achola J, Moses S, Plummer F A, Piot P 1992 Rapid increase of both HIV-1 infection and syphilis among pregnant women in Nairobi, Kenya. AIDS 6: 1181–1185

ter Meulen J, Eberhardt H C, Luande J, Mgaya H N, Chang-Claude J, Mtiro H, Mhina M, Kashaija P, Ockert S, Yu X et al 1992 Human papillomavirus (HPV) infection, HIV infection and cervical cancer in Tanzania, East Africa. Int J Cancer 51(4): 515–521

Thijs A, Janssen P G 1963 Pneumocystis in Congolese infants. Trop Geograph Med 15: 158–172

Thornton C, Latif A S 1989 Guillain-Barré syndrome in HIV infection: experience from an African centre. Fifth International Conference on AIDS, Canada. Abstr Th B P 214

Ulin P R 1992 African women and AIDS: negotiating behavioural change. Soc Sci Med 134(1): 63–73

UNICEF 1985 Children and women in Zimbabwe: a situation analysis. Government Printers, Harare, Zimbabwe

United Nations, Department of Internation Economic and Social Affairs 1987 The prospects of world urbanization, revised as of 1984–85. United Nations, New York

Van de Perre P, Rouvray D, Lepage P et al 1984 Acquired immunodeficiency syndrome in Rwanda. Lancet 2: 62–65

Van de Perre P, Clumeck N, Carael M et al 1985 Female prostitutes: a risk group for infection with human T-cell lymphotropic virus type III. Lancet 2: 524–526

Van de Perre P, Bakkers E, Batungwanayo J et al 1988 Herpes zoster in African patients: an early manifestation of HIV infection. Scand J Infect Dis 20(3): 277–282

Vandepitte J, Verwilghen R, Zachee 1983 AIDS and cryptococcus. Lancet 1: 925–926

Way P O, Stanecki K 1991 The demographic impact of an AIDS epidemic on an African country: application of the IWGAIDS model. Center for International Research, U.S. Bureau of the Census, Washington

Wofsy C B, Padian N S, Cohen J B, Greenblatt R, Coleman R, Korvick J A 1992 Management of HIV disease in women. In: Volberding P, Jacobson M A (eds), AIDS clinical review 1992. Marcel Dekker, New York

World Health Organization, Division of Family Health 1982 The prevalence and duration of breast-feeding: a critical review of available information. World Health Stat Q 35: 92–116

9. Terminal care for women with AIDS

Veronica A. Moss

INTRODUCTION

Sarah, a 28-year-old single mother, was admitted for terminal care. She had a diagnosis of chronic cryptosporidiosis with persistent diarrhoea, and also of pulmonary tuberculosis which was proving to be resistant to treatment. She had lost 10 kg in weight in the past few weeks and was suffering from chronic vaginal and oral candidiasis and her menstrual pattern had become irregular. She tended to focus on her gynaecological problems and she was depressed. She was anxious about her 10-year-old son's future and about who would take care of him as she had no family in the UK. Her husband had been killed in Africa and she had fled to the UK as a refugee with her son 3 years previously.

She had been struggling on at home refusing to be admitted because of Peter until she collapsed, dehydrated as a result of an acute exacerbation of diarrhoea, and was admitted to hospital. Her son had been nursing her at home and called the ambulance. He was taken into care, to the same foster mother with whom he had spent a previous admission and with whom Sarah had maintained contact.

Having been rehydrated, stabilized and reassessed at the acute hospital, Sarah was referred for terminal care to Mildmay where Peter continued to visit her daily. She was emaciated, depressed but in denial about her condition. She had not been able to discuss Peter's future in the event of her death – attempts by counsellors and social workers had met with denial or evasion of the problem. She was afraid to let any friends know the diagnosis, and she was afraid that Peter would be stigmatized at school should her status become known, although he was HIV-negative.

When Sarah was found to have a perianal abscess causing her severe pain and distress, she was referred for surgery. Her own acute centre was unable to find a surgeon who was willing to deal with it, and she was therefore referred to another centre to which she was admitted for a few days. Unfortunately, she developed a rectovaginal fistula. Sadly, Peter was not allowed to visit as it was felt it would be unsuitable for such a young child to see her in her condition postoperatively. Sarah became convinced that he had died and became acutely distressed and agitated. The psychiatrist who was called to see her did not understand her distress because of a language problem and diagnosed an acute psychosis, possibly relating to the general anaesthesia she had undergone.

When Sarah returned to Mildmay she was still acutely distressed, and wanted only to die. As soon as it became clear that she thought Peter was dead, arrangements were quickly made for Peter to visit. Peter had been very withdrawn and silent and he told the counsellor during his first visit that he had thought his mother had died since he could no longer visit her, and that everyone had been lying to him when they had reassured him.

Once Sarah and Peter were reunited, Sarah settled down. She continued to deteriorate, however, and it was felt that Peter should spend as much time as possible with her and he was allowed to stay with her on several occasions. Sarah began to be willing to explore issues relating to Peter's future with the nurses and the counsellor, and she also welcomed pastoral support from the chaplaincy team who arranged regular services of communion for her. Her physical symptoms of pain, nausea and diarrhoea were controlled and she died in peace and comfort, with her son by her side, and supported by the team. There had been some discussion about the distress to Peter of seeing other ill people on the ward, but Peter showed clearly that he coped well. He was happier helping to care for his mother than being separated from her. After Sarah's death, he returned to the foster mother who had supported him throughout.

Sarah's story illustrates a number of the issues surrounding terminal care for women with AIDS. These include some of the following:

- the clinical needs for palliation and/or acute treatment of distressing physical problems, some of which may be gynaecological in nature
- neuropsychiatric problems
- the social isolation and fear with which many live with little or no support from family
- the anxieties relating to child care and the future of orphans who may be left destitute in some societies
- the need to provide support in the community for women who are themselves ill, and mothers in particular. This includes provision for flexible respite care and fostering arrangements, keeping separation to a minimum for the sake of both, and yet recognizing that the mother will also need a break from the child from time to time
- the needs of women who are usually 'the carers' needing care themselves. Who will care for them when they are disabled or ill? or when they are dying?
- the need for ongoing financial support, or for income generation. In many instances the woman will have been the sole breadwinner
- emotional, spiritual and pastoral needs
- confidentiality for herself and her child/ children
- the responsibilities of the woman as a carer for husband, elderly parents, children, without in many countries, the power or right to make her own decisions and choices, even when it comes to matters of sexual intercourse, childbearing or the future of dependants.

CLINICAL PROBLEMS

In most Central African countries and in some pattern I countries, such as New York City, AIDS has become the leading cause of death for women aged 20–40 years (Chin 1990). Most will be dying with little or no access to medical help, perhaps even to palliative care. Even in pattern I countries, such as USA and other Western areas where medical care is more readily available to all, women tend to delay in coming forward for medical care for themselves (Triple Jeopardy: Panos 1990). They are likely, therefore, to present with more advanced immunosuppression, and in a state of chronic ill health or as acute emergencies, unless they are fortunate enough to have been identified at an early stage and have found medical and social support for themselves and their families.

Women with late-stage HIV disease or AIDS are subject to a range of gynaecological problems which may cause anxiety, discomfort and pain, and exacerbate the ill health or weakness the patient is already experiencing as a result of HIV. Common gynaecological problems are, of course, common in this group of patients too, and it may not be possible to attribute their presence specifically to the HIV infection but more to immunosuppression and general debility. These problems may include pelvic inflammatory disease, menstrual irregularities, genital warts and ulcers, chronic vaginal candidiasis and cervical dysplasia.

Candidiasis

Vaginal and oral or oesophageal candidiasis may cause severe debility and discomfort in someone who has advanced HIV disease. It may become increasingly difficult to control. Oral candidiasis will cause anorexia, loss of taste and in some cases soreness of oral mucosa with sensitivity to hot and cold liquids. This will cause loss of weight as the anorexia and loss of taste persist, thus increasing the debility. Oesophageal candidiasis may cause dysphagia and retrosternal discomfort with a burning sensation, not usually described as pain. Again, weight loss will become an increasing problem as nausea, vomiting, anorexia and dysphagia may be very troublesome.

Treatment of candidiasis, whether oral, oesophageal or vaginal, may be complicated by the need also to treat bacterial infections with antibiotics. The *Candida albicans* sometimes develops resistance to the usual drugs in patients with advanced disease, and even larger doses than normal may not then control the problems. Fluconazole is the treatment of choice in dosages which may range from 100–400 mg daily (Laine et al 1992). Ketaconazole 200–400 mg daily may also be used or, in some cases, Itraconazole 200 mg daily, which may also be taken as a liquid. Very occasionally, amphotericin B or fluconazole may have to be given intravenously in someone with resistant oesophageal candida in whom symptoms of dysphagia and burning are causing distress; burning and itching due to vaginal candidiasis may also be distressing.

Nystatin suspension may contribute to the control of oral candidiasis, but larger doses than those normally recommended are required in patients with severe immunosuppression. A dosage of 3–5 ml should be given every 2–4 h, and held in the mouth for as long as possible before swallowing. Unfortunately, some patients may develop diarrhoea as a side-effect, or may find the taste unpleasant. Nystatin or amphotericin pastilles may then be sucked instead. Miconazole tablets 250 mg, may also be sucked, and miconazole oral gel (Daktarin) which is sugarless may be more acceptable to some patients. In very resistant cases, clotrimazole (Canestan) vaginal tablets (100, 200 or 500 mg) taken orally and sucked once or twice daily may be effective in clearing plaques of oral candidiasis within 2–3 days; some patients find the taste and foaming of the tablets unpleasant in the mouth, but may be pleasantly surprised to find quick relief.

Vaginal candidiasis and candidal vaginitis may be similarly distressing and difficult to treat in severely immunosuppressed women. Systemic treatment with fluconazole or other drugs mentioned above will be necessary, with the application of clotrimazole cream to the vulva and clotrimazole vaginal tablets inserted as high as possible in the vagina; 500 mg tablets will be more effective than the lower dosages in controlling symptoms quickly.

Recurrences of infection are almost inevitable, and most patients will require prophylactic or maintenance treament with, for example, fluconazole;

in advanced disease, higher doses will be required to maintain control. Perianal *Candida* infections and other skin sites, such as groin, umbilicus or under breasts, may also require regular attention with clotrimazole or miconazole cream.

In the terminal care situation the patient may be unable to take oral medication. Here the administration of nystatin suspension or miconazole oral gel (with good mouth care) is even more important in order to maintain comfort. Vulvitis and vaginitis should not be forgotten as a possible cause of restlessness in a dying patient, or of dysuria and frequency, and treated appropriately. Natural yoghurt may be soothing when applied to the vulvae, and taken orally may help to control oral candidiasis.

Table 9.1 summarizes the presentation and treatment of candidiasis in women with advanced HIV disease.

Genital herpes simplex infections

Genital herpes infections become progressively more common as the CD4+ lymphocyte count falls, and there is a high rate of previous sexually transmitted diseases (Norman et al 1990). The association between genital ulcerative disease and HIV infection is well established (Cameron & Padian 1990, Plourde et al 1992).

Herpes ulceration may cause severe stinging and burning of the vulva or vagina, with dysuria. In patients with advanced disease, the lesions may be difficult to treat effectively. Acyclovir given orally in doses of 400 mg, five times daily, with the local application of acyclovir cream, where possible, will cause healing and relief within a week to 10 days when resistance has not developed. When the ulceration persists despite treatment, distress and agitation may become difficult to deal with, and patients may require analgesia in the form of morphine with an anxiolytic or sedative. (See further under symptom control issues.) Local anaesthetic gels may give temporary relief, but prolonged regular applications may cause local sensitivity reactions. Some patients will find relief from soaking in a mildly saline bath. Patients who are too weak even for this require careful and meticulous attention to hygiene by the nursing staff.

In patients who have well-advanced HIV disease

Table 9.1 Candidiasis in women with advanced HIV disease

Site	Problems	Recommended treatment
Oral	Anorexia, loss of taste, weight loss	*fluconazole 100–200 mg od *nystatin 3–5 ml 2/4 hourly *miconazole oral gel or tabs to suck *clotrimazole (vaginal) tabs 200 or 500 mg to suck bd ('live' natural yoghurt as part of diet)
Oesophageal	Dysphagia, retrosternal burning sensation, weight loss, anorexia, nausea, vomiting	fluconazole 200–400 mg daily (or ketoconazole or itraconazole) iv amphotericin B or fluconazole may be necessary nausea & vomiting may require maxolon, cyclizine and/or haloperidol, sometimes via syringe-driver
Vaginal	Vulvitis with burning, itching, dysuria and frequency; vaginitis with pain, itching and typical discharge; mixed infections may be common	fluconazole 150–400 mg daily clotrimazole or miconazole cream clotrimazole vaginal tablets (200–500 mg) treat other infections appropriately (live natural yoghurt applied locally)

* One or more of these may be necessary

with emaciation, weakness and immobility, pressure areas may break down and become infected with herpes, causing extensive ulceration of sacral or perianal areas or around the vulva. Severe distress and pain is the result and must be managed with good wound care, treatment of infection where possible, and regular and adequate analgesia with morphine and/or non-steroidal anti-inflammatory medications. A short-acting but effective analgesic, such as dextromoramide 5–10 mg, orally or by injection, may be given prior to wound dressings. Alternatively, if the patient is on a syringe driver with diamorphine, a boost may be given just before the procedure. Entonox (50% mixture of nitrous oxide and oxygen) may be helpful in some patients during painful procedures. (See also later under symptom-control issues, p. 113.)

Pelvic inflammatory disease

This is very common in women who are at risk of sexually transmitted diseases. It may cause severe lower abdominal pain, confusing the differential diagnosis of abdominal emergencies. In advanced AIDS, chronic problems may cause increasing debility and discomfort and should be managed so as to promote comfort and pain relief as far as possible. Constipation may also cause lower abdominal pain; this is particularly likely in someone on regular opioid analgesia, and should be prevented with regular stool softeners, such as lactulose.

Tuberculosis

In countries where tuberculosis is widespread, there is a marked association between HIV and tuberculosis, with a resurgence of multiple drug-resistant tuberculosis associated with problems in some Western countries, e.g. the USA (Fischl et al 1992). It is expected that pelvic tuberculosis will also increase (Norman et al 1990), as indeed will other pelvic inflammatory diseases. In end-stage disease, treatment with dexamethasone may reduce the pain or discomfort associated with pelvic and abdominal tuberculosis.

Intravenous drug users

As many HIV-infected women in the West are intravenous drug users, many of the problems they face are related to their drug use. These may be both social and medical. Patients with the weakness and debility associated with well-advanced AIDS or HIV disease often appear to become less dependent on the drugs as they become more dependent on nursing care. However, in treating the patient's pain it is important to bear in mind the past history and pattern of drug use and to adjust the dosages appropriately. For example, patients who have already been on opiates, albeit not prescribed, may need larger than the usual dosages to deal effectively with pain. The same applies to benzodiazepines such as diazepam or temazepam for anxiolysis or night sedation. In the terminal care situation it is more important to treat pain and other symptoms effectively than to be concerned about treatment or prevention of addiction. Maintenance doses of methadone will enable the patient to remain stable, while any pain problems should be treated separately and appropriate and adequate analgesia or adjuvant treatment given (see symptom-control issues).

Adjustment time

As women tend to present later for diagnosis and treatment, and maybe to have less easy access to care in some countries, it may be that immunosuppression through HIV infection has progressed further at the point of presentation in these women (Triple Jeopardy: Panos 1990). This may mean that some women will have a shorter time period in which to come to terms with their own losses and fears about the physical progress of the disease. The same applies to dealing with the many social issues and decisions which have to be faced (see later under social needs), in particular to planning for the future of any children.

Neuropsychiatric problems

A variety of neuropsychiatric problems occur in advanced AIDS which range from acute anxiety states to frank psychoses, extreme paranoia and dementia. Depression and anxiety are very common and may be masked by organic disease processes, including HIV encephalopathy. What role a developing HIV encephalopathy plays in the development of postmorbid psychiatric syndromes is not clear. One study in Zaire showed that 41% of HIV-seropositive patients showed evidence of neuropsychiatric abnormalities (Perriens et al 1992). One post-mortem study showed that nearly 90% of patients reviewed had cerebral abnormalities (Lantos et al 1989). An unpublished analysis of 100 patients admitted consecutively to a hospice unit (Midmay Mission Hospital) revealed that 22% had a significant psychiatric problem other than mild anxiety or depression. The same range of neurological problems occur in women as in men.

Women with psychiatric problems, who also have children, present special problems. It is distressing for the child to watch its mother behaving in bizarre and uncharacteristic ways, which may also be very frightening. Counsellors and social workers seeking to help the mother to deal with issues relating to her own impending death and her child's future may have difficulties with enabling her to reach meaningful resolutions. Great sensitivity, patience and an ability to work with children and other family members are essential.

Patients with advanced AIDS appear to be more sensitive than usual to psychotropic drugs, and smaller doses than those normally recommended for the treatment of psychiatric problems may be required to avoid serious sedation and extrapyramidal side-effects. However, in seriously disturbed or psychotic patients, it may be necessary to use high doses to achieve control. In a terminally ill patient methotrimeprazine or midazolam may be used in the syringe-driver to control severe agitation and restlessness (Back 1992).

Symptom control issues in advanced AIDS

The purpose of symptom control or palliation in AIDS, as in any terminal illness, is:

— to relieve distress or pain
— to enhance the quality of life as far as possible
— to enable the achievement of goals
— to facilitate a comfortable death with peace and dignity.

Prolongation of life would not be the main aim of palliation, but the achievement of relief from distressing symptoms may, in some cases, lead to a reawakening of the will to live, and an improvement in appetite. The outcome may then be, incidentally, that the patient lives longer with some quality of life. Some patients will even be able to achieve goals they had given up hope of being able to reach.

Patients with advanced AIDS will usually present with a similar range of problems to those found in a patient with advanced cancer or other life-threatening conditions (Table 9.2). These will include severe weight loss, anorexia, or nausea and vomiting. In addition they will have symptoms which are specifically related to HIV/AIDS, such

Table 9.2 Some symptoms commonly encountered in advanced AIDS

Symptom	Comment
General debility/weight loss	almost universal
Pain	60.4% in one sample ($n = 13$) with mean of 1.6 pains per patient, from one to four causes (Moss 1990)
Skin problems	extremely common; may be fungal or bacterial infections, scabies, molluscum contagiosum, psoriasis, folliculitis, drug-rashes etc.
Anorexia	often related to general disease process, drugs, candidiasis
Nausea and vomiting	may be related to drugs, candidiasis, cryptosporidiosis, constipation, anxiety
Diarrhoea	many treatable causes, but often no cause is found and only symptom control is possible
Confusion	may be drug-induced, due to infection or HIV-related encephalopathy; differential diagnosis very important
Depression	natural sadness due to losses and illness must be differentiated from clinical depression
Other psychiatric problems	may range from acute anxiety state to frank psychoses

as the pain of HIV-related peripheral neuropathy, or visual problems with retinitis caused by cytomegalovirus. Many symptoms are directly related to the common opportunistic infections; these infections should be treated whenever possible to give relief. For example, perianal ulceration caused by herpes simplex genitalis will cause intense pain, particularly on defaecation, possibly with tenesmus. The management here should aim first at treating the infection whenever possible with acyclovir. The symptoms of localized anal pain may require treatment with local anaesthetic applications for a few days and tenesmus may be relieved by chlorpromazine 25 mg, tds or nifedipine 10 mg stat. In some instances, especially when extensive ulceration is present, opioids may also be required. Constipation should also be guarded against in this case with the prescription of regular stool softening laxatives such as lactulose or co-danthromer. In

the terminal care situation, healing of ulceration may not be possible; relief of pain and distress certainly is.

A patient with AIDS usually has a number of coexisting diagnoses for which she may be taking a number of prophylactic or maintenance drugs. This frequently results in a degree of polypharmacy which may cause side-effects and symptoms which present problems for symptom control. Drug interactions may also cause difficulties. When a patient is entering the terminal phase, it may be possible to reduce the number of drugs being taken. This should not be done in such a way that the patient feels 'abandoned' – 'They've given up on me' or 'They can't do any more for me'. This may induce a sense of fear and hopelessness. It is never necessary to say 'We can do nothing more for you'. There is always something that can be done to relieve pain or distress, or to comfort.

Pain in advanced AIDS

This may have many causes. In one sample (see Table 9.2) 60.4% of patients had a significant painful problem. The causes include:

- Peripheral neuropathy – HIV-related
- Pressure sores
- Herpes simplex ulceration
- Epigastric or oesophageal pain – which may be due to candidiasis, herpes simplex or cytomegalovirus ulceration, lymphoma, Kaposi's sarcoma
- Visceral pain – which may be due to Kaposi's sarcoma, lymphoma, pelvic inflammatory disease and other gynaecological problems
- Joint pains – HIV-related arthropathy, septic arthritis
- Headaches – these may be caused by tension, or for example sinusitis, toxoplasmosis, meningitis, cerebral lymphoma.

'Total body pain' is a condition in which a patient is overwhelmingly distressed by a number of painful problems occurring at once. She may not be able to identify any of them at the time, and may present as being 'in shock'. In such cases the pain must quickly be relieved by morphine (orally in less severe cases) or diamorphine (subcutaneously or intravenously) plus an antiemetic such as haloperidol. Once the patient has relaxed, the components of the pain should be elucidated and treated appropriately.

Principles of pain control

The basic principle of good pain control when pain is chronic, persistent or recurring is to give a regular or 'prophylactic' analgesic or appropriate adjuvant (see Table 9.3). The patient should not

Table 9.3 Useful adjuvants in control of chronic pain

Type pf pain	Adjuvant indicated
Inflammatory, joint or bony pain	NSAIDs
Raised intracranial pressure	dexamethasone
Deafferentation pain (nerve destruction, burning pain, 'pins & needles')	tricyclic antidepressants and/or anticonvulsants, NSAIDs
Intermittent stabbing pain, e.g. post-herpetic neuralgia	anticonvulsant, e.g. carbamazapine or sodium valproate
Rectal and bladder or oesophageal spasm	chlorpromazine nifedipine
Muscle spasm pain	baclofen diazepam

NSAIDs = non-steroidal anti-inflammatory drugs

be left to request analgesia 'when necessary'. She will live in anxiety about the next period of pain when the analgesia has worn off, and may feel censured for 'needing' to ask for more pain relief, and so delay in asking until in considerable distress. The cycle is only perpetuated by this approach and frequently the perception of pain worsens with the fear.

Initially each pain should be identified and, where possible, a cause established. If a treatable cause is found this should, of course, be treated whenever possible. The severity or intensity of pain should be measured using a visual analogue scale such as simply, a line with 0 at one end for no pain, and 10 at the other end for the worst ever experienced (Fig. 9.1).

0	5	10
No pain	Moderate Pain	Worst ever pain

Fig.9.1 Visual analogue scale.

The starting point for treating pain with analgesics should be with simple non-opioids such as aspirin or paracetamol. Once a baseline has been established, the response to therapy can be monitored on a day to day basis. The World Health Organization analgesic ladder (Fig. 9.2) provides guidelines for progression from non-opioids to weak and then strong opioids for pain that persists or recurs. They should be combined, where appropriate, with adjuvants (see Table 9.3). The dosage interval for any regular medication should be determined by the length of time during which the drug is effective. Morphine sulphate given orally in elixir or tablet form for opioid-sensitive pain has an effective period of between 3 and 5 h; it is therefore usually administered or taken at 4-hourly intervals. The starting dose is usually 5–10 mg depending on debility, severity of pain or the previous drug history. The patient's response to treatment should be closely monitored and the treatment dose titrated upwards according to a preset incremental scale until good pain control is achieved (see Table 9.4 and Twycross & Lack 1990).

Table 9.4 Morphine and diamorphine conversion chart and 4-hourly dose equivalents

Oral morphine (mg)	Oral diamorphine (mg)	Injected diamorphine (mg)
5	2.5	2.5
10	7.5	5
20	15	7.5
30	20	10
45	30	15
60	40	20
90	60	30
120	90	40

Conversion ratios: 3 : 2 : 1

For the first few days after starting on morphine, the patient may require regular antiemetics such as prochlorperazine 4–6-hourly or haloperidol once or twice daily. The morphine-induced nausea usually subsides within a few days. Once good pain control has been achieved it should be maintained more conveniently for the patient with a sustained release formula (MST continuous) taken 12-hourly. The total dose over 24 h is divided by 2 to obtain the 12-hourly dose.

A troublesome side-effect of opioids is con-

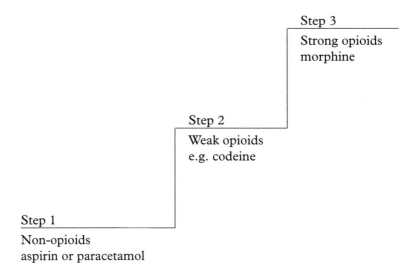

Fig. 9.2   WHO analgesic ladder for persistent or recurring pain.

stipation and it is usually necessary to prescribe regular doses of laxatives, preferably a stool softener such as lactulose, sometimes in combination with a stimulant such as senakot. Of course, if the patient suffers from chronic diarrhoea then the opioid is very useful as an antidiarrhoeal agent.

In non-opioid-responsive pains or only partially responsive pains a different approach using, for example, the adjuvant drugs shown in Table 9.3 may be used. It should also be remembered that non-drug approaches may be more effective or could be used in conjunction with appropriate drugs – for example, therapeutic massage, heat pads, transcutaneous nerve stimulation or acupuncture.

The addition of dexamethasone may achieve good results in some cases of intractable pain and may also improve mood, sense of well-being and appetite. Its risks for long-term therapy must be borne in mind, but in the terminal care situation it may be entirely appropriate to improve quality of life.

Nausea and vomiting

Nausea and vomiting may be very troublesome in many patients with advanced AIDS. They may be related to a number of causes, often in combination. These may include anxiety and fear; diar-

rhoeas caused by, for example, cryptosporidiosis; raised intracranial pressure; or may be the side-effects of drugs. The choice of treatment should depend on the likely cause or causes of the symptoms. When the symptom is a persistent or recurring one the approach should again be to take prophylactic action by prescribing regularly rather than on an 'as necessary' basis. In terminal care when oral medication may be difficult, or for intractable vomiting, a syringe-driver may prove a useful tool to achieve good control.

Anorexia

This may have a number of causes and these should be addressed where possible. For example, oral *Candida* may cause anorexia and is easily treatable. Megoestrol acetate 80–160 mg bd (von Roenn 1988) is a good appetite stimulant, as is dexamethasone.

Diarrhoea

Chronic or recurring diarrhoea is a common, and in some cases serious problem. Numerous causes of diarrhoea exist in AIDS and these should be treated whenever possible. HIV itself may cause diarrhoea, but the most troublesome to treat or control is the diarrhoea caused by cryptosporidiosis, with severe weight loss and debility. The diarrhoea is, typically, profuse with 10–20 bowel movements a day with the loss of up to 8–10 1 daily. Rehydration and nutrition are, of course, important, but control may be successfully achieved with loperamide – up to 32 mg in 24 h according to O'Neill (1992) – or an opioid preparation such as morphine sulphate as MST. This could be combined with an isphaghula husk preparation (Mulvenna & Moss 1992) to thicken the stool and sometimes an antispasmodic such as hyoscine butyl bromide (buscopan) may help (Sims & Moss 1990).

The use of the syringe-driver

The use of the syringe-driver is now well established practice in terminal care as well as in acute or postoperative pain management. It enables smooth and accurate delivery of a single drug or a combination of drugs to achieve effective symptom control. Drugs are usually delivered subcutaneously (or intravenously) through a fine needle which remains in situ for several days or until skin reaction prompts a change of site. Table 9.5 shows some of the more useful drugs for AIDS symptom control.

Table 9.5 Drugs commonly used in a syringe driver in terminal care in AIDS

Drug	Indications and comment
Diamorphine	Pain control, diarrhoea or dyspnoea More soluble than morphine
Hyoscine	Reduction of secretions in chest infections Control of diarrhoea, peristalsis in intestinal obstruction
Methotrimeprazine	Sedation in 'terminal restlessness' Powerful antiemetic Has analgesic properties
Midazolam	Anticonvulsant in those needing replacement for anticonvulsant therapy Sedative/tranquiliser for restlessness and agitation
Haloperidol	Antiemetic; particularly effective in drug-induced nausea and vomiting Agitation or psychosis
Metoclopramide	Antiemetic
Cyclizine	Antiemetic – use well-diluted to prevent precipitation; will precipitate in saline

May be used in combination (Johnson 1992)

SOCIAL NEEDS AND PROBLEMS

Someone to care for her

Women are usually the providers of care for husbands, children and elderly parents. The woman who has a partner willing to care for her when she herself is ill, disabled or dying is indeed fortunate. Sadly, there are many women who are deserted by their partner when they are no longer able to fulfil their usual role, or when the diagnosis becomes known. In cultures where the extended family system is strong, such as in Scotland or Uganda, the task of caring for the ill woman will usually fall to her mother. In some cultures the woman will be expected to move back into her parental home with her children if they are small. Thus, the grandmother will often become the surrogate mother for the children. Grandmothers are the main carers in many communities in Africa where large numbers of women of child-bearing age are dying as a result of AIDS. This places a huge burden on elderly women who may themselves be suffering from the problems of increasing age. In the West, with many women living far from their parents, often being themselves single parents, there may be no-one to care for the ill or dying woman who will end up in hospital unless community services can be set up to provide care in the home.

Delays in treatment

The responsibility for a child or children, and the resistance she may have to the child being taken into care, may cause the woman to delay in seeking help. The situation may then become an emergency and result in admission to hospital with the children taken into care amidst great trauma. Other reasons for delay may be guilt about a lifestyle such as drug misuse, guilt about 'being the cause' of the child's HIV status, guilt about 'not being able to cope' and a resultant feeling that she does not deserve help. In one study in New York, women were found already to be very ill when they presented for medical treatment. On average women suffered nearly 60 weeks of ill health before seeking medical care, compared with just 24 in men (Triple Jeopardy 1990).

Confidentiality

Other anxieties often relate to issues of confidentiality. Once her HIV status is known to social services, home help services, or her GP, to whom else will the knowledge be 'leaked'? What will be the result for her child? Will he/she be ostracized, stigmatized, and be thrown out of school or creche? What about the neighbours?

> One mother with AIDS attended a day centre to which she was given a lift by a car which had the name of an institution well known for its AIDS care. She would also be taken back and dropped off outside her home in a block of flats. She would then go to the nearby school to bring her daughter home from school. One day, as they approached their block, a bucket of water was thrown over them from an upstairs flat. Subsequent events convinced her that neighbours had observed the name on the car and put two and two together. She requested that the name be removed from the car to prevent similar problems happening to other people.

The fear of confidentiality being broken may have a profound effect on the woman's attitudes to her own need for medical help. Here fear of the reactions she or her child may provoke if the diagnosis becomes known may keep her isolated and lacking in the support and help that could be available to her.

The need for respite and support in the community

A woman who is herself debilitated, disabled or ill whilst still caring for a small child will suffer extreme fatigue and exhaustion at times, particularly as her condition advances. It is important to plan for support for her in the community or for flexible respite admissions with arrangements for the child to remain with the mother should she wish for this. Provision should then be made for the child to be cared for by, for example, nursery nurses during the day and perhaps also at night, to give the mother adequate periods of rest.

Other forms of support could include creche facilities for the child/children under age 5 years so that the woman can have several 'free' periods during the week. A flexible approach to this may also be helpful so that, if she feels particularly unwell one day, the child may be taken to the creche or to a foster mother. This may enable her to cope in the community for as long as possible, even when suffering chronic ill health.

Fostering and adoption

In Scotland an innovative approach to fostering has been developed to support mothers who have advanced AIDS. Prospective foster parents are trained in issues relating to HIV/AIDS and may be introduced to a mother soon after her first admission with an AIDS-related condition (Brettle 1990, personal communication). The foster mother is then allocated to that family 'on standby'. During subsequent admissions of the mother to hospital the child is then cared for by the same foster mother so that both mother and child become secure in the knowledge of the arrangements. As the mother's condition advances, discussion may then begin about arrangements for the child when she dies.

Similarly, prospective adoptive parents may also be given some training in regard to HIV/AIDS. For some mothers it is important to have an opportunity to meet the people who may adopt her child/children after her death. Others will not be able to cope with this, and in some cultures it is only felt to be appropriate for the child to go to a member of the extended family. For example, in Zimbabwe, some families will be unwilling to introduce into the 'family line' a child from an unrelated family as he/she may bring misfortune or 'a curse' upon the adoptive family. It is felt the child may be blamed for any subsequent problems which could arise. Thus, in this situation, some may prefer orphans to go into an orphanage. In Uganda, however, it is felt that the community should take responsibility for its orphans. Great sensitivity is needed in broaching the subject with an ill or dying woman, with some understanding of her cultural background.

EMOTIONAL AND SPIRITUAL CARE

Children, illness and death

Women who have lost a considerable amount of weight, who are disfigured, who have developed signs of HIV encephalopathy or who have psychiatric problems may cause a great deal of distress to their partner or children as their condition deteriorates. Some women will not wish their child to see them in this condition – they will wish the child to 'remember me as I was'. The partner and adult family members, of course, must make their own decisions about how much time they spend with the dying woman, and whether or not they wish to be present with her at the moment of death. It is to be hoped that their decision will relate to the woman's own need for supportive company.

However, a small child is in a different situation. Some mothers may make it clear that they do not wish the child to see them; others, like Sarah, will be very distressed by separation. Some children, like Peter, will be happier to be involved and will cope well. Great sensitivity is needed in supporting both the dying woman and the family through this time. Nursing, medical as well as social work, counselling and pastoral personnel will all be involved, and will need to work together to develop a common approach in each individual case.

Counselling

Counselling will, in most instances, focus around the issues already discussed. The woman who faces all the losses inherent in having advanced AIDS will require understanding support which enables her, where possible, to make meaningful decisions. In many cultures, particularly in developing countries, women are not empowered to make decisions for themselves about any major issues, including their children's future. They may therefore be unused to, or afraid of, broaching or discussing difficult emotional issues. In some Kenyan circles, for example, it is considered unacceptable to discuss someone's impending death as this, in itself, is seen as hastening or causing the death. A wife, therefore, who has the courage or temerity to raise the subject of her own or her husband's possible death with a view to making decisions about the children's future support, may be accused of causing the death. She may even be thrown out of the home and disinherited by the rest of the family. A counsellor faced with such a cultural background will have to be prepared to approach the whole subject in an indirect way and may need to be very patient, accepting the cultural inability of the ill woman to deal with the issue.

The question of wills may also cause similar problems. In the West, counsellors dealing with a woman in the terminal phase of her illness would naturally raise the issue and provide supportive help to someone seeking to complete 'unfinished business', such as the writing of a will. A woman would be encouraged to do this in the same way that a man would be.

However, in many cultures it would be seen as inappropriate for a woman to do so, and in some a will written by a woman would not be considered legally binding, in any case. She may not be able to own anything in her own name, and therefore will have nothing to leave. These issues are now being addressed in many developing countries where the writing of any wills has not been common. Tribal law will have dictated what happens to property or money after someone's death. For example, in Ugandan 'common' law, the husband's brothers inherit any property he leaves. In parts of Uganda, women lawyers are encouraging women to take control of their own situations and to seek legal advice about how to write a legally valid will. Women with AIDS, who have been able to set up income–generating projects, are opening accounts in the name of their child/children, to ensure some continuing financial support for them. Men are also being encouraged to plan ahead and to write wills which will provide ongoing support for their spouse and children. However, these are still new ideas for some communities and cannot be imposed.

Counsellors may therefore have to work with women to whom the whole idea of writing a will, and making decisions relating to their own death, may be very unfamiliar, even shocking. Emotionally, a woman may not be able to handle the issue and may therefore avoid or deny the need to do so.

Pastoral care

A woman's religious background may be, or become, very important at this time. Even someone with little or no religious affiliation will begin to ask questions which have spiritual significance, and some will discover a faith for the first time. It is vitally important that spiritual issues and questions relating to the meaning of life, suffering and death be taken seriously. Pastoral care should be available through a chaplaincy team, or contact made possible with religious leaders from the woman's own background. Religious rites and practices may take on a meaning and an importance they have not had until the woman became ill, particularly during the terminal phase.

The family, or the woman herself, may express strong wishes with regard to the funeral; a chaplain should be available to discuss these wishes, and to enable them to be fulfilled as far as possible.

It is also important to bear in mind that spiritual conflict or pain may have a profound effect on symptoms and on the response to symptom control measures. A woman who feels that her illness or pain is a punishment for something in the past is in great need of spiritual help. She may feel she should bear the pain stoically as a punishment, or that she does not deserve to be given any relief or help. She needs to feel forgiven by God, by the people she feels she has wronged, and also by herself. A woman who has an HIV-positive child may feel very guilty about having infected her child, or about leaving her family orphaned.

Anger or anxiety may also affect the response to proffered help, to medication and to the perception of symptoms. The anger may be directed at God, or at the religious community from which the woman comes; anxiety may be about what will/may happen after death. The reality and depth of these feelings must not be negated or ignored. Good teamwork between doctors, nurses and spiritual carers may result in resolution of fears and relief of problems or symptoms, leading to a death marked by peace instead of conflict.

CONCLUSION

In addition to the physical problems that anyone with AIDS faces, a woman may have gynaecological problems requiring urgent diagnosis and treatment. However, she will also be facing a number of issues that are of special concern to her – as a child-bearer, a mother, a wife and a daughter. As the disease process advances and death approaches, these issues become more acute. The question arises of who will care for her, the one who is usually the carer, when she is too weak to cope, or when acute illness or terminal problems overtake her. And who will care for those who she usually supports – her children, her elderly parents, her husband or partner, who may also be ill?

The memories with which the woman's family, partner and child or children are left will be profoundly coloured by the attitudes of the whole team at this crucial time. The medical and nursing problems and the distress or conflict in which she may die if appropriate, skilled support is not available will remain with them forever. In such a case, anger, bitterness or fear may be the legacy that a poorly managed death will leave with the survivors. On the other hand, when symtoms are well controlled, when anxiety or fear is alleviated, when appropriate plans are made with the woman, and when spiritual comfort and reassurance are available, the patient will be more likely to die with dignity and in peace. The memories then, even in the midst of grief, can bring comfort and strength for the future.

REFERENCES

Back I N 1992 Terminal restlessness in patients with advanced malignant disease. Pall Med 6: 293–298
Brettle R 1990 Personal Communication
Cameron W D, Padian N S 1990 Sexual transmission of HIV and the epidemiology of other sexually transmitted diseases. AIDS 4 (Suppl 1): S99–103
Chin J 1990 Current and future dimensions of the HIV/AIDS pandemic in women and children. Lancet 336: 221–224
Fischl M A, Uttamchandani R B, Daikos G L et al 1992 An outbreak of tuberculosis caused by multiple drug resistant tubercle bacilli among patients with HIV infection. Am Intern Med 117(3): 177–183
Johnson I 1992 Drugs used in combination in the syringe driver – a survey of hospice practice. Pall Med 6: 125–130
Laine W, Dretler R H, Conteas C N et al 1992 Fluconazole compared with ketoconazole for the treatment of candida

oesophagitis in AIDS – a randomised trial. Ann Intern Med 117(8): 655–660

Lantos P L, McLaughlin J E, Scholtz C L et al 1989 Neuropathology of the brain in HIV infection. Lancet 1 (8633): 309

Moss V A 1990 Palliative care in advanced HIV disease: presentation, problems and palliation. AIDS 4 (Suppl 1): S235–242

Mulvenna P, Moss V A 1992 (Corresp) AIDS related diarrhoea: a rational approach to symptomatic treatment. Pall Med 6: 261

Norman S, Studd J, Johnson M 1990 HIV infection in women. Br Med J 301: 1231–1232

O'Neill W 1992 AIDS related diarrhoea: a rational approach to symptomatic treatment. Pall Med 6: 61–64

Perriens J H, Mussa M, Luabeya M K et al 1992 Neurological complications of HIV scropositive internal medicine patients in Kinshasa, Zaire. J AIDS 5 (4): 333–340

Plourde P J, Plummer F A, Pepian J 1992 HIV-1 infection in women attending a sexually transmitted diseases clinic in Kenya. J Infect Dis 166(1): 86–92

Sims R, Moss V A 1990 Terminal care for people with AIDS. Edward Arnold, p, 53

Swerdlow M, Ventafridda V (eds) 1987. Cancer pain, MTP Press, UK

Triple jeopardy: women and AIDS 1990 The Panos Institute, p 41

Twycross R, Lack S 1990. Therapeutics in terminal cancer, 2nd edn, Churchill Livingstone.

von Roenn J H 1988 Megoestrol acetate for treatment of cachexia associated with human immunodeficiency virus infection. Ann Intern Med 109: 840–841

10. Community care and community support for women

G. O. Huby, E. R. van Teijlingen, J. R. Robertson and A. M. D. Porter

INTRODUCTION

Community care encompasses more than just clinical medicine. Health workers operating in the community trying to address the medical component of a patient's problem tend to find themselves involved in a wider range of issues than the purely medical. The following case history of a short consultation encountered by an Edinburgh family doctor exemplifies the complexity and magnitude of problems experienced by women living with HIV.

The woman was a 28-year-old mother of four, who was unknown to any specialist care services. She had only confided her HIV status to her family doctor, her social worker and a welfare rights worker. In an attempt to involve her in her own treatment she was asked to prioritize her problems. Her immediate anxiety centred round her court appearance scheduled for the following week. Second on the list was problems with her oldest two children: one had behavioural problems and the other had recently been assaulted. Her third problem was having to keep her HIV status a secret from legal authorities, because she was worried that her ex-husband would find out. Her fourth major concern was her 1-year-old toddler whose HIV status was still uncertain. Fifth on her list was her own health, which was something she had largely chosen to ignore for the very pragmatic reason that she felt she could not cope either mentally, in confronting her own problem, or practically, in attending clinics. Sixth on her list was panic attacks, which were largely related to her insecurity regarding her present HIV-positive

condition. The second last problem was a long-standing cervical smear abnormality for which she continued to receive letters from the hospital insisting and cajoling her to attend for laser treatment. Finally, her mother's illness was another issue that worried her greatly but which she had failed to confront.

In the experience of the above-mentioned family doctor, people living with HIV and AIDS by and large appreciate and depend heavily on hospital-based services, although, at the same time, they are very keen to spend most of their time at home (Acheson 1989).

In this chapter, we propose to move away from a definition of community care which is seen as an opposite, and a rival to, hospital care. Central to our ideas about care is the importance of care arrangements that are flexible and tailored to the individual's circumstances. Occasional spells of hospital care clearly play a part in these arrangements, depending on the patient's needs and the support available in the community.

At this stage in the discussion, we would like to draw attention to some features of our case history: first, the clinical management of the woman's HIV infection cannot be seen in isolation from the general support she needed to gain some control over her situation and to use available facilities to look after her own health. The woman's complex and interrelated concerns included responsibilities towards her mother and her children, and these responsibilities affected the way she was dealing with her own needs. Second, our case-study family doctor needed to liaise with social workers, paediatricians, psychologists, lawyers, gynaecologists, staff of voluntary organizations and perhaps geriatric community nursing help, in order effectively to support his patient.

We shall argue that women need flexible and user-led arrangements of care to look after their own health while at the same time meeting social and cultural expectations of how women should live and behave. Important among these expectations are women's roles as providers of care and support, whether or not they are ill themselves. In conclusion, we shall argue that flexible and user-led care requires mechanisms of interagency cooperation and communication. Care and support for women living with HIV and AIDS is thus a matter of planning, management and funding of services, as well as day-to-day service delivery.

WHAT IS SPECIAL ABOUT WOMEN'S EXPERIENCE OF HIV INFECTION AND AIDS?

Women as patients

HIV infection, AIDS and the risk of contracting or transmitting the virus affect relationships and areas of women's lives which are gender-defining and lie at the core of what 'being a woman' means, both to the women themselves, and to wider society. Murray (1991) considered the following aspects of HIV transmission that are particular to women:

- Heterosexual intercourse
  — There is a large pool of infected men
  — Women retain infected secretions while men do not
- Sexual partners of bisexual men
- Sexual partners of haemophiliac men
- Prostitution
- Rape
- Contraception
- Menstruation
- Female to female transmission
- Female intravenous drug users
- Female non-intravenous drug users
- Vertical transmission: mother to child.

Women's vulnerability to HIV infection and their potential role in transmitting the virus through heterosexual contacts seem to derive to a large extent from expectations of how a woman behaves

in personal relationships towards men as sexual partners (Wilson 1992a). Such expectations have proved formidable barriers to prevention of spread of HIV heterosexually (McKeganey & Barnard 1992). These expectations seem to apply to personal sexual relationships, as opposed to professional sexual relationships where sex is directly exchanged for cash. McKeganey and Barnard (1992) found in Glasgow that female sex workers 'saw condom use as part and parcel of the work', while condoms were rarely used in personal non-commercial relationships. Female sex workers seem to be able to set the terms of the commercial exchange of sex and money in a way which they are not expected to do in personal sexual relationships (Day et al 1988, Holland et al 1990).

Women's child-bearing and child-rearing roles also affect the care and support they receive for their HIV infection. The infection may prevent women from having children, not only because of physical factors, but also because pressure is exerted on HIV-positive women to terminate pregnancies. However, having children is often central to womanhood and adulthood, and the importance of children may increase with the prospect of a terminal illness. HIV infection is not perceived by women to be a main factor in their decision whether to terminate or proceed with a pregnancy (Johnstone et al 1990), and the risk of vertical transmission is not yet fully understood, but is far less than previously thought (see Ch. 16).

Because of unknown risks to unborn babies, women are generally excluded from drug trials, and little is therefore known about the effects of anti-HIV drugs on women (Bury 1992). At the same time, the trend towards an increase in heterosexually transmitted and vertically transmitted HIV infection places women as an important target group as far as clinical trials and measures of prevention are concerned. The implication of this is that some women feel that they are defined as carriers of the virus or carriers of babies, rather than as individuals affected by the virus, with their own needs.

Women as carers

Most care provided to people with chronic illnesses is provided by female family members. This is also true for people with HIV and AIDS. Richardson (1989) concluded that, 'While women do get AIDS themselves, it is as carers of people with AIDS that the disease has, so far, had its biggest impact on women's lives. This is because those who do most of the caring for the sick, both within the home and outside it, are women'.

Women act as carers for partners as well as children. In Tayside (Scotland) it was noted that of the carers with whom the community care team was involved, 80% were female and fell into two age-groups: those 24–29 years old, and those over 41 years of age (Carnegie & Rutter 1992). It is likely, considering the epidemiology of the disease, that the former group of women are caring as partners and/or mothers, and the latter group as mothers. The involvement of informal carers does not end with the death of a family member or a friend. Barter and Mansfield (1991) point out that support for bereaved partners, family and friends may be poor.

HIV infection affects women's careers and roles as mothers. Nurses working with mothers of haemophiliacs infected with HIV through contaminated blood products have reported that some feel guilty and at fault for their sons' haemophilia and HIV infection. Mothers and grandmothers in an area of Edinburgh with a high prevalence of both drug use and HIV are struggling to provide care for a whole generation of young people and, in turn, their children, who are affected by drug use and HIV infection (Foster 1992).

Women's caring roles often mean that they put their own health needs after the needs of others in the family (Butler & Woods 1992). Our case history brings out this point very strongly. Increased burdens of care reduce women's choice as to health-promoting strategies. Considering support and care for women, it is important to look at ways in which expectations and rules about what women are and how they behave condition their access to resources and behaviours which enhance health (Payne 1991). Women are an important community care resource, and community support and care for women must thus take into account their roles as providers of care, as well as their own needs for care.

The social environment of HIV

There is a growing awareness that HIV infection affects people in other areas of their lives than stigmatized behaviours such as drug use and certain sexual preferences. HIV infection affects people as parents, grandparents, spouses, children, friends, lovers. It is also clear that measures to halt the spread of HIV and support people already affected need to address factors beyond the individual psychological and physical circumstances. In the USA, about 73% of women who have received an AIDS diagnosis are coloured (Shayne & Kaplan 1991). A study in Dublin found that 'the women who were HIV positive ... were already among Irish society's most deprived sub groups' (Butler & Woods 1992). HIV is enmeshed in social and economic dynamics in a way that produces an association between prevalence of HIV and stigma and/or poverty, deprivation and lack of economic opportunity (Krueger et al 1990, Drucker 1990). Recognizing this fact implies looking at social and economic factors which structure behaviour and expose people to risks of HIV infection. Zwi and Cabral (1991) argue that analysis of and intervention against the spread of HIV infection focus too much on individuals and their behaviour. They suggest the introduction of a new term – 'high risk situations' – to describe 'the range of social, economic, and political forces that place groups at particularly high risk of HIV infection'. Supporting women affected by HIV infection means considering some of the ways political, social and cultural factors expose women to the risk of infection and condition their access to and use of care and support facilities.

Jackson (1992) points out that for families in Edinburgh with whom the health visitor works, 'HIV is just another thing to add to all the other horrible things in their lives. Quite often it's on the bottom of the list. Some of the partners of HIV-positive women have not even bothered to be tested themselves'. The needs of women living with HIV or AIDS may thus be complex, as our case history already suggested. This complexity becomes apparent in a community care context, to which we return after considering some of the clinical issues involved in community care.

AIDS AND HIV, A COMMUNITY COMMITMENT

Medical issues in community care

The initial medical response to the HIV and AIDS epidemic in Europe and North America has been the provision of hospital care for people infected. However, the longer the epidemic has been established in an area, the less use seems to be made of specialized hospital facilities and the more community services are called for (e.g. Greco et al 1991, Scitovsky et al 1990, Smits et al 1990). Advances in medical treatment have increased longevity and have offered people the prospect of a reasonable quality of life from a medical point of view. There is also a recognition of a large spectrum of HIV-related diseases (Stoneburner et al 1988), some of which require a longer-term and more comprehensive provision of care. HIV infection and related opportunistic diseases have become a long-term chronic condition, and it is recognized that people living with HIV and AIDS need the support of a well co-ordinated system of services addressing long-term clinical, psychological and social issues.

The generalist is often well placed to manage many of the long-standing and clinical manifestations of HIV infection. Primary care services providing contraception, counselling and support during pregnancy are easily adapted to providing care to women living with HIV. Good general recommendations on the prevention of the spread of HIV infection and advice about the use of barrier contraception in addition to the usual method of contraception (e.g. the oral contraceptive pill) are a useful development that could also reduce the prevalence of other sexually transmitted diseases.

Cervical cytology is particularly important in women with HIV infection or those at risk of HIV infection. It is known that patients with advanced disease have an increased incidence of cervical abnormalities and invasive carcinoma (McCarthy et al 1992, Clark et al 1992, Agarossi et al 1992). It is particularly important, therefore, that this group is carefully screened, and this may be carried out opportunistically in consultations initiated for other reasons.

Many clinical conditions common amongst people with HIV infection are not exclusive to that disease, but may manifest in a more florid and intractable form when the patient is immunosuppressed. Specific examples are seborrhoeic dermatitis, fungal skin and nail infections, psoriasis and herpetic oral and genital conditions. Standard preparations are, therefore, often useful although increasing doses may be required and long-term treatment may be necessary.

The other great strength of primary, generalist care, namely continuity and familiarity with a longer-term perspective of patients' requirements, allows for earlier intervention and better support during difficult stages of the disease. Early contact with a woman and her family could be argued to have medical and social benefits. However, if the intervention is specialist, this could lead to early stigmatization and go against the idea of letting the woman and her family maintain a normal life for as long as possible. It may be easier for a woman to call on non-specialist services at an earlier stage of her illness. The patient's fear of stigmatization by outsiders has also been used as an argument against providing care in that community. Community care requires more service providers to be informed about the patient's HIV infection and an increased interagency communication, which in turn increases the risk of outsiders finding out.

Psychological problems may be maximal during the discovery of HIV-positive status and towards the terminal phase of the disease, but there may be many other periods during which psychological difficulties are encountered. Decisions and worries about pregnancies, the death or illness of a partner or the welfare of a child are often major issues in a woman's life. Less specifically, it is likely that most women with HIV infection have recurring periods of stress and anxiety, often precipitated by comments and events reminding them of their situation. Easy access to an informal system of care might facilitate management of such conditions.

More specific management, such as the prescribing of established antiviral agents such as zidovudine, could, to a large extent, be provided effectively by primary care workers as long as specialist back-up is available. Furthermore, Moss (1992) noted that once stabilized on zidovudine, many patients preferred to go to their family doctor for their monthly full blood count rather than to attend the hospital.

What is community care?

The importance of community care in the provision of services to people with HIV and AIDS is well recognized – e.g. the theme of World AIDS Day 1992 was 'A Community Commitment'. However, community care is a term with many meanings. It is often used to describe all care which is not provided in hospital, although sometimes it is taken to mean care provided by hospital satellites near to people's homes. These definitions emphasize a division between hospital-based and other sources of care and articulate a competition for resources between different service sectors. In Britain, according to Ham (1985) there exists a considerable pressure to move towards community-based provisions at the 'expense' of hospital-based care. Long-term institutions are being closed down and former residents are moved out to a care setting comprising a range of agencies who are to co-ordinate their input into a comprehensive package of care.

Other definitions of community care emphasize flexibility of care arrangements and user control over non-institutionalized care. Slater (1990) describes community-based models of care as user-centred, which 'embrace all the needs of the person with HIV or AIDS in a community setting'. This use of the term implies a user-led service, involving a range of facilities, offering choice and control of the mix of care provided. The division between hospital-based and other services becomes redundant with this use of the term. Hospital services become one of several facilities a person might use in order to manage life with HIV or other chronic conditions.

Higgins (1989) goes as far as suggesting that the term 'community care' is redundant since it mystifies, rather than illuminates, issues of need and care provision. The term implies a continuum of services in terms of skills and intensity of care, from an informal home environment to a formal, institutional setting. This conceptualization of services structures illness careers whereby people are assumed to inevitably progress from low levels of impairment, requiring 'low intensity' community care, to high levels of disability needing institutional care. In reality, Higgins argues, levels of impairment and concomitant needs will fluctuate

and vary in persons living with a long-term disability or illness.

The term 'community care' also masks the large amount of care work that is being provided by unpaid family carers, mostly women (Corbin & Strauss 1990), and by primary care and generic services which take on extra work without extra funding. Gender issues in care cross over the provider/recipient divide, in that the 'coal face' personnel of care often are women: nurses, health visitors, social workers (Wilson 1992b).

According to Higgins (1989), care can be adequately classified and described using only two criteria: location of care, and the person providing the care. Specifying care in this way makes care and care costs visible. This way of classifying care also avoids the idea of a continuum of care to which people's illness careers are to adapt, and allows for arrangements of care which are flexible and tailored to people's changing needs.

Such care arrangements require mechanisms of coordination and monitoring. Various forms of case management are now being introduced in the care for people with HIV and AIDS as a way of meeting these requirements (Layzell & McCarthy 1992). The idea of case management has developed out of the debate about community care. Case managers appointed to individual clients are to ensure that service users have access to relevant services; that these services are co-ordinated, efficient and flexible; and that the service user has some control over decisions concerning care arrangements. Case management is often also introduced to ensure cost containment of care.

The literature about non-institutionalized care for people living with HIV and AIDS indicates that these issues, which various forms of case management attempt to address, are recurrent.

ISSUES IN NON-INSTITUTIONAL CARE FOR PEOPLE LIVING WITH HIV AND AIDS

Co-ordination of care

While it is perhaps tempting to assume that all people with HIV infection want home-based care, it is arguable that specialist provision evolved because some people prefer this kind of service.

Confidentiality is easier to maintain with fewer agencies involved, and staff in hospitals with a large specialist caseload of people with HIV infection may be better equipped and trained to provide a service to this group (Layzell & McCarthy 1992).

While specialist provision may ensure people get the services they need, they may be costly, and they may 'de-skill' generic, primary care workers. In Britain, general medical practitioners have reportedly been reluctant to become involved in the management of people with HIV and associated problems such as drug use (Naji et al 1989, King 1989). The prominent role of hospital-centred care in Britain is to some extent bypassing the general medical practitioner and perpetuating this lack of involvement (Bennet & Pettigrew 1991).

Co-ordinating specialist care, for example hospital services, with generic and primary care services is important in developing systems of service that offer people a realistic choice of care and support arrangements. Two studies of hospital-based and community-based provision for people with HIV infection and AIDS in Lothian (Scotland) point to separate networks of professionals, with perceptions of people's needs and appropriate support articulated differently in different care settings. While each opinion may be logical and justified in its own terms, a crucial question concerns the service user and his or her own perspectives. When so many professionals hold views and opinions about the same person, a crucial question concerns the opinions and priorities of the 'real' service user, and ways of arranging care packages that reflect overall and agreed views about a person's situation. This requires mechanisms where perspectives can be compared and negotiated, and we believe that it is crucial that the service user is in some ways involved in the negotiations.

Community care teams

Community care teams have been established as a way of supporting and training general, primary care medical services to become involved in the care of people with HIV (Smits et al 1990, Hjem-mebehandlingsteam for HIV/AIDS pasienter 1991). Community care teams vary in composition

from place to place. Usually, they consist of generic medical and, in some cases, social work personnel with a special interest and special skills in care for people with HIV and AIDS. The team organizes home care for people who need support after leaving hospital. The team may take on the home care themselves, or the care is delegated to primary care personnel who are supported in this task by the team. The teams also co-ordinate input of care and help service users gain access to important services. Jones (1992) argued that the membership of a primary care team should be determined by the task to be performed, not by a fixed structure. The same argument may apply to community care teams for people with HIV and AIDS.

Access

The access to services of people with HIV and AIDS will vary according to the general system of health and social care in different countries. In the USA with a large privately funded health care sector, the range of services may be varied, but people with HIV and AIDS are in some places denied services and benefits for which they are eligible, because of stigma and fear (Sonsel et al 1988). Many people with HIV and AIDS do not have private health insurance and this limits their access to services. In New Jersey, a care management programme has been established mainly as a way of ensuring that a population of intravenous drug users and people with HIV infection gain access to a wider range of services (Crystal et al 1990). In Fairfax County (Virginia) an HIV Case Management Programme for residents asymptomatically infected with HIV was started in 1987. The programme is designed to service mainly low-income, high-risk heterosexual populations, where access to services is an issue and intravenous drug use is an important HIV risk factor. The case management programme is an important measure to prevent the infection spreading to heterosexual partners of intravenous drug users (Payne et al 1992).

The role of the voluntary sector

The voluntary sector has had an important influence on the development of services for people living with HIV and AIDS, filling gaps in statutory provision brought about by lack of experience, skills, knowledge and confidence in managing the epidemic and its clinical and psychosocial effects on individuals. In New York the Gay Men's Health Crisis initiated a 'buddy programme' in 1983, providing people living with HIV and AIDS with a special friend to help with practical and emotional support (Perrow & Guillén 1990). In Britain, non-statutory organizations (such as The Terrence Higgins Trust and the London Lighthouse) have initiated innovations in provision of services, in empowering people with HIV and AIDS, and in representing their needs to the statutory sector (Grimshaw 1990). Self-help groups have proved to be of great importance in supporting women living with HIV.

While HIV health care is generally characterized by the involvement of voluntary groups, one of the current limitations of the services for people living with AIDS and HIV is that the services are too specific. Voluntary organizations focus, for example, on certain disease aspects, or services are still too much aimed at male drug users and gay men. Women-centred provisions are only slowly being incorporated into the existing medical and social services, and largely as a result of voluntary sector pressure groups.

MATCHING SERVICES TO NEEDS

Aiming services at women's needs

Smith and Gibbons (1990) concluded that 'women need to become more vocal, more visible and more assertive not only as carers but also in devising policy and in the appropriate deployment and management of resources for all people affected by AIDS'. Our case history showed that the agenda of the service provider may differ from that of the service user. The empowerment of women as patients, health workers and informal carers should be incorporated in the future developments of community care.

Good community support and care for women living with HIV and AIDS concerns ways in which service users are involved in decisions about care. A user-led service for women living with HIV means taking their views about vital concerns in their

life, be they contraception, pregnancy, housing, benefits, care of children and other dependants, into account, and providing assistance, information and advice which addresses the way in which women themselves prioritize their needs. It means helping to ensure that services are accessible to women and that clear and realistic advice is given, and helping women negotiate the support they need.

This might involve new forms of organizing services, an example being one-stop services which offer help with a range of social, psychological and medical problems in the same place, at the same time. In Glasgow, for example, the hospital obstetrics department runs several out-reach reproductive health clinics for women needing extra support because of social problems. These clinics offer not only reproductive health care, but also assistance and support with, for example, housing, benefits, emotional problems, drug use and child care. Since women can attend without an appointment and they can refer themselves to these clinics, they can access a relevant service as and when needs arise (Hepburn 1992a).

This out-reach service is funded partly from the HIV budget and partly from the routine maternity budget, with input from social service and local authority staff offering welfare rights, counselling, social services and medical services to women attending the clinics. The clinics also help generic staff build up expertise and skills in a specialized area. Weekly meetings between social work staff and clinics ensure that women's long-term social problems are being addressed appropriately (Hepburn 1992b).

However, if this kind of service is to be made available to larger numbers of women, the cost and cost efficiency of a specialist service must be compared to that of generalist, primary care services. Ultimately, it could be argued, a flexible, user-led service should be the aim of all primary care services and should benefit all users with their diverse needs. This will involve finding ways for service providers, be they doctors, social workers, nurses or non-statutory agency workers, to liaise and co-ordinate with other services on a practical level on a regular basis. This is only possible if structures and procedures exist for them to do so. Attempts to introduce case management as part of community care legislation in Britain illustrates some of the issues around interagency collaboration.

Case management

Concern about long-term care for elderly people has led to experiments in care management as a way of addressing problems of access and coordination for this group (Hughes 1985). Case management is increasingly being tried out in long-term care for people with HIV and AIDS (Layzell & McCarthy 1992).

Case management is the main feature of the Community Care Act which will be introduced in Britain over the next 2 years. Assessment and case management are to ensure that decisions about care are passed on to the service user, together with a care manager.

Evaluation of case management programmes in the USA indicates that service provision improves, as do service provider and user satisfaction. However, neither the cost of service provision nor the use of inappropriate services is reduced (Benjamin 1989).

In Britain, attempts to introduce case management as part of community care legislation have highlighted the uncertainty of what 'care management' means. Are care managers to act as 'brokers' of services for their clients? Are they to act as advocates, or to adopt key worker roles? Furthermore, there is uncertainty over the power the case manager will have over purchasing of services (Beardshaw & Towell 1990). Conflict of interest converges on case managers between cost containment and securing the best possible service for a client (Layzell & McCarthy 1992). Effective coordination or case management requires clearly articulated and agreed remits in terms of competence, responsibility and accountability between different workers and different agencies. This is a task for planners and managers of services.

It is also important that the local environment is considered and consulted when systems of care for women and men living with HIV infection are planned. The dynamics by which sociocultural factors interact with epidemiological and biological factors to produce a certain manifestation of the epidemic will vary from setting to setting.

No two care initiatives for women with HIV can therefore be exactly the same.

Cost implications of community care

Inevitably, community care is seen by administrations to be complex and overlapping between different disciplines – for example, health, social work, employment, housing, welfare rights, voluntary care and family care. Overall responsibility, therefore, is not assumed by any administering authority. The reality, however, is that long-term care requires substantial investment over a period of several years, the total cost of which must include periods of expensive intermittent high-technology hospital care. Cost implications of this are as yet poorly understood and there have been few attempts to quantify the investment required in individual cases or populations, although at least one study attempts to assess the effects of early treatment with zidovudine on the medical care costs of persons with HIV in the first 12 months (Scitovsky et al 1990). Clearly it is impossible to extrapolate from fairly simple studies of this nature to the overall provision of hospital care services, although an increasing number of patients requiring long-term care will force policy-makers to seriously contemplate alternative management strategies.

CONCLUSION: WHITHER COMMUNITY CARE?

We have argued that community support and care for women living with HIV and AIDS is not a matter of considering hospital-based vs home-based care, but of a political and social obligation to help people manage their life with a chronic, long-term illness. Providing care to women means considering special issues of access and availability in order to ensure that women make use of services to help look after their own needs.

Furthermore, we have argued that the provision of long-term, appropriate and effective services is a matter of sound planning and management of services, particularly of establishing procedures of interagency communication and collaboration. This involves service providers on all levels of organization. It also involves political will to fund and value initiatives which begin to address the association between prevalence of HIV and poverty, marginalization and lack of prospects.

This chapter suggests that general issues in care must be addressed when planning and delivering care and support to women living with HIV and AIDS. Focusing on HIV and special care for women infected should not detract attention from general issues of women and care – its agendas, its organization and financing, and ways in which women's perspectives are incorporated in these processes. HIV infection and AIDS provides a special example of care provision: AIDS has caught the imagination and concern of people to an extent other conditions have not (Frankenberg 1992). AIDS research and care are funded and prioritized. The need for interdisciplinary and intersectorial co-operation is acknowledged (Bennet & Pettigrew 1991). The voluntary sector has been involved in the debate and development of services and has advocated innovation in, and empowerment and user control of service provision (Grimshaw 1990). Providing support for women with HIV infection and AIDS is important in its own right; it may also produce models and examples of service provision for women which are more widely applicable.

ACKNOWLEDGEMENTS

The authors would like to thank Judy Bury for her very constructive comments on an earlier draft of this chapter. We would also like to thank all those providing services in Lothian who agreed to discuss their work with Guro Huby. Finally, we gratefully acknowledge the help from Lindsey Walls in getting the finished manuscripts in the post to the editors.

REFERENCES

Acheson D 1989 AIDS and community care. In: Beardshaw V (ed) AIDS: can we care enough? King's Fund Centre, London

Agarossi A, Muggiasca M L, Ravasi L et al 1992 HIV infection and C.I.N. VIII Int. Conf. on AIDS, Amsterdam. Abstract 3045: B94

Barter G, Mansfield S 1991 Community care of AIDS patients. Matern Child Health 16: 286–288

Beardshaw V, Towell D 1990 Assessment and case management: implications for the implementation of

'Caring for People'. Briefing Paper. King's Fund Institute no 10

Benjamin A 1989 Perspectives on a continuum of care for persons with HIV illnesses. In: LeVee L N (ed) New perspectives on HIV related illnesses: progress in health services research. National Center for Health Services, Rockville, USA

Bennet C, Pettigrew A 1991 Pioneering services for AIDS: the response to HIV infection in four health authorities (final report). Centre for Corporate Strategy and Change, University of Warwick, Warwick

Bury J 1992 Women and AIDS epidemic – some medical facts and figures. In: Bury J et al (eds) Working with women and AIDS: medical, social and counselling issues. Routledge, London

Butler S, Woods M 1992 Drugs, HIV and Ireland: responses to women in Dublin. In: Dorn N, Henderson S, South N (eds) AIDS: women, drugs and social care. Falmer Press, London

Carnegie A, Rutter J 1992 Growing concern. Nursing Times 88: 40–42

Clark R, Dumestre J, Pindaro C et al 1992 Gynecological findings in HIV + women in New Orleans. VIII Int. Conf. on AIDS, Amsterdam. Abstract 3045: B95

Corbin J, Strauss A 1990 Managing chronic illness at home: three lines of work. In: Conrad P, Kem R (eds) The sociology of health & illness: critical perspectives, 3rd edn. St Martin's Press, New York p 122–135

Crystal S, Merzel, C, Kurland, C 1990 Home care of HIV illness. Fam. Commun. Health 13: 29–37

Day S, Ward H, Harris J R W 1988 Prostitute women and public health. Br Med J 297: 1585

Drucker E 1990 Epidemic in the war zone: AIDS and community survival in New York City. Int J Health Serv 20: 601–615

Foster, C 1992 Personal communication

Frankenberg R 1992 The other who is also the same: the relevance of epidemics in space and time for prevention of HIV infection. Int J Health Serv 22: 73–88

Greco D, Declich S, Pezzotti P et al 1991 Hospital use by HIV patients in Italy: a retrospective longitudinal study. J Acq Immune Defic Synd 4: 471–479

Grimshaw J 1990 Introduction. In: Craig M, Hopper C(eds) HIV/AIDS services in the contracts culture. London Voluntary Service Council, London

Ham C 1985 Health policy in Britain 2nd edn. Macmillan, Houndmills

Hepburn M 1992a Pregnancy and HIV: screening, counselling and services. In: Bury J et al (eds) Working with women and AIDS: medical, social and counselling issues. Routledge, London

Hepburn M 1992b Personal communication

Higgins J 1989 Defining community care: realities and myths. Soc Pol Admin 23: 2–16

Hjemmebehandlingsteam for HIV/AIDS pasienter 1991 Statusrapport 1991. Ulleval Sykehus, Ulleval (Norway)

Holland J, Ramazanoglu C, Scott S et al 1990 Sex, gender and power: young women's sexuality in the shadow of AIDS. Social Health Illness 12: 336–350

Hughes S L (1985) Apples and oranges: a critical review of evaluations of community-based long term care. Health Serv Res 20: 461–488

Jackson C 1992 Waiting for the wave to break. Health Visitor 65: 262–263

Johnstone F D, Brettle R P, McCallum L R et al 1990 Women's

knowledge of their HIV antibody state: its effect on whether to continue their pregnancy. Br Med J 300: 23–24

Jones R V H 1992 Teamwork in primary care: how much do we know about it? J Int Professional Care 6: 25–29

King M B 1989 London general practitioners' involvement with HIV infection. J R Coll Gen Pract 39: 280–283

Krueger L E, Wood R W, Diehr P H et al 1990 Poverty and HIV seropositivity: the poor are more likely to be infected. AIDS 4: 811–814

Layzell S, McCarthy M 1992 Community-based health services for people with HIV/AIDS: a review from a health services perspective. AIDS Care 4: 203–215

McCarthy K H, Johnson M A, Norman S G et al 1992 Abnormal cervical cytology and frequency of cervical infections in 35 HIV positive women related to severity of disease. Poster Abstracts VIII Int. Conf. on AIDs/III World Congress Amsterdam. Poster 3045: B96

McKeganey N, Barnard M 1992 AIDS, drugs and sexual risk. Open University Press, Buckingham

Moss A 1992 HIV and AIDS: management by the primary care team. Oxford University Press, Oxford

Murray E 1991 Women: unique HIV transmission risks. Nurs Stand 5: 34–35

Naji S A, Russell I T, Foy G J W, Gallagher M, Rhodes T, Moore M P 1989 HIV infection and Scottish general practice: knowledge and attitudes. J R Coll Gen Pract 39: 284–288

Payne F J, Sharrett C S, Poretz D N et al 1992 Community-based case management of HIV disease. Am J Public Health 82: 893–894

Payne S 1991 Women, health and poverty: an introduction. Harvester, London

Perrow C, Guillén M F 1990 The AIDS disaster. The failure of organisations in New York and the nation. Yale University Press, New Haven

Richardson D 1989 Women and the Aids crisis, 2nd edn. Pandora, London

Scitovsky A A, Cline M W, Abrams D I 1990 Effects of the use of AZT on the medical care costs of persons with AIDS in the first 12 months. J Acq Immune Defic Synd 3: 904–912

Shayne V T, Kaplan B J 1991 Double victims: poor women and AIDS. Women Health 17: 21–37

Slater C 1990 An integrated approach to HIV and AIDS. Practice Nurse 3: 75–78

Smith C, Gibbons C 1990 The role of women in the care of people with HIV/AIDS. Matern Child Health 15: 322–325

Smits A, Mansfield S, Singh S 1990 Facilitating care of patients with HIV infection by hospital and primary care teams. Br Med J 300: 241–243

Sonsel G E, Paradise F, Stroup S 1988 Case management practice in an AIDS service organisation. Soc Casework 69: 388–392

Stoneburner R L, Des Jarlais D C, Benezra D et al 1988 A larger spectrum of severe HIV-1-related disease in intravenous drug users in New York City. Science 242: 916–918

Wilson J 1992a Offering safer sex counselling to women from drug using communities. In: Bury J et al (eds) Working with women and AIDS: medical, social and counselling issues. Routledge, London

Wilson J 1992b Women as carers. In: Bury J et al (eds) Working with women and AIDS: medical, social and counselling issues. Routledge, London

World AIDS News 1992 The Newspaper of the Harvard–Amsterdam Conference, (29 July), Amsterdam

Zwi A B, Cabral A J 1991 Identifying 'high risk situations' for preventing AIDS. Br Med J 303: 1527–1529

11. Drug use in HIV-infected women

Loretta P. Finnegan, Katherine Davenny and Diana Hartel

INTRODUCTION

The field of substance abuse treatment has been severely challenged with the advent of the epidemic of the acquired immune deficiency syndrome (AIDS). The first cases of AIDS reported in the USA in 1981 were noted in homosexual or bisexual men, but soon cases were identified in injecting drug users (Centers for Disease Control 1981, Gottlieb et al 1981, Selik et al 1984). Since the early 1980s, therefore, the evolution of the AIDS epidemic and the dynamics of transmission of human immunodeficiency virus (HIV) have been closely associated with the phenomenon of injection drug use (Selik et al 1984, Haverkos & Edelman 1988, Des Jarlais & Friedman 1988, Brickner et al 1989, Centers for Disease Control 1989b).

Injecting drug users now account for an increasing number of AIDS cases not only in North America, but also in Europe (Moss 1988, Centers for Disease Control 1989b, WHO 1990). In parts of southern Europe and in certain areas in northeastern United States, current or newly reported AIDS cases show that the largest proportion are drug users (Moss 1988, Centers for Disease Control 1989c, WHO 1990, Downs et al 1990; New York City Department of Health 1990, Department of Health New Jersey 1990). HIV infection associated with drug use has now been documented world-wide, including Australia, parts of Latin America, Thailand and Myanmar (formerly Burma) (Wodak et al 1987, Pan American Health Organization 1988, Sato et al 1989, Vanichseni et al 1989, Government of Burma 1990).

AIDS cases associated with injection drug use have been involved in heterosexual and perinatal transmission (Haverkos & Edelman 1988, Centers for Disease Control 1991b). With more than two-thirds of all AIDS cases among women in the United States involving drug-using women or the female sexual partners of male drug users, it is clear that, especially among women, AIDS and drug use are virtually inseparable (Selwyn 1992). Unfortunately, attention to HIV infection in women has lagged behind that given to the disease in men. This may be due to several factors, including the lack of recognition of the disease in women at the outset of the epidemic, the relatively small total number of women with the disease in comparison to men, or because women are politically weaker as a group. In spite of their lower number, the rate of increase in new cases of AIDS among women is higher than among men. AIDS is now the leading cause of death among women 25–44 years of age in New York City (Heagarty & Abrams 1992).

Rosser (1991) has commented on issues of women and AIDS. She states that, in our culture, the institutionalized power, authority and domination of men frequently result in acceptance of the male world view as the norm. AIDS, therefore, represents a prime example of a disease in which women are placed at a disadvantage for diagnosis, treatment and care. Gender differences have been ignored and research on AIDS has concentrated on prostitutes and pregnant women. Rather than studying AIDS in prostitutes in an attempt to understand the manifestations and progression of the disease in women, the focus of these studies has been epidemiology and the heterosexual transmission of AIDS to men (Cohen et al 1988). Comparable discussion about heterosexual transmission to women whose male partners have multiple sexual encounters has not been aired in the literature. Studies demonstrate that the source of AIDS infection for most prostitutes is IV drug use, rather than sexual encounters (Anastos & Marte 1989). Failure to study the impact of the 'crack' epidemic and its associated hypersexuality in crack houses where many women and adolescent girls exchange sex for drugs with men (many of whom may be older IV drug users) will provide incomplete information about heterosexual transmission from men to women. Studies of crack houses using the traditional male world view approach considering women as prostitutes who are only vectors for transmission to men are likely to overlook important information on AIDS and women (Rosser 1991).

Although there is much to learn about drug use and its effects upon women, especially when complicated by HIV infection, this chapter will attempt to delineate the most current information that can be substantiated by the available literature. The sections in this chapter include: HIV infection transmission and the social background of women drug users, the effect of drug use on progression of HIV disease, and the management of drug-dependent women who are HIV-infected.

HIV INFECTION TRANSMISSION AND THE SOCIAL BACKGROUND OF WOMEN DRUG USERS

Despite the fact that most injection drug users are males, the epidemic of HIV among injection drug users in the United States has had a greater relative impact on women compared to men. Over 50% of AIDS cases among women reported to the Centers for Disease Control have been attributed to injection drug use (CDC 1991a). The percentage of AIDS cases among men associated with injection drug use is close to one-half the percentage among women. These reported cases likely underestimate the importance of injection drug use to AIDS among women. In general, AIDS is under-diagnosed in women to a greater degree than among men (Anastos & Marte 1989, Schoenbaum et al 1992). For both men and women, there is under-reporting of injection drug use in medical and other records used for AIDS surveillance (Schoenbaum et al 1992, Hartel et al 1992). In

addition, injection drug users are more likely than any other AIDS risk group to die of non-AIDS causes before reaching an AIDS diagnosis (Guinan & Hardy 1987, Selwyn et al 1988, Hartel et al 1992). All reporting biases associated with injection drug use are likely to have a greater impact on female AIDS cases than on male AIDS cases due to the greater importance of injection drug use to HIV disease among women relative to men.

The second most common risk category for AIDS in women is heterosexual contact with an HIV-infected male; 32% of female AIDS cases are attributed to heterosexual transmission (CDC 1991b). Only 2% of male AIDS cases have been attributed to heterosexual transmission. Overwhelmingly, the cases of heterosexual AIDS in women have been associated with male injection drug users. However, the hierarchical classification system used for surveillance data in the USA and elsewhere obscures the fact that the vast majority of injection drug-using women have more than one risk factor (Moss 1987, Anastos & Marte 1989, Cohen et al 1989). Most female injection drug users are also sex partners of male injection drug users (Cohen et al 1989, Mondanaro 1990).

The AIDS case data described above can only roughly indicate trends in HIV infection transmission for women relative to men. Due to the long latency for HIV infection, a median of 8–11 years from first infection to AIDS diagnosis (Munoz et al 1989), AIDS cases likely result from risk behaviour which occurred, on average, 10 years ago. In recent HIV seroprevalence and seroincidence studies, it has become clear that heterosexual transmission is of increasing importance to the future of the HIV epidemic – even among injection drug users (Thomas et al 1988, Chin 1990, Vlahov et al 1990, Schoenbaum et al 1990, Nicolosi et al 1992). In sexual transmission, however, drug use remains an important risk behaviour. In a wide number of studies, drug use, including alcohol, has been associated with failure to employ safer sex practices by men and women (McCoy & Khoury 1990, Vermund et al 1990, Chiasson et al 1991). In the sections which follow, the extent of different types of HIV risk behaviours and factors which facilitate transmission among drug-using women are assessed.

Needle use

Women at highest risk of HIV are those who share non-sterile injection equipment, especially if there is frequent change in needle-sharing partners or change in needle-sharing networks (Schoenbaum et al 1989b, Cohen et al 1989, Nicolosi et al 1992). However, women use the injection route far less frequently than men, and even fewer share needles in high-risk settings such as shooting galleries (Cohen et al 1989, Kane 1991). Estimates of the numbers of women who are injection drug users are generally deemed unreliable, as are estimates of the injection drug user population as a whole (Spenser 1989, Blower & Hartel 1990). The most recent estimate of 1.8 million injection drug users in the USA was based on several different projection techniques (Office of Technology Assessment 1990). The ratio of women to men injection drug users has been estimated to be 1:3 (Drucker 1986). Female injection drug users may number as many as 500 000 in the United States (Cohen et al 1989; Cohen 1991). Injection drug users represent the most extreme end of the spectrum of women who are dependent on pyschoactive drugs (Worth 1991). Despite the high numbers of estimated injection drug users, the percentage of the population which employs this method is relatively small: under 1% of the general population.

The majority of women who inject drugs are also sexual partners of men who inject drugs; 50–80% of female sex partners of male injecting drug users, however, do not inject drugs (Cohen et al 1989, Mondanaro 1990). Typically, women are introduced into injection drug use by male partners, resulting in a life of prostitution to support their drug habit and, most often, that of their sex partner (Wofsy 1992). More recently, women have reported initiating each other into drug use, including injection techniques (Worth et al 1989). Heroin is the most common drug injected among both male and female injecting drug users not enrolled in drug treatment in the USA. In a sample of 5232 injection drug-using women enrolled in the National AIDS Demonstration Research Project, only 21% injected drugs other than heroin or heroin in combination with cocaine (speedball) (Weissman 1991b, 1991c). Women in this study as in others (Kane 1991) were more likely than

men to share needles within small groups or with sex partners only.

Most studies indicate that intravenous drug users are more likely to change injection behaviour than sexual risk behaviour (Sasse et al 1989, Robert et al 1990). Over time, lower levels of needle-sharing and greater practice of needle hygiene have been reported in several studies (Vermund et al 1990). A recent investigation of new recruits into injection drug use reports a high degree of safer needle practices than was the case before the AIDS epidemic (Vlahov et al 1991). Continued reduction of high-risk needle use, however, requires long-term public health educational programmes plus provision of accessible, acceptable and effective drug addiction treatment. Women, who tend to be under-enrolled in drug treatment and tend to drop out once enrolled to a higher degree than men, require programmes which are tailored to their specific needs (Mondanaro 1989, 1990; Finnegan et al 1991, Finnegan 1991b, 1991c). (See sections below on barriers to risk reduction and also on management of HIV-infected women.)

Sexual risk

Increasingly, for all drug-using women including women who inject drugs, heterosexual risk behaviour is the most important mode of HIV infection acquisition (Moss 1987, Schoenbaum et al 1989b, Nicolosi et al 1992). While there appears to be no gender difference in the risk of acquiring HIV infection through needle-sharing (Hahn et al 1989), women who are injection drug users have a higher overall infection risk than men who are injectors (Vlahov et al 1990). There are several factors which may underlie these observations. There has been widespread reduction in high-risk needle use (Vermund et al 1990, Ickovics & Rodin 1991). There may be greater use of condoms among males compared to females (Catania et al 1992). In addition, the natural transmission dynamics of the HIV epidemic have resulted in removal of the highest risk needle-using individuals, primarily males, through disease and death (Blower et al 1991).

In general, heterosexual transmission risks are greater for women than for men. In industrialized countries, HIV transmission appears to be more efficient from an infected male to an uninfected female than the reverse (Haverkos & Edelman 1988, Handsfield 1988, European Study Group 1989). There is considerable controversy regarding the magnitude of gender-based differences in transmission efficiency (Haverkos et al 1992) and factors accounting for such differences. HIV is likely to be more concentrated in semen than in vaginal secretions. In addition, the female genital tract is conducive to passage of virions through tissue to CD4 + cell receptors (Ickovics & Rodin 1991). Other factors include undiagnosed sexually transmitted infections, especially ulcerative processes such as syphilis and chancroid (Holmes & Kreiss 1988, Johnson & Laga 1988, Holmberg et al 1989, Vermund et al 1990, Holmes et al 1990, Nelson et al 1991). While most sexually transmitted diseases are not gender–specific, women are more likely to have undiagnosed and untreated conditions. Oral contraceptives are associated with cervical fragility and may be a transmission cofactor as well. There are other hypothesized cofactors currently under investigation which may contribute to gender differences in sexual transmission of HIV, including viral antigenic variations and altered immune function (Vermund et al 1990).

Heterosexual transmission studies often suffer from methodological problems, particularly an inability to measure cofactors accurately. In many studies, there is no ability to distinguish behaviour which occurs just prior to infection from that which occurs after infection. Mathematical modelling studies have been useful in identifying factors which may be crucial to HIV infection transmission dynamics (Blower & Medley 1991). These studies indicate that female predominance in heterosexually acquired HIV late in the epidemic may be attributed, in part, to differences in sexual partner mixing patterns (Blower et al 1991; LePont & Blower 1991). Women are more likely than men to encounter an infected injection drug-using sex partner due to the larger numbers of male injection drug users infected early in the epidemic.

Women who associate with injection drug users are also more likely than other women to engage in high-risk sexual behaviour (e.g. frequent partner change, unprotected vaginal or anal intercourse) (Donoghoe et al 1989). A great deal of attention has been devoted to women with the most extreme numbers of sex partners – prostitutes. While at any given time the majority of drug-using women are in long-term partnerships or married (including common-law marriage), many must engage in sex work or practice survival sex (sex in exchange for rent or food) (Wofsy 1992). Since the late 1980s, there have been many reports of sex risk associated with crack/cocaine among prostitutes – the high numbers of partners, the decreased vigilance regarding safer sex practices, and the desperate circumstances of women who use crack/cocaine heavily (Worth, 1989, Chiasson et al 1991). Some women have reported higher pay for unprotected vaginal intercourse. For most prostitutes, previous needle use is likely the primary risk factor but it is highly correlated with the number of sex partners. (Schoenbaum et al 1989a, Wofsy 1992). Moreover, prostitutes are much more likely to require condoms or use other safer sex practices with their clients than they and nearly all women do with their primary sexual partners.

While the problems of sex workers are important, they have received disproportionate attention from researchers and the media (Treichler 1988). The net result has been an HIV risk prevention message for women to reduce the numbers of sex partners. However, the literature on heterosexual transmission has not clearly indicted frequent partner change as a central feature of high risk behaviour (Vermund et al 1991). The greatest infection risk for all women appears to be repeated unprotected sex with an infected steady sex partner, especially an injection drug user. In data collected among drug users, non-drug users and sex partners of drug users, condom use was primarily reported for casual sex partners only but rarely with primary sex partners (Weissman 1991a, 1991b, 1991c; Centers for Disease Control 1991b, Catania et al 1992).

Barriers to reduction of sexual risk behaviour and treatment access

In data from a national probability sample of heterosexuals, men were more likely than women to report safer sex practices (Catania et al 1992). For all women, whether they sell sex for drugs or have a single primary sex partner, the overwhelming problem in reduction in sexual risk of HIV is male control over safer sex practices such as condoms. There is an extremely limited interpersonal forum between most men and women for discussing or negotiating safer sex (Worth 1989, Kane 1990, Stein 1990, Cohen 1991). Initiation of condom use into heterosexual relationships often places unrealistic pressures on women to assert themselves in a situation in which they frequently have little power. In addition, a woman's request to use condoms may be tantamount to an accusation of infidelity on the part of the male partner (Cohen 1991).

There are sometimes serious consequences to discussing safer sex and HIV risk with male sex partners. Dissolution of the partnership and, in some cases, a violent assault on the woman may result (Amaro et al 1990). For many women, fear of violence or abandonment ensures their silence (Warren 1992). Few HIV prevention programmes are prepared to deal with the unique problems of women substance users, as many as 75% of whom have experienced abuse in childhood and/or adulthood (Bollerud 1990). HIV prevention programmes which are specifically designed for women who are drug users and partners of drug users are relatively recent. In these programmes, male domination of sexual roles and the potential for violence have emerged as the greatest barriers to HIV risk reduction (Cohen et al 1992, Brown et al 1992). For drug-using women, a history of childhood abuse, particularly sexual abuse, is common (Leach 1990). Such histories have been hypothesized to be important to initiation and maintenance of substance abuse problems, as well as contributing to a tendency to remain in abusive relationships (Mondanaro 1989, 1990). Intervention is particularly difficult if substance abuse is a means to alleviate psychological distress associated with childhood abuse.

The literature on violence toward women and methods of dealing with potentially violent partners is relatively recent. As information has accrued, it has become obvious that the problem is pervasive, occurring in nearly all social classes and cultures (Klein 1981). McKinnon (1989) views rape and other violent acts toward women as 'indigenous to women's social condition', anal-

ogous to lynching of African-American males when racism was at its peak. In the USA, the numbers of women battered each year are estimated to range from 1.6 million to 12 million. Data indicate that between 21 and 30% of the population of adult women have been assaulted by a sex partner at least once (Helton et al 1987). Pregnancy is an especially high risk period for assault (Surgeon General 1988), with injuries directed to the abdomen, breast and genitals (Helton et al 1987). There is gross under-detection of episodes of battering (Briere & Zaidi 1989, Randall 1990, Guinan 1990, Harlow 1991) although there has been a move toward education of emergency care clinicians to identify and refer these women to counselling and other needed services (McLeer & Anwar 1989, McIlwaine 1989, Randall 1990, Guinan 1990). In general, the consequences of violence are more severe among those with limited resources, as women do not have access to alternative housing or sources of sustenance and cannot readily escape a violent partner (Amaro et al 1990).

All of the above problems may be exacerbated by psychoactive substance use. Women are more likely to be attacked while one or both partners are under the influence of psychoactive substances – most commonly, alcohol (Kantor & Straus 1989, Amaro et al 1990). In a large-scale study of non-injecting women sex partners of injection drug users, only 16% had *not used drugs* within 6 months of interview (Weissman 1991a, 1991b, 1991c). Women who regularly abuse drugs are likely to view HIV infection risk as a low priority relative to drug procurement, daily subsistence, and the needs of their sexual partners – most often themselves chemically dependent. The majority of women drug users are likely to be isolated, clinically depressed, and in a dysfunctional relationship (Brown et al 1992). For many women, the psychoactive effects of drugs, particularly cocaine and alcohol, are known to increase HIV sexual risk behaviour through disinhibition, life-style destabilization or impairment of judgement (Gawin & Ellinwood 1988, McCoy & Khoury 1990, Chiasson et al 1991).

Most programmes which deliver substance abuse treatment are prime examples of the failure to recognize the status of women with its associated violence as an underlying issue in treatment. Aggressive, male-centred techniques are commonly employed in drug treatment; these methods are not effective for women, especially for those with a history of physical abuse (Mondanaro 1989, 1990). In many instances women are placed in group counselling sessions with males who have a history of attacking their own sexual partners. There is little chance of examination of early childhood abuse history or for improving the mental health of abused women in such settings. For most chemically-dependent women, early programme dropout is typical. Model programmes are currently under development which directly address problems of abuse and lack of empowerment of women as a fundamental step in drug treatment (Mondanaro 1989, 1990; Bollerud 1990, Weissman 1991b, 1991c; see section on care of HIV-infected women).

Male sex partners may indirectly obstruct health care access for HIV-positive, drug-using women. Disclosure of HIV status and risk history to male sex partners is often a necessary first step to obtaining medical treatment for HIV infection (Hartel 1992). For many women, disclosure of HIV status is perceived as so dangerous that it is delayed until serious manifestations of HIV disease appear (Lang 1991, Hartel 1992, Perkins et al 1992). Ethical–legal debates on HIV partner notification have recently recognized the importance of violence toward women as an outcome of notification of HIV infection status (North & Rothenberg 1990, Rothenberg 1991). Partner notification programmes must be cognizant of the possibility of placing a woman in danger of a violent attack as a result of notification.

EFFECT OF DRUG USE ON HIV PROGRESSION

Early in the HIV epidemic in injecting drug users it was recognized that drug injection might influence the progression of HIV disease, either by increased vulnerability of the immune system to HIV infection or by alterations to the immune system subsequent to HIV infection which would potentiate or accelerate the disease process. It has long been known that injecting drug users are prone to other infectious disease processes, and that drug users have high background levels of infections such as bacterial pneumonia, tuberculosis and hepatitis. It is also well-established that immune dysfunction is associated with drug use. The potential impact of drug injection on the immune system involves the effects of using preparations and equipment which are unsterile and/or contaminated with allogeneic blood, the effects of drug preparations contaminated with adulterants, and the effects of immunomodulation more directly due to the illicit drug compounds themselves. With the advent of the HIV epidemic in injecting drug users it was hypothesized that drug injection would heighten the risk of immunosuppression characteristic of HIV (Zagury et al 1986, Des Jarlais et al 1987), speeding progression to AIDS.

As has been pointed out by others (Hankins & Handley 1992), much of the published research on development of HIV disease and risk factors for progression has been performed in large cohorts of homosexual men. In contrast to homosexual men, knowledge of the natural history of HIV in injecting drug users is less well characterized. Most HIV, drug use and disease progression studies are occurring in mixed cohorts of male and female in-treatment injecting drug users, and thus far there has been little focus on gender differences except as they relate to pregnancy. Those studies which have focused on HIV in drug-using women in relation to pregnancy have directed attention towards the risks of drug use as they relate to maternal–infant transmission. Virtually no published research is available which has assessed gender differences as they may relate to the impact of drug use and HIV on immunopathology and consequent HIV disease development in women. The key factors of HIV disease in women who are drug users have not yet been well determined (Hankins & Handley 1992). Such factors may include gender-specific disease manifestations or gender-specific factors which determine the progression of HIV disease. Other factors might differentially affect survival of HIV-infected women who use drugs. Neuroendocrine and immune system interactions may influence women's vulnerability to drug immunomodulation and hence to specific disease entities such as HIV. Only recently has a concerted effort been undertaken to investigate gender differences of HIV in women, with particular effort directed at those who are drug users.

No studies of HIV in drug users have definitively answered questions related to the impact of drugs and drug-using behaviours on progression of HIV disease. Information can be extrapolated from prospective studies of HIV in injecting drug users, comparisons of HIV disease progression in homosexual men with disease progression in drug users, comparative studies of immune parameters in healthy controls with HIV-seronegative and -seropositive drug users, animal models of the impact of drugs on the immune system, and in vitro studies of immunomodulation by drugs. In general, clinical studies of injecting drug users have been deficient in providing more definitive answers regarding drug use, immune function and disease, in part due to the extraordinary logistical and methodological difficulties inherent in studying this population. As has been pointed out by Kreek (1990), to understand the direct and indirect effects of drugs on the immune system requires rigorous clinical studies of drug users which control for a complicated set of variables, including those related to treatment history (e.g. status, treatment variation in drug treatment settings, treatment dose and duration of treatment), drug use history (e.g. duration and frequency of drug use, injection frequency, polydrug use, verification of self-report), and medical history (e.g. the presence of chronic infection and measures of immune status).

Studies of drugs, HIV and the immune system

Studies of immune parameters in drug users prior to the HIV epidemic had accumulated evidence of abnormalities in both cellular and humoral immunity in association with active drug use, particularly as these issues related to heroin use. In the last decade, studies of cocaine have also been undertaken. While results from this accumulated research have left many unanswered questions regarding the effects of drug use on the immune system, they have provided a base from which to investigate the role of drug use in the development of HIV disease.

The early observations of abnormalities in the immune system were thought to be related to the high background levels of bacterial and viral infections, particularly viral hepatitis, common to chronic drug users, as well as to the consequences of repeated antigenic stimulation of the immune system via adulterated and contaminated drug injections (Brown et al 1974, Kreek et al 1972). Assessment of the impact of drug use has also been complicated by polydrug use, which often includes such drugs as marijuana and alcohol which are known to suppress immune function.

Studies of the reactivity of sera from heroin users early on identified various serological abnormalities. Heroin users were found to have a higher than normal proportion of biological false-positive tests for syphilis (Cherubin & Millian 1968). Researchers also observed differences in immune parameters between street injecting drug users and those receiving methadone treatment. Elevated IgM was observed in untreated heroin users (Nickerson et al 1970, Grieco & Chuang 1973), while studies of methadone-maintained heroin users found increased levels of IgG and diminished levels of IgM during methadone treatment (Cushman & Grieco 1973), further complicating use of syphilis serology. Defects were also observed in cellular immunity, including abnormal T-lymphocyte rosetting and diminished reactivity of cultured lymphocytes to mitogen stimulation (Brown et al 1974). Abnormal proportions, both increased and decreased, of circulating B lymphocytes, and diminished T lymphocyte subpopulations were observed in methadone-maintained heroin users (Cushman et al 1977). Studies of peripheral blood lymphocytes from street opiate users also found a significant depression in the absolute number of total T lymphocytes, without significant alterations in the absolute number of B lymphocytes or total white blood count (McDonough et al 1980). Lymphocytosis (Kreek et al 1972) and increased expression of the CD4+ receptor (Donahoe et al 1986) have also been observed in injecting drug users. Identification of opiate-binding sites on T lymphocytes (McDonough et al 1980, Madden et al 1987) has established both direct and indirect routes for potential immunomodulation in drug users, as well as a basis for a more direct interaction between HIV and opiates (Donahoe 1990). Recent in vitro studies of both cocaine and morphine in human peripheral blood mononuclear cells have shown that these agents can affect the growth of HIV (Peterson et al 1990, Peterson et al 1991). These studies provided in vitro evidence that morphine and cocaine may act as cofactors in HIV pathogenesis. Morphine was observed to stimulate the growth of HIV in co-culture in a dose–response relationship, suggesting that morphine may promote the growth of HIV by triggering an opiate receptor which stimulates production of cytokines, thus promoting replication of HIV; alternatively, morphine may suppress production of HIV inhibitory cytokines (Peterson et al 1990). Cocaine has been found to potentiate the replication of HIV in human peripheral blood monocyte co-cultures through a mechanism which is thought to involve stimulation of transforming growth factor β (Peterson et al 1991).

More recently, population-based data have become available from studies which have assessed immune parameters in injecting drug users with known HIV serostatus. Comparisons of several immune parameters from HIV-infected and uninfected injecting drug users (Zolla-Pazner et al 1987) showed significant differences in HIV-seronegative values as compared with values from a normal blood donor population. In this study, which did not assess the impact of specific drug-use variables on the immune parameters being measured, HIV-seronegative drug users had lower mean CD4/CD8 ratios (due mainly to an increase in CD8 + cells), elevated mean IgG, IgA, and IgM; and elevated mean serum β2 microglobulin levels compared with normal values. A cross-sectional study of HIV seropositive and seronegative injecting drug users investigating the impact of drug use on immune parameters (Mientjes et al 1991) assessed injection frequency relative to total numbers of lymphocytes and total numbers of T lymphocyte subpopulations, as well as T lymphocyte reactivity. Based on self-reported drug use behaviours in the 4–6 months preceding laboratory assays, neither drug type (mainly methadone, cocaine, heroin, or cocaine/heroin) nor frequency of injection was found to affect results of quantitative assays of lymphocytes or lymphocyte subsets in drug users. However, functional assays indicated diminished reactivity: the lymphoproliferative response to anti-CD3 monoclonal

antibody was significantly diminished in frequent injectors, regardless of HIV status. The response to stimulation was noticeably diminished in those whose injection frequency was $\geqq 50$ times per month. The mean response to anti-CD3 monoclonal antibody in HIV-seronegative non-injectors was found to be comparable to that in healthy uninfected homosexual men. In HIV-seronegatives, T cell reactivity declined as injection frequency increased. T lymphocyte reactivity was 40–50% lower in both HIV-infected and uninfected users who had injected a mean of three times per day in the preceding 4–6 months, compared with those who had not injected. Except for higher mean CD4 + cells in women, there was no correlation of gender with any other immune parameter. A history of bacterial infection in the prior 4–6 months did not affect values of any of the immune parameters studied. Age > 30 years was associated only with lower mean CD4 + cells in HIV-seropositives.

Studies of these indicators in injecting drug users with and without HIV infection provide presumptive evidence for some impact of chronic drug use and frequent injection on the immune system, without necessarily suggesting a more direct effect of specific drugs on the immune system. However, while abnormalities in baseline immune parameters in injecting drug users may increase vulnerability to HIV infection, they may not measurably affect progression to disease once infection is established.

Studies of HIV disease progression in injecting drug users

Sources for prospective data regarding the impact of injection drug use on HIV disease progression are sparse, and come mainly from a few prospective studies of HIV in cohorts of injecting drug users. Cross-comparisons among these studies are complicated by differences in study protocols and methodologies, measurement, unstandardized drug and behavioural variables, validation of self-report, as well as by potential background confounders such as gender, race/ethnicity, and provision of health care. Definitive results are slowed by problems of relatively small numbers in individual studies and the long duration of study time necessary to measure time-dependent events. Studies which have analysed data regarding drug use and its association with risk of progression of HIV disease have varied in methods of analysis and length of observation. Stratification by detailed drug use variables is often not possible given small study samples.

In published prospective studies the most powerful predictor of HIV disease progression in injecting drug users is absolute number of CD4+ cells (Des Jarlais et al 1987, Fernandez-Cruz et al 1990, Italian Seroconversion Study 1992, Margolick et al 1992, Munoz et al 1992, Selwyn et al 1992). The presence of p24 antigenaemia, proportion of CD4+, elevated serum neopterin, low response to pokeweed mitogen, two or more constitutional symptoms, pyogenic bacterial infections, pulmonary tuberculosis, oral candidiasis, and older age, have also been associated with risk of disease progression and AIDS in various studies (Fernandez-Cruz et al 1988, Italian Seroconversion Study 1992, Munoz et al 1992, Selwyn et al 1992). In contrast to studies in homosexual men, serum β 2 microglobulin, a marker of immune activation, has not been found to be a strong predictor of progression in drug injectors (Fernandez-Cruz et al 1990, Munoz et al 1992, Selwyn et al 1992), most likely due to the high background levels observed in HIV-seronegative injectors due to chronic liver disease and/or chronic antigenic stimulation. To date, gender differences in rates of disease progression have not been observed (Munoz et al 1992, Selwyn et al 1992). Generally, studies have observed progression of disease rates similar to those rates derived from studies of homosexual men (Rezza et al 1989, 1990, Munoz et al 1991, Margolick 1992, Selwyn et al 1992). An early study of New York City HIV-infected injecting drug users indicated that those who reduced or ceased drug use were less likely to manifest signs of disease progression (Des Jarlais et al 1987). Injecting drug users from methadone treatment and drug detoxification programmes were followed for a mean of 9 months. Those who did not develop AIDS demonstrated statistically significant declines in total lymphocytes, CD4+ and CD8+ cells and B cells, as well as significantly elevated IgG. Analysis of the effect of drug injection on CD4+ cell decline

indicated a combined effect of continued and prior drug injection. Of variables which were potential cofactors for disease progression, such as alcohol and marijuana, methadone, and age, only drug injection remained a significant predictor of CD4+ count in HIV-seropositives. There was no effect related to cocaine or heroin as the main drug of choice. These findings were similar in part to data from Scotland which showed that clinical progression did not differ by whether or not drug use continued, but those who continued injecting had a steeper decline in CD4+ cells (Brettle et al 1989). However, in a Bronx, NY study of former and continuing injectors no difference was observed in the rate of CD4+ decline by injection status (Schoenbaum et al 1989a). More recent studies with longer observation time have not confirmed this association. No significant association of injection with risk of progression to AIDS was observed in two large cohort studies with many months of observation (Munoz et al 1992, Selwyn et al 1992). In these two studies, clinical events and CD4+ cell counts were the only independent predictors of progression. A study in Italy which enrolled both homosexual men and injecting drug users compared the risk of developing AIDS in seroconverters from these two groups, in an attempt to determine whether continued drug injection was associated with a higher incidence rate of AIDS (Rezza et al 1990). The risk of developing AIDS 4 years after seroconversion was not significantly different in the two groups: 14% in intravenous drug users and 16% in homosexual males. After 2 and 3 years post-seroconversion, similar proportions of intravenous drug users and homosexual men remained AIDS-free. In addition, the risk of AIDS increased significantly in both groups after 24 months post-seroconversion. A broad-based study to evaluate HIV disease in women receiving adequate primary care compared the rate of decline in CD4+ cells in those classified as heterosexual partners of injecting drug users with those having a history of drug injection. Although the observation period for this study was insufficient to definitively determine whether there was differential disease progression relative to infection risk group, results from 20 months of follow-up demonstrated no significant difference in the rates of decline of CD4+ cells when stratified by risk group (Carpenter et al 1991).

A study of drug use as a potential cofactor was performed in a multicentre cohort of HIV-infected and uninfected homosexual and bisexual men. No evidence for accelerated immuno-deficiency was observed in HIV-infected men who used alcohol, marijuana, cocaine, and opiates prior to study enrollment or among those who continued to use drugs over 18 months (Kaslow et al 1989). No increased risk for developing AIDS was observed in those who had used drugs within 2 years of study entry, or in those who continued to use drugs during the study period. There was no increased risk of AIDS associated with increased frequency of drug use, nor was there a significant difference in the risk of AIDS between injectors and non-injectors. When stratified by low CD4+ cell counts, no significant association was found for alcohol or drug use and the development of AIDS. Similarly, no significant differences in risk were observed in HIV-related manifestations or in the decline of CD4+ cells over 18 months, and continued drug or alcohol use was not associated with a greater mean decline in CD4+ cells.

While these results have implications for the impact of drug use in the presence of HIV infection, research issues specific to injecting drug users remain to be addressed, and the consequences of HIV infection in conjunction with long-term, chronic drug abuse and its sequelae remain to be clearly defined. As there continues to be concern among clinicians regarding drug use and acceleration of HIV disease, the evidence to date, albeit sparse, does not so far indicate a significantly increased risk of disease progression. Treatment of substance abuse and its attendant social and health problems remains critical to prevention of HIV infection and to the management of HIV disease in drug-using women.

MANAGEMENT OF DRUG-DEPENDENT WOMEN WHO ARE HIV-INFECTED

Many concerns and limitations exist within the available research relating to HIV infection in drug-using women; however, it is evident that, if these women are to receive appropriate services, the clinician must be knowledgeable in four inter-connected areas. These include:

- Drug abuse-related medical problems
- HIV-related medical problems
- Psychiatric disorders associated with drug abuse and HIV infection
- Drug abuse treatment issues.

Medical complications related to drug abuse and to HIV infection

The clinician involved in the care of the HIV-infected drug user must attempt to distinguish between the manifestations of HIV infection and the effects of drug use and its acute and chronic sequelae. Certain infectious diseases commonly seen among injecting drug users may be more frequent or severe in the setting of HIV infection. Infectious complications of injection drug use may be mistaken for manifestations of HIV infection and vice versa. The possibility of coexisting morbidity from HIV disease and the medical complications of drug use is an ever-present consideration.

Concomitant with infectious complications and other related syndromes, a number of constitutional symptoms often seen in HIV-infected patients can overlap with symptoms due to acute or chronic drug use, and the physician must differentiate between the symptomatology of drug use or withdrawal and that of HIV. Symptoms of HIV, for example, can include fever, weight loss, fatigue, malaise and diarrhoea (Centers for Disease Control 1986), and several of these symptoms meet the diagnostic criteria for HIV-related wasting syndrome (Centers for Disease Control 1987a). However, among active injecting drug users, fever, fatigue, malaise and diarrhoea are not uncommon. Weight loss is also a common finding among street addicts, especially among cocaine users in whom anorexia and a hypermetabolic state are related directly to the pharmacological effects of the drug (Sapira 1968; Jaffe 1990). Smoked freebase cocaine or crack use has been associated with pulmonary oedema, barotrauma, bronchospasm and other pulmonary manifestations (Kissner et al 1987, Leitman et al 1988,

Hoffman & Goodman 1989) and dyspnoea on exertion or at rest is often reported by such patients. Dyspnoea without a productive cough or other obvious signs of pneumonia is one of the most common symptoms in the onset of *Pneumocystis carinii* pneumonia in HIV-infected patients (Glatt & Chirgwin 1990). Crack use is frequently associated with heavy cigarette smoking which may present similar symptoms. Patients and clinicians may often mistakenly attribute cough or dyspnoea simply to excessive smoking (especially in the absence of fever or other signs of pneumonia), when in fact these symptoms may indicate the gradual onset of *P. carinii* pneumonia. The presence of generalized lymphadenopathy, often found in HIV-infected patients, may at times be confused with the finding of multiple palpable lymph nodes due to lymphatic drainage from sites of drug injection, localized soft tissue infection, oral pathology or other conditions commonly seen in injecting drug users (Sapira 1968, Centers for Disease Control 1986). Therefore, among drug users, the sites most specific for HIV-related lymphadenopathy are the posterior cervical chains, which in the absence of scalp lesions, are sites least likely to reflect lymph node enlargement due merely to local skin and soft tissue pathology.

Table 11.1 lists the medical complications seen in intravenous drug users (Novick 1992). The specific treatment of each one of these entities is beyond the scope of this publication. Additionally, medical complications particularly associated with cocaine use are listed in Table 11.2. Some of the medical complications will be highlighted and these include: bacterial infections, tuberculosis, sexually transmitted diseases, hepatitis B, neurological manifestations and malignancies.

The most common complications seen in drug users with HIV infection are serious bacterial infections, especially bacterial pneumonia, endocarditis and bacterial sepsis. It has been suggested that bacterial infections not only occur more commonly in HIV-infected drug users than in their HIV-seronegative counterparts, but also that they may be more severe, with higher case fatality rates and more lengthy hospitalizations (Selwyn et al 1988). In one New York study, the HIV-seropositive group showed a fourfold increased risk of bacterial pneumonia, compared with the serone-

Table 11.1 Medical complications of intravenous drug users

Cardiovascular	*Neuromuscular*
Arrhythmia	Stroke
Mycotic aneurysm	Brain abscess
Thrombophlebitis	Epidural or subdural abscess
	Anoxic encephalopathy
Gastrointestinal	Peripheral neuropathy
Constipation	Horner's syndrome
Diarrhoea	Mytosis
Hepatic	*Pulmonary*
Acute and chronic hepatitis	Pulmonary oedema
Cirrhosis	Pneumothorax
	Pneumomediastinum
Infections	
Bacterial endocarditis	*Renal*
Pneumonia	Glomerulonephritis
Cellulitis	Renal failure
Cutaneous abscesses	
Osteomyelitis	*Miscellaneous*
Septic arthritis	Anaemia
Sexually transmitted diseases	Overdose
Tuberculosis	Allergic reaction
Tetanus	Pyrogenic reaction
HIV infection	Trauma
HTLV-I/HTLV-II infection	Needle embolus
Hepatitis A, B, C and D	Amenorrhoea
viruses	Hormonal abnormalities
	Thrombocytopenia
Immunological	
Generalized	
lymphadenopathy	
Elevated serum	
immunoglobulins	
False-positive serologic tests	
Lymphocytosis	
Increased lymphocyte subset	
cell numbers	
Reduced responsiveness of	
lymphocytes to mitogens	
Reduced natural killer cell	
activity	

Adapted from Novick D M 1992 In Lowinson J, Ruiz J, Millman R (eds) Substance abuse: a comprehensive textbook, 2nd edn. Williams and Wilkins, Baltimore, MD, p 657–674

gative group (Selwyn et al 1988). The predominant pathogenic organisms identified have been encapsulated bacteria, such as *Streptococcus pneumoniae* and *Hemophilus influenzae*. Most theories indicate that pneumococcal pneumonia is one of the most common entities seen in HIV-seropositive patients with bacterial infections (Simberkoff et al 1984, Polsky et al 1986, Witt et al 1987, Schrager 1988, Selwyn et al 1988, Gilks et al 1990). Therefore, it has been suggested that pneumococcal polysaccharide vaccine be considered for drug users and other individuals with HIV infection.

Table 11.2 Medical complications seen in cocaine abusers

Cardiovascular	*Pulmonary*
Myocardial infarction	Decreased diffusing capacity
Arrhythmia	Pneumomediastinum
Aortic rupture	Pulmonary oedema
Hypertension	
Cardiomyopathy	
Gastrointestinal	*Miscellaneous*
Intestinal ischaemia	Acute hepatic necrosis
Colitis	Hyperpyrexia
	Loss of sense of smell
Neurologic	Perforated nasal septum
Stroke	Loss of eyebrows, eyelashes
Subarachnoid haemorrhage	Sexual dysfunction
Seizures	Motor vehicle accidents
Fungal meningitis	Trauma
Headache	Sudden death
	Endocarditis
Psychiatric	HIV infection
Psychosis	
Depression	
Personality changes	
Delusions of parasitosis	

Adapted from Novick D M 1992 In: Lowinson J, Ruiz J, Millman R (eds) Substance abuse: a comprehensive textbook, 2nd edn. Williams and Wilkins, Baltimore, MD, p 657–674

Another important condition that has been noted among HIV-infected populations is tuberculosis. It has been suggested that pulmonary tuberculosis, like bacterial pneumonia, may be more likely to occur prior to an AIDS-defining illness in HIV-infected patients, since *Mycobacterium tuberculosis* is an organism that is comparatively more virulent than those causing the major AIDS-defining opportunistic infections, and indeed affects individuals with normal immune systems as well (Louie et al 1986, Selwyn & Iezza 1990, Theuer et al 1990).

In the USA, tuberculosis in HIV-infected patients is concentrated primarily among injecting drug users and minority populations (Sunderam et al 1986, Centers for Disease Control 1987b, 1989a, Selwyn et al 1989b, Theuer et al 1990). The association between the two infections has been shown most strikingly in certain cities in the northeastern and southeastern United States, where HIV seroprevalence studies have found HIV infection as high as 40% among patients treated at tuberculosis clinics (Centers for Disease Control 1989a). It should be noted that tuberculosis has been a common condition among drug users even before the AIDS epidemic (Reichman et al 1979).

Specifics with regard to the diagnosis and treatment of tuberculosis are well detailed in other publications (Selwyn 1992). Isoniazid prophylaxis is recommended in all patients with HIV infection and a positive turberculin skin test. HIV-infected, tuberculin-negative patients should have a three-antigen panel applied to test for the presence of anergy (Selwyn 1992). Multidrug chemotherapy can be given effectively to those in whom the diagnosis is strongly suspected. Good compliance with therapy is possible to maintain within the setting of drug treatment programmes, particularly in the situation of methadone maintenance, where the tuberculosis medications can be given along with the patient's daily methadone doses (Reichman et al 1979, Selwyn et al 1989b).

Injecting drug users historically have been found to be at increased risk of sexually transmitted diseases, presumably related both to sexual behaviours associated with drug use and to engagement in prostitution as a means of supporting the cost of addiction (Sapira 1968, Stoffer 1968). It has been reported in several studies that, under certain circumstances, drug users have adopted safer drug-using practices in order to reduce the risk of HIV transmission. Generally, such changes have not been noted in their sexual behaviour (Des Jarlais & Friedman 1987, 1988; Office of Technology Assessment 1988). Moreover, the recently described relationship between cocaine use and sexually transmitted diseases – either through a drug-specific disinhibition of sexual behaviour or the more formal exchange of sex for money or drugs – underscores the importance of addressing sexually transmitted diseases in the care of drug users with, or at-risk for, HIV infection (Stall et al 1986, Coates et al 1988, Goldsmith 1988, Guydish & Coates 1988, Centers for Disease Control 1988, Cates 1990, Fullilove et al 1990, Rolfs et al 1990).

Initial assessment of drug-using patients with known or suspected HIV infection should include a thorough history regarding other sexually transmitted diseases. Some of the more commonly seen are herpes simplex, syphilis and human papillomavirus (HPV) infection (Greenspan et al 1988, Byrne et al 1989, Henry et al 1989, Feingold et al 1990, Friedman 1989). Herpes simplex and syphilis in the presence of HIV infection may be more severe, more difficult to treat, and possibly accelerated in their courses. HPV may cause extensive or recurring genital or oral warts that may be difficult to treat. Moreover, HPV infection has been strongly linked with an increased risk of cervical cytologic abnormalities in HIV-infected women, including dysplasia and frank carcinoma (Byrne et al 1989, Henry et al 1989, Friedmann et al 1990, Feingold et al 1990). The degree of malignant cytologic change appears to increase as women become more immunosuppressed in the course of HIV infection (Friedmann et al 1990, Feingold et al 1990).

Although it has been suggested that HIV-infected women may be at increased risk of severe or refractory pelvic inflammatory disease, no prospective studies have addressed this. However this diagnosis should be considered in drug-using women presenting with abdominal pain, especially in patients who are known to be at high risk for sexually transmitted diseases (Kloser et al 1988, Chu et al 1990, Hoegsberg et al 1990).

An important challenge for clinicians who deal with drug users with HIV infection is the distinction between HIV-associated neurological disease and that which results from acute or chronic substance abuse and its effects on the nervous system. This distinction is particularly important since many of the neurological syndromes seen in HIV-infected patients may be treatable, but successful treatment depends on an accurate identification and differentiation of both the underlying and immediate problems. Clinicians in drug treatment settings who are unfamiliar with HIV disease may assume that a patient's cognitive or behavioural disturbances reflect a resumption of alcohol or drug use behaviour, when in fact these findings may indicate a central nervous system (CNS) opportunistic infection or HIV-dementia or encephalopathy. On the contrary, clinicians in AIDS treatment units may respond to a patient who develops lethargy, dysarthria, and pin-point pupils by performing an emergency computerized tomographic brain scan and lumbar puncture, when a simple urine toxicology would have detected evidence of illicit opiate use. The most important CNS manifestation of HIV infection is the entity called AIDS dementia complex, also described as subacute encephalitis or AIDS encephalopathy. This clinical syndrome is believed to result from the direct effects of HIV and/or additional factors related to the local response of the central nervous system to HIV infection (Navia et al 1986, Rowbotham 1990, Dalakas et al 1989).

Hepatitis B virus infection was commonly known to occur in injecting drug users long before the AIDS epidemic (Stimmel et al 1975, Mangia et al 1976, Kreek 1978). More than 50% of chronic drug users show evidence of prior hepatitis B exposure. Most of these patients are seropositive for antibody to hepatitis B surface antigen and/or antibody to hepatitis B core antigen, with a small percentage exhibiting chronic hepatitis B surface antigenaemia. The use of hepatitis B vaccine is recommended for susceptible injecting drug users and medical personnel providing care to such patients both as a clinical intervention and to help minimize occupational acquisition of hepatitis B virus (HBV) from patients who show greater or more prolonged infectivity with HBV due to a greater burden of circulating virus (Selwyn 1992).

Although heterosexual drug users with HIV infection have been found to be at low risk for Kaposi's sarcoma as compared with homosexual men, the occurrence of malignant lymphomas among HIV-infected drug users has been documented (Barbieri et al 1986, Tirelli et al 1987, Vazquez et al 1989, Beral et al 1990). The common occurrence of HPV co-infection in HIV-infected drug-using women requires clinical vigilance for cervical dysplasia and carcinoma. Concomitant HIV-related medical complications such as *pneumocystis carinii* pneumonia, toxoplasmosis, candidiasis, and cytomegalovirus infection will be described in other chapters in this publication.

It is evident from the above that primary medical care is vital for drug users in general, and particularly for those with HIV infection. There is a great need for comprehensive integration of drug abuse treatment into mainstream medical care. In order to provide effective treatment for drug abusers with HIV infection, a primary care physician must co-ordinate all of the services along with various specialists, in order to properly manage the numerous medical complications related to drug abuse and those related to HIV infection.

Psychiatric disorders in drug abusers with HIV Infection

The frequent co-occurrence of psychiatric disorders in HIV infection has been described in drug-using populations in which the background prevalence of psychopathology is already likely to be elevated and the need for psychiatric intervention is often compelling in many cases (Silberstein et al 1987, Sorenson et al 1989, O'Dowd et al 1989, Ross et al 1988, Batki 1991). Conventional drug abuse treatment programmes may find it difficult to treat these patients since they may be unprepared to address the psychiatric problems that can complicate treatment.

Batki and others (Batki et al 1988) have described a number of psychological problems seen in drug users who are HIV-positive which include denial, anger, depression and isolation. Patients who must cope with both substance abuse and medical problems associated with AIDS may experience denial. One outcome may be that patients attempt to employ one problem to defensively deny the other. They may use the medical problems as a rationalization for taking drugs. Patients may seek to maintain the illusion of health by maintaining their drug use and the life-style associated with it.

Anger about having HIV infection can be expressed as non-compliance with substance abuse treatment rules and as defiance of limits set by the treatment staff. Non-compliance may also occur regarding other medical treatment, by failure to keep clinic appointments or by misuse of medications. Anger can coexist with depression and may be the first sign of a mood disorder.

Depression is one of the most common psychiatric problems among substance abusers, particularly opiate addicts. It may be universal among AIDS patients who abuse substances but may surface only after denial and defiance are exhausted. Depression can also appear after addicts stop self-medicating with intravenous drugs. Suicidal ideation is often present. Depression and a sense of loneliness in AIDS patients can be reinforced since they are frequently stigmatized and isolated. Drug users with AIDS are at risk of being ostracized by the 'straight' society and by other drug users. This is particularly true with regard to women. Drug users with AIDS are more likely to have psychiatric problems than other drug users or other AIDS patients and they are likely to require more mental health services due to the complex way in which their problems interact.

Drug abuse treatment

Although most physicians can conjure up appropriate compassion and knowledge in order to treat the individual suffering from HIV infection, many physicians show pejorative attitudes towards patients with drug abuse problems. They frequently believe that they cannot contribute to treating such patients and their attitudes preclude them from doing so (Dole & Nyswander 1967, Levine & Novick 1990). Since substance abusers may show a high relapse rate, they are not easy to treat. Physicians, therefore, have a low expectation of treatment success and frequently are discouraged. Many physicians only see substance abusers in limited settings such as hospital emergency units. Many of these patients have frequent relapses to substance abuse and poor compliance with the medical treatments prescribed. Unfortunately, some physicians feel that substance abusers are responsible for their addiction and hence their medical problems (Chappel & Schnoll 1977, Stimmel 1989). Many barriers exist within the potential for treatment of substance abusers including the lack of knowledge by many physicians, the attitudes as mentioned above, the lack of insurance coverage, lack of substance abuse treatment facilities, and the fear of economic loss by physicians due to malpractice suits. Moreover, specific treatment for women has not been readily available, in spite of the fact that many guidelines exist at this time (Finnegan et al 1991, Finnegan 1991a).

In today's world of medical practice, a careful diagnostic approach and an effective therapeutic effort must be applied to chemical dependency problems as well as the many medical complications. Health care providers should realize that substance abuse can be treated successfully and should be regarded as a disease that may have a metabolic basis (Dole 1967), rather than as a moral weakness. Providers should be aware of the fact that negative attitudes may contribute to treatment failures.

There is no question that the treatment of addicted women has been a challenge for the last several decades for treatment providers and researchers. Although comprehensive services for women in general, as well as women with dependent children, have been described since the early 1970s, considerable impediments have been evident in providing such a comprehensive model. It has been well documented that treatment for substance-abusing women should include a wide range of co-ordinated and comprehensive services. Treatment programmes should adopt a flexible and integrated model in which all of the diverse needs are acknowledged and addressed holistically. Treatment for women requires that providers recognize the contribution to addiction of biological, psychological and social variables while providing culturally, racially, and ethnically sensitive psychotherapy. Additionally, the comprehensive treatment model should emphasize the reduction of socio-economic and political barriers which impede the effectiveness of treatment. (Finnegan et al 1991, Finnegan 1991a)

Issues of gender, culture, sexual orientation, economics, medical status, education, child care, transportation, ethnicity and race are among the many variables that have been neglected in the treatment of women substance abusers. Physicians who treat women with substance abuse and HIV infection must override the impediments to the delivery of an adequate comprehensive multisystem treatment model. Table 11.3 describes the many services that need to be developed for women who are substance abusers. The comprehensive services should include the following components: medical, psychological, socio/cultural, psychological/behavioural; and in those who have dependent children, the mother/infant and early childhood development issues must be addressed.

Outreach services should be an integral part of any treatment approach. Utilizing workers indigenous to the neighbourhood and to the culture of the women facilitates overall understanding of the impact of diversity in treatment. These workers can serve as a conduit between addicted women and a treatment facility in order

Table 11.3 Drug abuse treatment schema for HIV-infected drug-dependent women

Outreach services	*Biological/physiological/medical*
Community liaison	For potential infections
indigenous workers	assess complications of
mobile van	drug abuse and HIV
distribution of prevention	infection: tuberculosis,
and educational	hepatitis, CMV
information	assess various organ
work with community	systems: hepatic, renal,
organizations, churches,	cardiovascular
recreational centres, etc.	pulmonary, GI, CNS
Immediate access to	assess for STDs
treatment	assess immunologic status
provide transportation	
co-ordinate intake	Pharmacological
medical	methadone maintenance
drug abuse treatment	psychotropic medication
psychiatric evaluation	antibiotics for bacterial
	infections
	HIV drug treatment
	clinical trials
Psychological/behavioural	*Demographic/sociocultural*
Life-skills management	Survival management
defining and accessing	housing
problems associated	clothing
with addiction	food
attitudes, beliefs,	financial and budgetary
knowledge and	Sociological considerations
expectation	gender
modification	race
problem-solving	social class
coping mechanisms	economics
relapse prevention	culture
social skills competence	
Psychological	
psychiatric assessment	
HIV counselling	
nutritional counselling	

STD, sexually transmitted disease; GI, gastrointestinal; CMV, cytomegalovirus; CNS, central nervous system

to provide transportation and co-ordinate intake with regard to medical, psychiatric or drug treatment. They will be able to act as case managers in linking social service systems with other services. Moreover, AIDS prevention issues can be discussed. Medical treatment and psychiatric treatment have been previously described. Other psychological management should include problem-solving, coping mechanisms, social skill competence, relapse prevention and a host of educational issues to include nutrition and health preservation techniques (Finnegan et al 1991).

Substance abuse treatment issues must also address issues of survival management, including housing, clothing, food and the ability to finance the above, as well as health care needs of the HIV-infected women. If women have drug-dependent children, treatment within the substance abuse centre must be family centred. Specifics concerning the assessment and management of children born to HIV-infected women, and follow-up with regard to HIV disease and psychosocial considerations are described elsewhere in this volume (Finnegan et al 1991, Finnegan 1991b).

The most common form of long-term treatment of opiate dependence is methadone maintenance treatment (MMT). MMT can play an important role in both AIDS prevention and reduction of HIV-related morbidity through diminishing drug use, promoting a healthier life-style, and providing direct medical and psychiatric care (Ferrando & Batki 1991, Finnegan 1991b).

MMT is an effective treatment strategy for opioid addiction uncomplicated by HIV infection. MMT reduces opioid use as well as criminal behaviour and improves employment and overall health status (Ball et al 1988). MMT has a high retention rate compared to other forms of treatment such as outpatient detoxification and residential therapeutic communities (Zweben & Payte 1990). Therefore, MMT has been proposed as a preferred method of treatment for the HIV-infected opioid user (Batki 1988, Cooper 1989, Ball et al 1988). From the medical perspective, continued opioid use, in addition to cocaine, marijuana and alcohol (which are common secondary drugs of choice among opioid addicts) may increase the risk of HIV disease progression through direct immune suppression (Zagury et al 1986, MacGregor 1988). Continued drug use may also increase the exposure to opportunistic infections. Concern was expressed with regard to providing methadone to HIV-infected addicts due to the fact that various opioids have been found to suppress immune function in vitro. However, evidence indicates that, for some immune parameters, opioid users in MMT have better functioning immune systems than do street heroin addicts (Kreek 1981, Lazzarin et al 1984, Falek et al 1986). Moreover, MMT can offer a valuable treatment environment for a group of patients who are poorly compliant with medical treatment, as it

can provide ready access to medical care as part of an integrated treatment plan.

There are a number of special issues which must be considered when providing drug abuse treatment to HIV-infected individuals. These include pain management, drug interactions and self-medication. Patients with HIV infection frequently require analgesia for pain resulting from specific opportunistic infections or their complications. Physicians may be concerned about the possibility of drug-seeking behaviour or manipulation by drug users with regard to narcotics or other psychotropic medications. However, this concern may be inappropriate if the physician withholds or underuses strong analgesics in situations in which they are medically indicated. A common misconception is that patients maintained on methadone do not require additional narcotics for analgesia or that analgesia can be achieved, if necessary, simply by increasing the patient's daily methadone dose. On the contrary, methadone maintenance patients quickly develop tolerance to the drug's analgesic effects and have not been found to have blunted perception of noxious stimuli (Ho & Dok 1979, Kreek 1983). Due to individual tolerance to narcotic drugs, patients require at least the standard, and, at times higher than standard doses of short-acting narcotic analgesics, such as oxycodone, hydromorphone, meperidine and codeine, when indicated for pain relief. The drugs must be administered on a more frequent dosing schedule than in non-tolerant patients because of their rapid elimination in narcotic addiction. Additional problems of undermedication may result in a typical pattern of confrontation and acting out among drug users, with the frequent result of poor patient outcomes and increased frustration and/or dissatisfaction among medical staff. In spite of the need for these medications, clinicians should provide small quantities at a time for outpatients and renew prescriptions on a fixed schedule. They should taper such medication gradually before discontinuation (Selwyn 1992).

Of special relevance to the care of HIV-infected opioid addicts, especially those on methadone maintenance, are the potential drug interactions. The most important of these interactions is between rifampin and methadone (Kreek et al

1976). Another medication frequently used in the care of HIV-infected drug users is phenytoin, since seizures may occur as a complication of certain HIV-related central nervous system infections or malignancies. Both these drugs have an effect on methadone metabolism, presumably through a comparable effect involving the hepatic microsomal enzyme system. In the case of phenytoin, the effect is less dramatic and usually occurs more slowly, often over the course of several weeks as opposed to the first few days following initiation of therapy with rifampin (Tong et al 1981). Although methadone dose increases are often necessary to prevent opiate withdrawal in patients on methadone maintenance who are placed on phenytoin, these increases generally need not be as great or as rapid as in the case of rifampin. However, the clinician must be aware that these drugs cause an increase in the elimination of methadone and reduce plasma levels. This effect results clinically in the onset of typical opiate withdrawal symptoms. The physician will need to increase the daily methadone dose usually by 10mg and titrate the dose up, depending on the symptoms of each individual patient. In the case of rifampin, the increased methadone dose could be as much as 50% greater than the original maintenance dose before the patient reaches a new stable steady state. Specifics of the management of these drug interactions are more fully described in other references (Tong et al 1981, Mandell & Sande 1990).

Preliminary data from two studies from Edinburgh and New York have indicated that there may be pharmacokinetic interaction between zidovudine and methadone or other opiate drugs. Results from both of these studies suggest that the clearance of zidovudine may be reduced and plasma levels increased in patients taking opiate drugs concurrently (Brettle et al 1989, Schwartz et al 1990). The effect was not consistently seen in all study patients and the mechanisms for this putative effect have not been fully elucidated. Clinical observations have not noted that MMT patients who receive zidovudine exhibit greater toxicity from the latter drug and the preliminary data that do exist have not resulted in any recommendation for an alteration in zidovudine dosage schedules for opiate-dependent patients with HIV infection. It also does not appear that

zidovudine therapy affects the metabolism of methadone and there is no biological or pharmacological evidence to suggest that methadone dosage must be modified in patients initiating zidovudine therapy.

The use of non-prescribed antibiotics available through the street market or 'antibiotic abuse' has been described among injecting drug users, independent of the AIDS epidemic (Novick & Ness 1984, Crane et al 1986). In one study reported from Detroit, a risk factor noted was for methicillin-resistant *Staphylococcus aureus* infection among drug users hospitalized for bacterial endocarditis (Crane 1986). Antibiotic abuse is of particular relevance to the management of HIV-infected drug users, who may present with acute illness due to partially treated bacterial infections. Anecdotal evidence also now suggests that certain AIDS-related medications such as zidovudine, acyclovir and ketoconazole, in addition to standard antibiotics, are also available on the street and such medications may be taken sporadically in an unsupervised manner as a form of self-treatment (Selwyn & Iezza 1990). In a case report of zidovudine overdose in a female intravenous drug user (Selwyn & Iezza 1990), the patient showed no symptomatic effects that could be specifically linked to zidovudine, and minimal, if any, haematological toxicity was noted. Other cases of zidovudine overdose showed no consistent pattern of symptoms of apparent haematological toxicity, although possible acute neurological side-effects have been described. The possibility of increasing numbers of HIV-infected drug users being treated with zidovudine highlights the importance of the potential misuse of such medication in this population. However, zidovudine can be used sucessfully in a carefully monitored methadone maintenance programme, with high rates of compliance and follow-up.

From the above regarding the management of drug-dependent women who are HIV-infected, one can perceive that careful and precise co-ordination of the multitude of issues is mandatory if we are to successfully manage such patients. A vast amount of knowledge must be available to the clinician, not only with regard to the many medical issues, but also regarding the psychological and drug abuse issues. Knowledge of the clinician, coupled with the appropriate consultants, as well as compassion for women as individuals and women with many complicating issues, will provide the best possible outlook for drug-dependent women who are also HIV-infected.

REFERENCES

Amaro H, Fried L E, Cabral H, Zukerman B 1990 Violence during pregnancy and substance use. Am J Public Health 80: 575–579

Anastos K Marte C 1989 Women – the missing persons in the AIDS epidemic. Health/PAC Bull 19(4): 6–13

Ball J C, Lange R W, Myers P C Friedman S R 1988 Reducing the risk of AIDS through methadone maintenance treatment. J Health Soc Behav 29: 214–226

Barbieri D, Gualandi M, Tassinari M C et al 1986 B-cell lymphomas in two HIV-seropositive heroin addicts. Lancet 2: 1039

Batki S L 1988 Treatment of intravenous drug users with AIDS: the role of methadone maintenance. J Psychoact Drugs 20(2): 213–216

Batki S 1991 Drug abuse, psychiatric disorders, and AIDS: dual and triple diagnosis. West J Med 152: 547–552

Batki S L, Sorenson J L, Faltz B, Madover S 1988 AIDS among intravenous drug users: psychiatric aspects of treatment. Hosp Commun Psychiatry 39: 439–441

Beral V, Peterman T A, Berkelman R L, Jaffe H W 1990 Kaposi's sarcoma among persons with AIDS: a sexually transmitted infection? Lancet 335: 123–128

Blower S M, Hartel D 1990 HIV, drugs and ecology (letter). Science 246: 1236

Blower S M, Hartel D, Dowlatabladi H, Anderson R, May R 1991 Drugs, sex and HIV: a mathematical model for New York City. Phil Trans R Soc Lond B231: 171–187

Blower S M, Medley G 1992 Epidemiology, HIV and drugs: mathematical models and data. Br J Addict 87: 371–379

Bollerud K 1990 A model for the treatment of trauma-related syndromes among chemically dependent inpatient women. J Sub Abuse Treat 7: 83–87

Brettle R P, Jones G A, Bingham J et al 1989 Pharmacokinetics of zidovudine in injection drug use-related HIV infection. V International Conference in AIDS, Montreal, June 1989. Abstract WB03

Brickner P W, Torres R A, Barnes M et al 1989 Recommendations for control and prevention of human immunodeficiency virus (HIV) infection in intravenous drug users. Ann Intern Med 110: 833–837

Briere J, Zaidi L Y 1989 Sexual abuse histories and sequelae in female psychiatric emergency room patients. Am J Psychiatry 146: 1602–1606

Brown S, Stimmel B, Taub R N et al 1974 Immunologic dysfunction in heroin addicts. Arch Intern Med 134: 1001–1006

Brown V, Melchior L, Reback C, Huba G J 1992 Partner notification: psychosocial issues. NIDA technical review on partner notification for injection drug users and partners of injection drug users, Oct 1–2, 1992, NIDA, Rockville, MD

Byrne M A, Taylor-Robinson D, Munday P E, Harris J R W 1989 The common occurrence of human papillomavirus infection and intraepithelial neoplasia in women infected by HIV. AIDS 3: 379–382

Carpenter C C J, Mayer K H, Stein M D et al 1991 Human immunodeficiency virus infection in North American women: experience with 200 cases and a review of the literature. Medicine 70: 307–325

Catania J, Coates J, Stall R, et al 1992 Prevalence of AIDS-related risk factors and condom use in the United States. Science 258: 1101–1106

Cates W Jr 1990 Acquired immunodeficiency syndrome, sexually transmitted disease, and epidemiology. Am J Epidemiol 131: 749–758

Centers for Disease Control 1981 Pneumocystis pneumonia – Los Angeles. MMWR 30: 250–252

Centers for Disease Control 1986 Classification system for human T-lymphotropic virus type III lymphadenopathy-associated virus infection. MMWR 35: 334–339

Centers for Disease Control 1987a Revision of the CDC surveillance case definition of acquired immunodeficiency syndrome. MMWR 36 (suppl 1S): 1–18S

Centers for Disease Control 1987b Tuberculosis and acquired immunodeficiency syndrome – New York City. MMWR 36: 785–795

Centers for Disease Control 1988 Relationship of syphilis to drug use and prostitution – Connecticut and Philadelphia. MMWR 37: 757–764

Centers for Disease Control 1989a Tuberculosis and human immunodeficiency virus infection: recommendation of the advisory committee for the elimination of tuberculosis (ACET). MMWR 38: 236–250

Centers for Disease Control 1989b First 100 000 cases of acquired immunodeficiency syndrome – United States. MMWR 38: 561–563

Centers for Disease Control 1989c Update: acquired immunodeficiency syndrome – United States, 1981–1988. MMWR 38: 229–236

Centers for Disease Control 1990 National HIV seroprevalence surveys: summary of results, data from serosurveillance activities through 1989. US Department of Health and Human Services, Public Health Service, Centers for Disease Control, Atlanta, HIV/CID 19–90/006

Centers for Disease Control 1991a HIV/AIDS surveillance report, November 1–18

Centers for Disease Control 1991b Drug use and sexual behaviors among sex partners of injecting drug users. MMWR 40: 855–860

Chappel J N, Schnoll S H 1977 Physician attitudes: effect in the treatment of chemically dependent patients. JAMA 2318–2319

Cherubin C E, Millian S J 1968 Serologic investigations in heroin addicts: I. Syphilis, lymphogranuloma venereum, herpes simplex, and Q fever. Ann Int Med 69: 739–742

Cherubin C E, Millian S J 1969 Serologic investigations in narcotic addicts. From the Division of Epidemiology, Columbia School of Public Health and Administrative Medicine; and the Virus Diagnostic Laboratory, Bureau Laboratories, New York City Dept of Health, New York, NY

Chiasson M A, Stoneburner R L, Hildebrandt D, Ewing W E, Telzak E E, Jaffe H 1991 Heterosexual transmission of HIV-1 with the use of smokable freebase cocaine (crack). AIDS 5: 1121–1126

Chin J 1990 Epidemiology: current and future dimensions of the HIV/AIDS pandemic in women and children. Lancet 336: 221–224

Chu S Y, Buehler J W, Berkelman R L 1990 Impact of the human immunodeficiency virus epidemic on mortality in women of reproductive age. United States. JAMA 264: 225–229

Coates T J, Stall R D, Catanca J A, Kegeles S M 1988 Behavioral factors in the spread of HIV infection. AIDS 2 (Suppl 1): S239–246

Cohen J et al 1988 Prostitutes and AIDS: Public policy issues. AIDS Public Pol J 3: 16–22

Cohen J B, Hauer L B, Wofsey C B 1989 Women and IV drugs: parenteral and heterosexual transmission of human immunodeficiency virus. J Drug Issues 19: 39–56

Cohen J B 1991 Why women partners of drug users will continue to be at high risk for HIV infection. J Addict Dis 10: 99–110

Cohen J B, Derish P A, Dorfman L E 1992 AWARE: a community-based research and peer intervention program for women. In: Van Wright (ed) Community-based research, AIDS prevention and services, Praeger Press, New York, p 79–88

Coleman R M, Curtis D 1988 Distribution of risk behavior for HIV infection among intravenous drug users. Br J Addict 83: 1331–1335

Cooper J R 1989 Methadone treatment and acquired immunodeficiency syndrome. JAMA 262: 1664–1668

Crane L R, Levine D P, Zervos M J, Cummings G 1986 Bacteremia in narcotic addicts at the Detroit Medical Center. I. Microbiology, epidemiology, risk factors, and empiric therapy. Rev Infect Dis 8: 364–373

Cushman P, Grieco M H 1973 Hyperimmunoglobulinemia associated with narcotic addiction. Am J Med 54: 320–326

Cushman P, Gupta S, Grieco M H et al 1977 Immunological studies in methadone maintained patients. Int J Addict 12(2–3): 241–253

Dalakas M, Wichman A, Sever J 1989 AIDS and the nervous system. JAMA 261: 2396–2399

Department of Health 1990 State of New Jersey. AIDS surveillance report, October 31

Des Jarlais D C, Friedman S R 1987 HIV infection among intravenous drug users: epidemiology and risk reduction. AIDS 1: 67–76

Des Jarlais D C, Friedman S R, Marmor M et al 1987 Development of AIDS, HIV seroconversion, and potential cofactors for T4 cell loss in a cohort of intravenous drug users. AIDS 1: 105–111

Des Jarlais D C, Friedman S R 1988 HIV and intravenous drug use. AIDS 2 (Suppl 1): S65–69

Des Jarlais D C, Friedman S R, Stoneburner R L 1988 HIV infection and intravenous drug use: critical issues in transmission dynamics, infection outcomes, and prevention. Rev Infect Dis 10: 151–158

Dole V P, Nyswander M E 1967 Heroin addiction – a metabolic disease. Arch Intern Med 120: 19–24

Donahoe R M 1990 Drug abuse and AIDS: causes for the connection. In: Pham P T K, Rice K (eds) Drugs of abuse: chemistry, pharmacology, immunology, and AIDS. National Institute on Drug Abuse Research Monograph No 96, DHHS publication number (ADM) 90–1676, National Institute on Drug Abuse, Rockville, MD

Donahoe R M, Nicholson J, Maddan J et al 1986 Coordinate and independent effects of heroin, cocaine and alcohol abuse on T-cell rosette formation and antigenic marker expression. Clin Immunol Immunopathol 41: 254–264

Donoghoe M C, Stimson G V, Dolan K A 1989 Sexual behavior of injection drug users and associated risks of HIV infection from non-injecting sexual partners. AIDS Care 1: 51–58

Downs A M, Ancelle-Park R A, Costagliola D C et al 1990 J-B. Monitoring and short-term forecasting of AIDS in Europe. VI International Conference on AIDS, San Francisco. Abstract FC220

Drucker E 1986 AIDS and addiction in New York City. Am J Drugs Alcohol Abuse 12: 165–181

European Study Group 1989 Risk factors for male-to-female transmission of HIV. Br Med J 298: 411–415

Falek A, Madden J J, Shafer D A, Donahue R M 1986 Individual differences in opiate-induced alterations at the cytogenetic, DNA repair, and immunologic levels: opportunity for genetic assessment. In: Braude M C, Chao H M (eds) Genetic and biological markers in drug abuse and alcoholism. National Institute on Drug Abuse Research Monograph 66. National Institute on Drug Abuse, Rockville, MD, p 11–24

Feingold A R, Vermund S H, Burke R D et al 1990 Cervical cytologic abnormalities and papillomavirus in women infected with human immunodeficiency virus. J Acq Immune Defic Synd 3: 896–903

Fernandez-Cruz E, Fernandez A M, Gutierrez C et al 1988 Progressive cellular immune impairment leading to development of AIDS: two-year prospective study of HIV infection in drug addicts. Clin Exp Immunol 72: 190–195

Fernandez-Cruz E, Desco M, Garcia Montes M et al 1990 Immunological and serological markers predictive of progression to AIDS in a cohort of HIV-infected drug users. AIDS 4: 987–994

Ferrando S J, Batki S L, 1991 HIV-infected intravenous drug users in methadone maintenance treatment: clinical problems and their management. J Psych Drugs 23: 217–224

Finnegan L P, 1991a Perinatal substance abuse: comments and perspectives. In: Creasy R K, Warshaw J B (eds) Seminars in perinatology. W A Saunders, Philadelphia, PA, vol 15, no 4, p 331–339

Finnegan L P 1991b Treatment issues for opioid-dependent women during the perinatal period. J Psychoact Drugs 23 (2): 191–202

Finnegan L P, Hagan T, Kaltenbach K 1991 Opioid dependence: foundations for clinical practice. In: Pregnancy and substance abuse: perspectives and directions. Bulletin of the New York Academy of Medicine. New York, NY, vol 67, no 3, p 223–239

Friedmann W, Schafer A, Schwartlander B 1990 Cervical neoplasia in HIV-infected women. V International Conference on AIDS, Montreal. Abstract WCP53

Fullilove R E, Fullilove M T, Bowser B P, Gross S A 1990 Risk of sexually transmitted disease among black adolescent crack users in Oakland and San Francisco, California. JAMA 263: 851–855

Gawin F H, Ellinwood E H 1988 Cocaine and other stimulants. N Engl J Med 318: 1173–1182

Geller S A, Stimmel B 1973 Diagnostic confusion from lymphatic lesions in heroin addicts. Ann Int Med 78: 703–705

Gilks C F, Brindle R J, Otieno L S et al 1990 Life-threatening bacteremia in HIV-1 seropositive adults admitted to hospital in Nairobi, Kenya. Lancet 336: 545–549

Glatt A E, Chirgwin K 1990 Pneumocystis carinii pneumonia in human immunodeficiency virus-infected patients. Arch Intern Med 150: 271–279

Goldsmith M F 1988 Sex tied to drugs = STD spread. JAMA 260: 2009

Gottlieb M S, Schroff R, Schanker H M et al 1981 Pneumocystis carinii pneumonia and mucosal candidiasis in previously healthy homosexual men. N Engl J Med 305: 1425–1431

Government of Burma Ministry of Health 1990. Official report on HIV infection and AIDS in Burma on file at WHO (reference A20/422/2BUR)

Greenspan D, de Viliers E M, Greenspan J S, Desouza Y G, zur Hausen H 1988 Unusual HPV types in oral warts in association with HIV infection. J Oral Pathol 17: 482–487

Grieco M H, Chuang C Y 1973 Hypermacroglobulinemia associated with heroin use in adolescents. J Allergy Clin Immunol 51: 152–160

Guinan M E 1990 Domestic violence. Physicians a link to prevention. J Am Women Med Assoc 45: 231

Guinan M E, Hardy A 1987 Epidemiology of AIDS in women in the United States. JAMA 257: 2039–2042

Guydish J, Coates T J 1988 Changes in AIDS-related high risk behavior among heterosexual men. IV International conference on AIDS, Stockholm. Abstract 4074

Hahn R A, Onorato I M, Jones T S, Dougherty J 1989 Prevalence of HIV infection among intravenous drug users in the United States. JAMA 261: 2677–2684

Handsfield H 1988 Heterosexual transmission of human immunodeficiency virus. JAMA 260: 1943–1944

Hankins C, Handley M 1992 HIV disease and AIDS in women: current knowledge and a research agenda. J Acq Immune Defic Synd 5: 957–971

Harlow C W 1991 Female victims of violent crime. US Govt Pub No NCJ 126826, US Dept Justice Wash. DC

Hartel D 1992 Report on NIDA technical review on partner notification for injection drug users and partners of injection drug users, Oct 1–2, 1992. NIDA, Rockville, MD

Hartel D et al 1992 Gender differences in drug use and mortality among injection drug users (abstract). 8th International Conference on AIDS, Amsterdam

Haverkos H W, Edelman R 1988 The epidemiology of acquired immuno-deficiency syndrome among heterosexuals. JAMA 260: 1922–1929

Haverkos H W, Battjes R J, Phillips A, Johnson A, Padian N, Shiboski S, Jewell N 1992 Female-to-male transmission of HIV (letters). JAMA 268: 1855–1857

Heagarty M C, Abrams E J 1992 Caring for HIV-infected women and children. N Engl J Med 326: 887–888

Helton A S, McFarlane J, Anderson E T 1987 Battered and pregnant: a prevalence study. Am J Public Health 77: 1337–1339

Henry M J, Stanley M W, Cruikeshank S, Carson L 1989 Association of human papillomavirus infection and cervical intraepithelial neoplasia. Am J Obstet Gynecol 160: 352–353

Ho A, Dole V P 1979 Pain perception in drug-free and in methadone-maintained human ex-addicts. Proc Soc Exp Biol Med 162: 392–395

Ho D D (moderator), Bredesen D E, Vinters H V, Daar E S 1989 The acquired immunodeficiency syndrome (AIDS) dementia complex. Ann Intern Med 111: 400–410

Hoegsberg B, Abulafia O, Sedlis A et al 1990 Sexually transmitted diseases and human immunodeficiency virus infection among women with pelvic inflammatory disease. Am J Obstet Gynecol 163: 1135–1139

Hoffman C K, Goodman P C 1989 Pulmonary edema in cocaine smokers. Radiology 172: 463–465

Holmberg S D, Horsburgh C R, Ward J W, Jaffe H W 1989 Biologic factors in the sexual transmission of HIV. J Infect Dis 160: 116–125

Holmes K, Karon J M, Kreiss J 1990 Am J Public Health 80: 858–863

Holmes K, Kreiss J 1988 Heterosexual transmission of HIV. Am J Public Health 80: 858–863

Ickovics J R, Rodin J 1991 Women and AIDS in the United States: epidemiology, natural history and mediating mechanisms. Health Psychology 11: 1–16

Italian Seroconversion Study 1992 Disease progression and early predictors of AIDS in HIV-seroconverted injecting drug users. AIDS 6: 421–426.

Jaffe J H 1990 Drug addiction and drug abuse. In: Gilman A G, Rall T W, Nies A S, Taylor P (eds) The pharmacological basis of therapeutics, 8th ed. Pergamon Press, New York, p 522–573

Johnson A M, Laga M 1988. Heterosexual transmission of HIV. AIDS 2: S49–56

Kane S 1990 AIDS, addiction and condom use: sources of sexual risk for heterosexual women. J Sexual Res 27: 427–444

Kane S 1991 Heroin and heterosexual relations. Soc Sci Med 32: 1037–1050

Kantor G K, Straus M A 1989 Substance abuse as a precipitant of wife abuse victimizations. Am J Drug Alc Abuse 15: 173–189

Kaslow R, Blackwelder W C, Ostrow D et al 1989 No evidence for a role of alcohol or other psychoactive drugs in accelerating immunodeficiency in HIV-1-positive individuals. JAMA 261: 3424–3429

Kissner D G, Lawrence D W, Selis J E, Flint A 1987 Crack lung: pulmonary disease caused by cocaine abuse. Am Rev Resp Dis 136: 1250–1252

Klein D 1981 Violence against women: some considerations regarding its causes and its elimination. Crime Delinquincy 27: 64–80

Kloser P, Grigorin A, Kaplia R 1988 Women with AIDS: a continuing study. IV International Conference on AIDS, Stockholm, June 1988. Abstract 4065

Kreek M J 1978 Medical complications in methadone patients. Ann NY Acad Sci 311: 110–134

Kreek M J 1981 Medical management of methadone-maintained patients. In: Lowinson J H, Ruiz P (eds) Substance abuse: clinical problems and perspectives. Williams & Wilkins, Baltimore, p 181–201

Kreek M J 1983 Health consequences associated with the use of methadone. In: Cooper J R, Altman F, Brown B S, Chzechowicz D (eds) Research on the treatment of narcotic addiction. Treatment research monograph series. DHHS publication no. (ADM) 83–1281. National Institute on Drug Abuse, Rockville, MD, p 456–482

Kreek M J 1990 Immune function in heroin addicts and former heroin addicts in treatment: pre-and post-AIDS epidemic. In: Haverkos H, Hartsock P (eds) Drugs of abuse: chemistry, pharmacology, immunology, and AIDS. Research Monograph series No. 96. DHHS publication no. (ADM) 90–1676. National Institute on Drug Abuse, Rockville, MD, p 192–219

Kreek M J, Dodes L, Kane S et al 1972 Longterm methadone maintenance therapy: effects on liver function. Ann Int Med 77: 598–602

Kreek M J, Garfield J W Gutjahr C L, Guisti L M 1976 Rifampin-induced methadone withdrawal. N Engl J Med 294: 1194–1206

Lang N G 1991 Stigma, self-esteem, and depression:

psychosocial responses to risk of AIDS. Hum Organization 50: 66–72

Lazzarin A, Mella L, Trombini M et al 1984 Immunological status in heroin addicts: effects of methadone maintenance. Drug Alcohol Dep 39: 161–166

Leach C L 1990 The abused woman and her family of origin. Perspect Psychiatric Care 26: 14–20

Leitman B S, Greengart A, Wasser H J 1988 Pneumomediastinum and pneumopericardium after cocaine abuse. Am J Radiol 151: 614

LePont F, Blower S M 1991 The supply and demand of sexual behavior: implications for heterosexual HIV epidemics. J AIDS 4: 987–999

Levine C, Novick D M 1990 Expanding the role of physicians in drug abuse treatment: problems and perspectives. J Clin Ethics 1: 152–156

Louie E, Rice L B, Holzman R S 1986 Tuberculosis in non-Haitian patients with acquired immunodeficiency syndrome. Chest 90: 542–545

McCoy C B, Khoury E 1990 Drug use and the risk of AIDS. Am J Behav Sci 33: 419–431

McDonough R J, Madden J J, Falek A et al 1980 Alteration of T and null Lymphocyte frequencies in the peripheral blood of human opiate addicts: In vivo evidence for opiate receptor sites on T lymphocytes. J Immunol 125: 2539–2543

MacGregor R R 1988 Alcohol and drugs as cofactors for AIDS. In: Siegel L (ed) Aids and substance abuse. Harrington Park, New York, p 59–63

McIlwaine G 1989 Women victims of domestic violence. Br Med J 299: 995–996

McKinnon C A 1989 Rape: on coercion and consent. In: McKinnon C A (ed) Toward a feminist theory of state. Harvard Univ Press, Cambridge, MA, p 120–151

McLeer S V, Anwar R 1989 A study of battered women presenting in an emergency department. Am J Public Health 79: 65–66

Madden J J, Donahoe R M, Zwemer-Collins J et al 1987 Binding of naloxone to human T lymphocytes. Biochem Pharmacol 36: 4103–4109

Mandell G I, Sande M A 1990 Antimicrobial agents: drugs used in the chemotherapy of tuberculosis and leprosy. In: Gilman A G Rall T W, Nies A S, Taylor P (eds) The pharmacological basis of therapeutics, 8th edn. Pergamon Press, New York, p 1146–1164

Mangia J L, Kim Y M, Brown M R et al 1976 HB-Ag and HB Ab in asymptomatic drug addicts. Am J Gastroenterol 65: 121–126

Margolick J B, Munoz A, Vlahov D et al 1992 Changes in T-lymphocyte subsets in intravenous drug users with HIV-1 infection. JAMA 267: 1631–1636

Mientjes G H, Miedema F, van Ameijden E J et al 1991 Frequent injecting impairs lymphocyte reactivity in HIV-positive and HIV-negative drug users. AIDS 5: 35–41

Mondanaro J 1989 Chemically dependent women assessment and treatment. Lexington MA, Lexington Books.

Mondanaro J 1990 Community-based AIDS prevention interventions: special issues of women intravenous drug users. In Leukefeld C G, Battjes R J, Amsel Z (eds) AIDS and intravenous drug use: future directions for community-based prevention research. NIDA Research Monograph series no 93. DHHS publication no 89–1627 National Institute on Drug Abuse, Rockville, MD, p 68–82

Moss A R 1987 The real heterosexual epidemic. Br Med J 294: 389–390

Moss A R 1988 Epidemiology of AIDS in developed countries. Br Med Bull 44: 56–67

Munoz A, Wang M-C, Bass S et al 1989 Acquired immunodeficiency syndrome (AIDS) – free time after human immunodeficiency virus type 1 (HIV-1) seroconversion in homosexual men. Am J Epidemiol 130: 530–539

Munoz A, Vlahov D, Solomon L et al 1992 Prognostic indicators for development of AIDS among intravenous drug users. J AIDS 5: 694–700

Navia B A, Jordan B D, Price R W 1986 The AIDS dementia complex: I. Clinical features. Ann Neurol 19: 517–524

Nelson K, Vlahov D, Cohn S et al 1991 Sexually transmitted diseases in a population of intravenous drug users: association with seropositivity to HIV. J Infect Dis 164: 457–463

New York State Department of Health Bureau of Communicable Disease Control 1990 AIDS surveillance quarterly update, October. NY Department of Health

Nickerson D S, Williams R C Jr, Boxmeyer M et al 1970 Increased opsonic capacity of serum in chronic heroin addiction. Ann Intern Med 72: 671–677

Nicolosi A, Leite M L C, Musicco M, Molinari S, Lazzarin A 1992 Parenteral and sexual transmission of human immunodeficiency virus in intravenous drug users: a study of seroconversion. Am J Epidemiol 135: 225–233

NIDA 1991 National household survey on drug abuse: population estimates. DHHS pub no ADM 92–1887. ADAMHA, Rockville MD

North R L, Rothenberg K H 1990 The duty to warn 'dilemma': a framework for resolution. AIDS Public Pol J 4: 133–141

Novick D M, Ness G L 1984 Abuse of antibiotics by abusers of parenteral heroin or cocaine. South Med J 77: 302–303

Novick D M 1992 The medically ill substance abuser. In: Lowinson J, Ruiz P, Millman R (eds) Substance abuse: a comprehensive textbook, 2nd edn. Williams and Wilkins, Baltimore, MD, p 657–674

O'Dowd M A, Natali C, McKegney F P 1989 Establishment of an HIV-related psychiatric clinic in an area of high substance abuse. V International Conference on AIDS, Montreal. Abstract WBP 217

Office of Technology Assessment 1988 How effective is AIDS education? Office of Technology Assessment, Washington DC

Office of Technology Assessment 1990 Sisk J E, Hatziandreu E J, Hughes R (eds) The effectiveness of drug abuse treatment: implications for controlling AIDS/HIV infection. OTA, Washington DC

Pan American Health Organization 1988 AIDS situation in the Americas 1988. Epidemiol Bull 9: 1–11

Perkins K, Hartel D, Wilson M 1902 HIV-infected women's experience and knowledge of clinical drug trials. Am Public Health Assoc Meeting, Washington DC, Abstract Session 2066

Peterson P K, Sharp B, Gekker G et al 1990 Morphine promotes the growth of HIV-1 in human peripheral blood mononuclear cell cocultures. AIDS 4: 869–873

Peterson P K, Gekker G, Chao C C et al 1991 Cocaine potentiates HIV-1 replication in human peripheral blood mononuclear co-cultures. Involvement of transforming growth factor beta. J Immunol 146: 81–84

Polsky B, Gold J W M, Whimbey E et al 1986 Bacterial pneumonia in a patient with acquired immunodeficiency syndrome. Ann Intern Med 104: 38–41

Randall T 1990 Domestic violence begets other problems of which physicians must be aware to be effective. JAMA 264: 940–944

Reichman L B, Felten C P, Edsall J R 1979 Drug dependence a possible new risk factor for tuberculosis disease. Arch Intern Med 139: 337–339

Rezza G, Lazzarin A, Angarano G et al 1989 The natural history of HIV infection in intravenous drug users: risk of disease progression in a cohort of seroconverters. AIDS 3: 87–90

Rezza G, Lazzarin A, Angarano G et al 1990 Risk of AIDS in seroconverters: a comparison between intravenous drug users and homsexual males. Eur J Epidemiol 6: 99–101

Robert C F, Deglon J J, Wintsch J, Martin J, Perrin L, Bowquin M, Gabriel V, Hirschel B 1990 Behaviour change in intravenous drug users in Geneva. AIDS 4: 657–660

Rolfs R T, Goldberg M, Sharrar R G 1990 Risk factors for syphilis: cocaine use and prostitution. Am J Public Health 80: 853–857

Ross H E, Glaser F B, Germanson T 1988 The prevalance of psychiatric disorders in patients with alcohol and other drug problems. Arch Gen Psychiatry 45: 1023–1031

Rosser S V 1991 Perspectives – AIDS and women, AIDS Education and Prevention, 3: 230–240

Rothenberg K H 1991 The 'duty to warn' dilemma and women with AIDS. Courts, Health Sci & Law 2: 90–98

Rowbotham M C 1990 Neurologic aspects of cocaine abuse. West J Med 323: 699–704

Sapira J D 1968 The narcotic addict as a medical patient. Am J Med A45: 555–588

Sasse H, Salmasa S, Conti S 1989 Risk behavior for HIV-1 infection in Italian drug users. JAIDS 2: 486–496

Sato P A, Chin J, Mann J M 1989 Review of AIDS and HIV infection: global epidemiology and statistics. AIDS 3 (Suppl 1): S301–307

Schoenbaum E E, Hartel D, Selwyn P A et al 1989a Lack of association of T-cell subsets with continuing intravenous drug use and high risk heterosexual sex, independent of HIV infection. V International Conference on AIDS, Montreal, Abstract ThAP101

Schoenbaum E E, Hartel D, Selwyn P A, Klein R S, Davenny K, Rogers M, Feiner, C 1989b Risk factors for human immunodeficiency virus infection in intravenous drug users. N Engl J Med 321: 874–879

Schoenbaum E E, Hartel D, Friedland G H 1990 Crack use predicts HIV seroconversion abstract. 6th International Conference on AIDS, San Francisco

Schoenbaum E E, Alcabes P, McLaughlin S et al 1992 Participation in a needle exchange program in NY City by injecting drug users (IDU) enrolled in a prospective study of HIV. 8th International Conference on AIDS, Amsterdam, Abstract PoC4801

Schrager L K 1988 Bacterial infections in AIDS patients. AIDS 2(Suppl 1): S183–189

Schwartz E L, Brechbuhl A-B, Kahl P et al 1990 Altered pharmacokinetics of zidovudine in former IV drug-using patients receiving methadone. VI International Conference on AIDS, San Francisco. Abstract SB 432

Selik R M, Haverkos H W, Curran J W 1984 Acquired immune deficiency syndrome (AIDS) trends in the United States, 1978–1982. Am J Med 76: 493–500

Selwyn P A, Feingold A R, Hartel D et al 1988 Increased risk of bacterial pneumonia in HIV-infected intravenous users without AIDS. AIDS 2: 267–272

Selwyn P A, Hartel D, Wasserman W, Drucker E 1989a Impact of the AIDS epidemic on morbidity and mortality among intravenous drug users. Am J Public Health 79: 1358–1362

Selwyn P A, Hartel D, Lewis V A et al 1989b A prospective study of the risk of tuberculosis among intravenous drug users with HIV infection. N Engl J Med 320: 545–550

Selwyn P A, Hartel D, Schoenbaum E E et al 1990 Rates and predictors of progression to HIV disease and AIDS in a cohort of intravenous drug users, 1985–1990. VI International Conference on AIDS, San Francisco, Abstract F.C. 111

Selwyn P A, Iezza A 1990 Zidovudine overdose in an intravenous drug user. AIDS 4: 822–824

Selwyn P A 1992 Medical aspects of human immunodeficiency virus infection and its treatment in injecting drug users. In: Lowin J, Ruis R, Millman R (eds) Substance abuse: a comprehensive textbook, 2nd edn Williams and Wilkins, Baltimore, MD, p 744–774

Selwyn P A, Alcabes P, Hartel D et al 1992 Clinical manifestations and predictors of disease progression in drug users with human immunodeficiency virus infection. N Engl J Med 327: 1697–1703

Silberstein C H, McKegney F P, O'Dowd M A et al 1987 A prospective longitudinal study of neuropsychological and psychosocial factors in asymptomatic individuals at risk for HTLV-III/LAV infection in a methadone program: preliminary findings. Int J Neurosci 32: 669–676

Simberkoff M S, El Sadr W, Schiffman G, Rahal J J Jr 1984 Streptococcus pneumoniae infections and bacteria in patients with acquired immune deficiency syndrome, with a report of pneumococcal vaccine failure. Am Rev Resp Dis 103: 1174–1176

Sorenson J L, Constantini M F, London J A 1989 Coping with AIDS: strategies for patients and staff in drug abuse treatment programs. J Psychoactive Drugs 21: 435–440

Spenser B D 1989 On the accuracy of estimates of the numbers of injection drug users. In: Turner C F, Miller H G, Moses L E (eds) AIDS: sexual behavior and intravenous drug use. National Academy of Sciences Press: Wash DC

Stall R, Mckusick L, Wiley J et al 1986 Alcohol and drug use during sexual activity and compliance with safe sex guidelines for AIDS: the AIDS behavioral research project. Health Educ Q 13: 359–371

Stein Z A 1990 HIV prevention: the need for methods women can use. Am J Public Health 80: 460–462

Stimmel B, Vernace S, Schaffner F (1975) Hepatitis B surface antigen and antibody. A prospective study in asymptomatic drug abusers. JAMA 243: 1135–1138

Stimmel B 1989 Unlimited entitlement to health care: the dilemma of narcotic dependency. Mt Sinai J Med 56: 176–179

Stoffer S S 1968 A gynecologic study of drug addicts. Am J Obstet Gynecol 101: 779–783

Sunderam G, McDonald R J, Maniatis T et al 1986 Tuberculosis as a manifestation of the acquired immunodeficiency syndrome (AIDS). JAMA 256: 362–366

Surgeon General 1988 Surgeon General's workshop on violence: recommendations on spouse abuse. US Surgeon General's Office, Washington, DC

Theuer C P, Hopewell P C, Elias D et al 1990 Human immunodeficiency virus infection in tuberculosis patients. J Infect Dis 162: 8–12

Thomas P A, O'Donnell R, Williams R, Chiasson M A 1988 HIV infection in heterosexual female intravenous drug users in New York City. N Engl J Med 319: 374

Tirelli U, Rezza G, Lazzarin A et al 1987 Malignant lymphoma related to HIV infection in Italy: a report of 46 cases. JAMA 258: 2046

Tong T G, Pond S M, Kreek M J et al 1981 Phenytoin induced methadone withdrawal. Ann Intern Med 94: 349–351

Treichler P 1988 AIDS, gender and biomedical discourse. In Fee E, Fox D (eds) AIDS. The burdens of history. Univ CA Press, Berkeley, p 190–266

Vanichseni S, Sonchai W, Plangsringarm K et al 1989 Second seroprevalence survey among Bangkok's intravenous drug addicts. V International Conference on AIDS, Montreal. Abstract TGO 23

Vazquez M, Rotterdam H, Sidhu G 1989 Malignant neoplasms in surgical specimens of different AIDS risk groups. V International Conference on AIDS, Montreal. Abstract MBP 239

Vermund S H, Shoen A R, Galbraith M A, Ebner S C, Fisher R D 1991 Transmission of the human immunodeficiency virus. In Koff W C, Wong-Staal F, Kennedy R (eds) Annual Review of AIDS Research 1: 81–135

Vlahov D, Munoz A, Anthony J, Cohn S, Celentano D, Nelson K 1990 Association of drug injection patterns with antibody to HIV type-1 among intravenous drug users in Baltimore, MD. Am J Epidemiol 132: 847–856

Vlahov D, Anthony J C, Celentano D, Solomon L 1991 Trends of HIV-1 risk reduction among initiates into intravenous drug use 1982–1987. Am J Drug Alc Abuse 17: 39–48

Warren D 1992 Doctoral dissertation. Johns Hopkins School of Public Health, Epidemiology

Weissman G 1991a Working with pregnant women at high risk for HIV infection: outreach and intervention. NY Acad Med 67: 291–300

Weissman G 1991b Working with women at risk: experience from a national prevention program. Plenary address, 1st Annual Training Institute, CHAMHEP, Detroit, MI

Weissman G 1991c Preventing HIV among women at high risk through drug abuse: a national demonstration research program. PHS task force on children, adolescents, women and HIV. Office of the Surgeon General, Wash DC

Witt D J, Craven D E, McCabe W R 1987 Bacterial infections in adult patients with acquired immune deficiency syndrome (AIDS) and AIDS related complex. Am J Med 82: 900–906

Wodak A, Dolan K, Imrie A et al 1987 Antibodies to the human immunodeficiency virus in needles and syringes used by intravenous drug abusers. Med J Aust 147: 275–276

Wofsy C 1992 Transmission of HIV by prostitutes and prevention of spread. In: Cohen P, Sandel M A, Volberding P A (eds) The AIDS knowledge base. Univ CA Press, Berkeley, 1.2.5: 1–3

World Health Organization Collaborating Centre on AIDS 1990 AIDS surveillance in Europe. Quarterly Report No. 26, Paris

Worth D 1989 Sexual decision-making and AIDS: why condom promotion among vulnerable women is likely to fail. Studies Fam Plan 20: 297–307

Worth D 1991 American women and polydrug abuse. In Roth P (ed) Alcohol and drugs are women's issues. Scarecrow Press, London

Worth D, Drucker E, Eric K, Chabon B, Pivnik A, Cochrane K 1989 An ethnographic study of high-risk sexual behavior in 96 women using heroin, cocaine and crack in the Bronx. V International Conference on AIDS, Montreal, Canada

Wybran J, Appelboom T, Famey J P, Govaerts A 1979 Suggestive evidence for receptors for morphine and methionine-enkephalin on normal human blood T lymphocytes. J Immunol 123: 1068–1070

Zagury D, Bernard J, Leonard R et al 1986 Long-term cultures of HTLV-III-infected cells: a model of cytopathology of T-cell depletion in AIDS Science 231: 850–853

Zolla-Pazner S, Des Jarlais D C, Friedman S R et al 1987 Nonrandom development of immunologic abnormalities after infection with human immunodeficiency virus: implications for immunologic classification of the disease. Proc Nat Acad Sci 84: 5404–5408

Zweben J E, Payte T 1990 Methadone maintenance in the treatment of opioid dependence: a current perspective. West J Med. 152: 588–599

12. Does pregnancy accelerate disease progression in HIV-infected women?

Laurent Mandelbrot and Roger Henrion

INTRODUCTION

Nearly a decade ago, reports of pregnancy-related deaths of HIV-infected women (Wetli et al 1983, Rawlison et al 1984) raised concern that pregnancy may have an adverse effect on the progression of HIV infection. AIDS has now become the major cause of pregnancy-related mortality in major cities of the United States (Mertz et al 1992), and accounts for 90% of all deaths among child-bearing urban Rwandan women (Lindan et al 1992). The immune changes associated with pregnancy may alter the host-virus relationship. However, the fact that HIV-related complications may occur during, or following, pregnancy does not necessarily imply that there exists a cause-and-effect relationship. The potential for disease progression exists in all HIV-infected individuals, regardless of their gender or pregnancy status. A growing body of immunologic and epidemiologic data refers to the interaction between infection with HIV type 1 and pregnancy. However, because of considerable methodologic difficulties, a large-scale prospective study is lacking to determine the impact of pregnancy on progression rates from asymptomatic to symptomatic infection, and on survival with AIDS.

PREGNANCY-RELATED CHANGES IN IMMUNE REGULATION

Because pregnancy is known to have an impact on various infections, as well as autoimmune diseases, it has the potential to influence disease progression in several ways. Pregnancy may favour virus replication either directly, or by depressing cell-mediated immunity. It may predispose to non-specific infectious morbidity. It has been shown that repeated challenges to the cell-mediated immune system stimulate HIV replication.

Pregnancy has been viewed as a period in which the immune system is down-regulated. Historically, this interpretation was grounded on the observation that some infectious diseases carry a worse prognosis in pregnant than in non-pregnant women. For many years, it was believed that maternal tolerance for the fetal allograft involved a decrease in the maternal immune response. More recently, it has been suggested that cell-mediated immunity, and in particular CD4 lymphocyte counts, are depresssed during pregnancy.

Infectious morbidity

Pregnancy appears to increase the incidence and/or severity of various bacterial, viral, parasitic, and fungal infections such as malaria, poliomyelitis and viral hepatitis. However, there may be a general tendency to overestimate maternal infectious morbidity (Feinberg & Gonik 1991). Most reports have been retrospective, based on case studies from hospitalized patients. For instance, an association between pregnancy and pneumonia during influenza and varicella infections has been reported, leading to maternal deaths from adult respiratory distress syndromes. However, prospective studies failed to demonstrate a relation between pregnancy and influenza-related death (Saltzman & Jordan 1988). Furthermore, a benign course of infection in the mother may be overshadowed by concern about transmission to the fetus. Infections such as rubella, *Toxoplasma gondii*, cytomegalovirus, herpes and *Listeria monocytogenes* may lead to severe perinatal complications, without having any serious effect on the mother. Finally, opportunistic infections have not been reported in pregnant women, in the absence of immunosuppressant therapy or HIV infection.

A pregnancy-related increase in the incidence of some infectious diseases may be related to factors other than depressed immunity. For instance, vaginal candidiasis and urinary tract infections are frequent in pregnancy, but involve various local changes independent of cell-mediated immunity.

Autoimmune disorders

Autoimmune disorders offer potential for interaction between the immune changes of pregnancy and those observed during infection with HIV. Clinical and biological manifestations of diseases such as systemic lupus erythematosis, immune thrombocytic purpura, thyroiditis, myasthenia gravis, and herpes gestationis, are often exacerbated during pregnancy. Thrombocytopenia, anticardiolipin antibodies and lupus anticoagulant have been reported in patients with symptomatic and asymptomatic HIV infection. However, these disorders do not necessarily have prognostic significance for HIV disease progression (Boué et al 1990). During pregnancy, thrombocytopenia may be secondary to a number of disorders, independently from HIV infection. Moderate third trimester thrombocytopenia is usually without pathologic significance. Therefore, it is difficult to evaluate the relative impact and possible interactions of HIV and pregnancy on thrombocytopenia. Similarly, although Johnstone and colleagues (1992a) found a quarter of a group of 55 pregnant women with HIV infection to have anticardiolipin antibodies, this biological abnormality did not appear to have any clinical impact.

Biological changes

The measurable systemic changes occurring in pregnancy are at most moderate (Feinberg & Gonik 1991). In vivo changes in immune regulation during pregnancy may be difficult to explore by standard techniques, since many of these changes occur locally within the placenta. Contrary to the classical hypothesis that maternal tolerance of the semi-allogeneic fetal graft involves immune suppression, more recent data suggest that maternal recognition of fetal (paternal) antigens is necessary for maintaining pregnancy. Numerous immunoregulatory substances and suppressor cells of maternal or fetal origin have been described, which may act at the maternal–fetal interface. Most of the available data concern cross-sectional comparisons, and are therefore subject to intra- and inter-assay variability inherent to bioassay evaluation.

Pregnancy does not appear to alter antibody-mediated immunity. Immunoglobulin G, A and M levels, B lymphocyte levels and function, and antibody responses to various vaccines are maintained throughout gestation. Although the absolute number of natural killer (NK) cells remains constant, a fall in NK activity has been reported (Delfraissy et al 1992). Reduced NK activity may contribute to increased HIV replication. Antibody-dependent cellular cytotoxicity is not altered.

Modifications in the production of certain cytokines, such as interleukin-1, interleukin-6, tumour necrosis factor, GM-CSF, M-CSF, β TGF and a-interferon have been reported (Delfraissy et al 1992). These cytokines or growth factors may be produced in the pregnant uterus and play a role in the regulation of placental function (Dudley et al 1990) and parturition (Witkin & McGregor 1991). Lymphokine production during pregnancy could theoretically play a role in stimulating HIV replication. In vitro, they lead to increased production of infective virions in peripheral blood mononuclear cells containing the latent provirus (Delfraissy et al 1992). Conversely, HIV may stimulate lymphokine production; however, there are no in vivo data on this point (Reuben et al 1991).

There is conflicting evidence as to whether cell-mediated immunity is depressed in pregnancy (Weinberg 1984). Although antigen-specific immunosuppression may occur, systemic T cell function appears to be maintained. However, hormonal factors may have an indirect impact on immune regulation. For instance, progesterone has been shown to enhance receptor expression involved in the activity of cytotoxic CD8 lymphocytes (Delfraissy et al 1992).

Lymphocyte subset counts

Because CD4 lymphocyte counts are used as a prognostic marker in HIV infection, it is of interest to study their variations in HIV-negative pregnancies. To date, no large-scale study has related lymphocyte subset variations in pregnancy to baseline values before pregnancy. In several small studies, postpartum subset counts were assumed to reflect baseline values. A decrease in CD4 lymphocytes has been reported, particularly during the second and third trimesters (Sridama et al 1982, Biggar et al 1989, Castilla et al 1989, Ravizza et al 1990). However, the decrease in trend is less marked when lymphocyte subsets are expressed as a percentage, to account for physiologic plasma volume expansion in pregnancy. Biggar et al (1989) observed an absolute and relative decrease in CD4 counts in the second trimester (Fig. 12.1). Expressed as a percentage of all lymphocytes, to adjust for the physiologic decrease in the total lymphocyte count, the decline in CD4 levels was approximately 10%. However, others have observed no decrease in CD4 lymphocyte counts in normal pregnancies (Lapointe et al 1991, Biedermann et al 1992).

Concerning CD8 counts, one study reported an increase during pregnancy (Biggar et al 1989), one reported a slight decline after delivery (Chiphangwi et al 1991), whereas another observed steady levels during pregnancy, with an increase after delivery (Lapointe et al 1991).

An increase in T cell activation, as reflected by a rise in CD45 lymphocytes and the presence of the soluble interleukin-2 (IL-2) receptor in serum has been reported (Delfraissy et al 1992). This finding has considerable implications for the interaction between HIV infection and pregnancy, because lymphocyte activation is thought to play a key role in accelerating HIV replication.

IMMUNE CHANGES IN HIV-INFECTED WOMEN DURING PREGNANCY

Most studies have compared CD4 counts in pregnancy between HIV-infected and HIV-negative women, rather than comparing HIV-positive pregnant women with non-pregnant HIV-positive controls (Brettle 1992). Several authors have suggested there is a minor trend towards a decline in CD4 counts during pregnancy in HIV-infected women (Chiphangwi et al 1991, Biedermann et al 1992), but others found no decline in the CD4 count during pregnancy in asymptomatic mothers (Ciraru-Vigneron et al 1992).

Biggar and colleagues (1989) suggested that the loss of CD4 lymphocytes accelerates with pregnancy (Fig. 12.1). CD4 and CD8 lymphocyte counts were monitored during pregnancy and through 12 months postpartum in 37 asymptomatic HIV-seropositive women and 63 HIV-negative controls. In HIV-positive women, as in controls, the CD4 count decreased in the midtrimester and increased prior to delivery. However, CD4 counts levelled off after delivery, whereas they increased in seronegative controls. The CD4/CD8 ratio was lower in the HIV-positive than the HIV-negative group, but it did not significantly change through pregnancy and postpartum in either group. Among seropositive women, HIV-related destruction of CD4 lymphocytes occurred throughought pregnancy and postpartum at an average rate of 2% per month. This decline appeared more rapid than that reported in the literature for cohorts of haemophiliacs or homosexual men. In a recent study by Biedermann and associates (1992), CD4 and CD4/8 ratios decreased significantly during pregnancy in 75 seropositive women, whereas they were maintained in 34 controls.

In our own experience, CD4 lymphocyte counts and CD4/CD8 ratios were followed over a total of 133 pregnancies in a cohort of 128 women, only seven of whom had HIV-related symptoms (Mandelbrot et al, submitted for publication). The mean CD4 lymphocyte count ($\pm$ SE) was 531 ($\pm$ 34) in the first trimester, 478 ($\pm$ 28) in the second trimester, 520 ($\pm$ 32) in the third trimester, increased slightly to 593 ($\pm$ 36) at delivery, and levelled at 490 ($\pm$ 48) in the postpartum period.

CD8 counts in HIV-positive pregnancies appear to be elevated during pregnancy, if postpartum levels are considered to reflect baseline values (Biggar et al 1989, Ravizza et al 1990, Chiphangwi et al 1991).

In a prospective study by Berrebi and colleagues (1990), outcome in asymptomatic HIV-infected women was compared between those who had

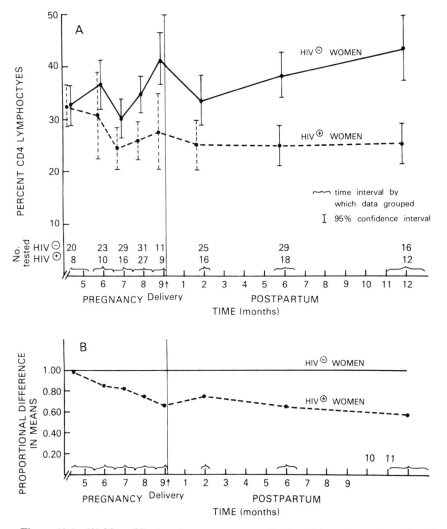

Figure 12.1 (A) Mean CD4 lymphocyte percentages (95% confidence intervals are shown) in HIV-positive (broken line) and HIV-negative (solid line) women. Braces indicate time intervals by which data are grouped. A levelling of postpartum values is observed in HIV-positive women. (From Biggar et al 1989, with permission from the publisher.) (B) Comparison of CD4 lymphocyte percentages in HIV-positive (broken line) and HIV-negative (solid line) women (calculated as (HIV-positive minus HIV-negative)/HIV-negative), showing a declining trend in CD4 lymphocytes in HIV-positive pregnancies

pregnancies and matched controls. The decline in CD4 lymphocyte counts and CD4/CD8 ratios over 3 years was equivalent in patients who delivered, in those who had pregnancy terminations, and in those who were not pregnant. There was also no difference among the three groups in the rate of decrease of serum total IgA levels. In another prospective study (Delfraissy et al 1989), over 2 years of follow-up, the absolute decline in CD4 counts

was significantly greater among women who had been pregnant (215 ± 85 cells/mm^3), than among those who had not been pregnant (97 ± 59 CD4 cells/mm^3).

Little information is available on changes during pregnancy for other prognostic markers of HIV infection, such as β2-microglobulin and neopterin (Brettle 1992, Delfraissy et al 1992). There are at present no data concerning modifications in cytokine release, T cell activation, or NK cells in HIV-positive pregnancies.

No data have been reported on the impact of pregnancy on CD4 counts in women with advanced disease, i.e. low baseline counts and/or HIV-related symptoms.

A possible direct approach to determine the short-term effect of pregnancy on HIV infection might be to measure variations in viral load. The viral load has been shown to correlate with disease progression in non-pregnant individuals (Schnittmann et al 1990). The effect of pregnancy on viral replication is not yet known. Some small studies have found an increase in P24 antigenaemia during mid-trimester (Delfraissy et al 1992). We have not observed such an increase in our own cohort, covering 133 pregnancies (Mandelbrot et al, submitted for publication). However, p24 antigenaemia is a surrogate marker, which lacks sensitivity and specificity. Ehrnst and co-workers (1991) found, in a small series of patients, that the proportion with positive plasma viraemia increased from 30% in the first trimester to 52% in the second trimester, and 67% in the postpartum period. However, since baseline results before pregnancy were not available, these findings may be misleading. Regarding long-term changes following pregnancy, Berrebi and colleagues (1990) observed no difference in the appearance of positive p24 antigenaemia in 3 years of follow-up after delivery, compared with non-pregnant controls.

SURVIVAL AND DISEASE PROGRESSION IN HIV-INFECTED WOMEN

When considering the impact of pregnancy on HIV infection, it cannot be assumed that the natural history and presentation of disease are the same for women as those reported for men. Intercurrent pregnancies are major events that distinguish women from men; however, there are a number of other demographic differences. Until recently, data on progression were based on studies of male cohorts, such as the San Francisco homosexual cohort, which now covers 12 years. HIV transmission to women is related to intravenous drug use, heterosexual contact or blood transfusions.

Data are now available on cohorts of transfusion-related cases and intravenous drug users of both sexes. Differences in life-style, psychological and hormonal environment offer potential for a unique evolution in women. Among AIDS-defining illnesses, Kaposi's sarcoma is less frequent in women than in men, creating a potential confounding factor in comparing rates of progression as well as survival rates in AIDS patients. Conversely, HIV infection influences the course of gynaecological problems such as vaginal moniliasis, pelvic inflammatory disease and especially cervical intraepithelial neoplasia, which do not appear in clinical classifications of HIV-infected patients.

In a large cohort study from Kigali, Rwanda (Lindan et al 1992), the 2-year mortality among HIV-infected women by Kaplan-Meier survival analysis was 7% overall (95% confidence interval, 5–10%), and 21% (CI, 8–34%) for those who had AIDS at entry into the study.

Most retrospective analyses as well as cohort studies suggest that rates of progression to AIDS are not related to gender (Ellerbrock et al 1991, Carpenter et al 1991, Szabo et al 1992, Melnick et al 1992, Benson et al 1992, Creagh et al 1992, Brettle et al 1992). In a large cohort study of 1816 HIV-infected persons from Bordeaux, France (Morlat et al 1992), progression rates did not differ significantly between men and women. Among 228 women who were asymptomatic at inclusion and had adequate follow-up, the cumulative probability of developing AIDS was 4.4% at 1 year, 9.1% after 2 years, 13.7% after 3 years and 17.5% after 4 years. In a crude comparison, these rates were actually lower than those for the 613 men enrolled in the study. When adjusting for CD4 count and age at entry, the probability of developing AIDS for men was not significantly higher than for women (adjusted relative risk 1.3; 95% confidence interval 0.8–2.2; $p = 0.26$).

Other studies suggested that survival with AIDS is shorter in women than in men (Rothenberg et al 1987, Reeves & Overton 1988, Lemp et al 1990, Friedland et al 1991). However, the apparent difference may be explained by the fact that most of these studies are from the United States, where HIV-infected women have poorer access to health care than do men (Minkoff & Dehovitz 1991). This is illustrated by the fact that more women died at the time they first presented with a diagnosis of AIDS (Araneta et al 1991).

One of the major difficulties in studying the natural history of HIV-infection is that the timing of infection is often unknown. Most precise data on incubation periods have been obtained in transfusion-related cases. One study actually suggested a trend towards a longer latency period in women (Medley et al 1987). In a Swedish cohort of people infected through blood transfusion, the progression rate was not related to gender (Blaxhult et al 1990). The Italian seroconversion study (1992) followed 468 intravenous drug users, 127 of whom were women, with known dates of seroconversion. The progression rates to AIDS were the same among men and women. In a recent update of the Edinburgh cohort (Brettle et al 1992), timing of HIV infection was known for 306 patients. The rates of progression from seroconversion to CD4 counts under 200, to AIDS, or to death were not influenced by gender.

Another area of concern has been the interpretation of CD4 levels, which could have a different prognostic value in women than in men. It has been suggested from preliminary work that women with HIV infection may have a poorer prognosis than men at comparable baseline levels (Creagh et al 1992); however, this has not been apparent in other cohort studies (Fernandez-Cruz et al 1990, Brettle et al 1992).

Among demographic characteristics, advanced age stands out as relating to more rapid disease progression, but gender does not appear to influence the natural history of infection with HIV-1. As concerns HIV-2 infection in women, a cohort study from Dakar, Sénégal, observed progression and death rates to be significantly less in women infected with HIV-2 than with HIV-1 (Siby et al 1992). There are at present no published data comparing the natural history of infection with HIV type 2 between men and women.

HIV PROGRESSION IN PREGNANCY

The above evidence indicates that the natural history of HIV infection in women is similar to that described for men. The lack of excess progression in women, despite intercurrent pregnancies, suggests in itself that pregnancy does not markedly accelerate HIV disease. Few studies have specifically focused on the impact of pregnancy on the course of infection. The available sources of data are retrospective studies and prospective studies, each containing inherent methodological limitations. Among the prospective studies, several are unmatched cohort studies, some compare HIV-positive mothers with HIV-negative controls, and very few have a control group of non-pregnant HIV-infected women.

Retrospective studies

The first report suggesting an adverse effect of pregnancy on HIV infection was a retrospective study from Miami (Scott et al 1985) on 15 mothers whose infants were followed for AIDS. All mothers had been asymptomatic during pregnancy; 80% had progressed to Centers for Disease Control (CDC) class IV disease within 30 months. The progression rate was clearly greater than would be expected in an unselected CDC group II population.

In a study from New York City (Minkoff et al 1987), among 34 women identified by the birth of an affected child, 44% developed symptomatic disease within a mean follow-up period of 27.8 months.

Gloeb and colleagues (1988) followed the clinical course of 50 HIV-infected women antepartum, intrapartum and/or postpartum. Three patients died of complications related to AIDS; two of these were asymptomatic when first seen in the course of their pregnancies. Two developed *Pneumocystis carinii* pneumonia and died during pregnancy and the third developed *Toxoplasma gondii* encephalitis at 18 weeks' gestation and died 4 months after delivery. Another two patients developed AIDS-related symptoms in the third trimester. An additional four developed oral candidiasis; three of these had CD4 counts under 160/mm^3 at delivery.

Retrospective studies are more likely to enroll patients whose children are followed for HIV infection, or who themselves enter the study because of symptomatic disease. The selection bias towards overestimating progression is obvious.

Descriptive pregnancy cohort studies

Gloeb and associates (1992) described survival and disease progression among 103 HIV-seropositive women, following an index delivery. At the time of delivery, 79.6% were asymptomatic (CDC group II), 12.6% had lymphadenopathy syndrome (group III), and eight had symptomatic (group IV) disease, of whom six fulfilled criteria for AIDS. Patients who were asymptomatic (group II) on entry into the study had mean cumulative probabilities of developing AIDS (mean ± SE) of 2.6% (± 1.8%) at 1 year and 21.2% (± 5.7%) at 3 years. Unexpectedly, the probability of developing AIDS was significantly greater in patients who had lymphadenopathy syndrome on entry: 24% (± 12.1%) at 1 year and 73.4% (± 15.6%) at 3 years. Another factor significantly associated with disease progression was herpes genitalis during pregnancy. The relationship between disease progression and CD4 lymphocyte counts was not studied, because subset counts were not routinely performed. Survival was also examined with Kaplan-Meier analysis. The cumulative probability of survival (mean ± SE) in group II patients was 97.4% (± 1.8%) 1 year postpartum, decreasing to 83.6% (± 5.2%) at 3 years. Survival rates were also significantly lower for patients with lymphadenopathy syndrome (group III) (Fig. 2). In cohorts of (mostly male) non-pregnant individuals, survival rates have been shown to be equivalent between patients in CDC groups II and III. The poor prognosis in pregnant group III patients may be indirect evidence for pregnancy-related disease progression. Covariates, such as ethnicity, age, gravidity and zidovudine therapy were controlled for. However, the authors acknowledged several limitations to the study. In particular, patients had HIV antibody testing on the basis of criteria, not as a routinely offered prenatal test. Most importantly, the loss to follow-up was relatively high – 21.4% by 1 year postpartum and 39.8% by 2 years. Nevertheless, this publication is particularly useful, since it is the first to report disease progression and survival in an obstetrical population using life-table analysis.

Similar results have been observed in our institution, the Port Royal Maternity in Paris. A cohort of 128 women, accounting for 133 deliveries between 1987 and 1992, was followed during preg-

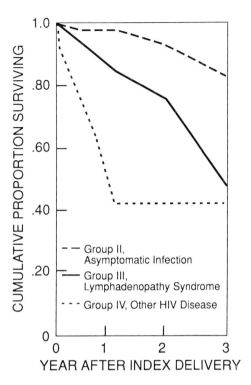

Figure 12.2 Cumulative survival (Kaplan-Meier method) over 3 years, following an index delivery in women who had asymptomatic HIV infection (group II, broken line) lymphadenopathy syndrome (group III, solid line) or symptomatic disease (group IV, dotted line). Lymphadenopathy was associated with poorer outcome than was asymptomatic disease, contrary to findings from cohorts of non-pregnant individuals. (From Gloeb et al 1992, with permission from the publisher)

nancy and afterwards (Mandelbrot et al, submitted for publication). Only seven (5.5%) had HIV-related symptoms, the remaining 121 being asymptomatic (CDC groups II and III); the mean CD4 lymphocyte count was 531/mm^3. Over a mean observation period of 23 months from the last menstrual period, 15 women progressed from asymptomatic to CDC group IV disease. The most frequent AIDS-defining illness was *Pneumocystis carinii* pneumonia (seven cases). There were six AIDS-related deaths. The cumulative survival, from the last menstrual period, calculated by the life-table method, was 99.2% (95% confidence interval: 95.6–99.8%) at 2 years and 73.6% (95%CI: 46.5–89.9%) at 4 years.

Several cohort studies compared seropositive mothers with seronegative pregnant controls.

Minkoff and colleagues (1990) compared the incidence of serious infectious morbidity in 56 HIV-infected and 76 seronegative controls through pregnancy and the immediate postpartum period. Controls were matched for intravenous drug use, Haitian origin and referral by an agency for HIV testing. There was no serious infectious morbidity in the seronegative group. In the HIV-infected group, there were five serious HIV-related infections, all in mothers with low CD4 counts. The difference was statistically significant.

In a prospective cohort of intravenous drug users, Selwyn and associates (1989) reported pregnancy outcomes in 97 women. Among those carrying pregnancies past 24 weeks, 24 were seropositive (only one with symptomatic disease), and there were 40 seronegative controls. Among HIV-infected women, 24% were hospitalized for non-AIDS-defining infectious diseases, versus 5% for seronegative controls. The relative risk for bacterial pneumonia was 11.5 ($p = 0.05$). However, in this small cohort, none of the seropositives developed AIDS during a mean of 19 months follow-up (range 3–27 months).

Cohorts of HIV-positive women

Few of the available cohort studies of HIV-infected individuals have investigated the relationship between pregnancy and disease progression among the enrolled women. In the Edinburgh, UK cohort, 107 women were followed from seroconversion through 6 to 54 months (MacCallum et al 1989). Intercurrent pregnancies did not appear to modify progression rates.

Prospective cohorts theoretically offer the best comparison, but there may be confounding elements. Women with children are followed longer and more regularly, especially in hospitals offering perinatal care. Patients who deliver may differ from those who abort, and from those who do not become pregnant, in many ways, such as age, socio-economic level, ethnic origin, transmission group, psychological state and disease status. Patients with poor prognostic factors may be more likely to forgo pregnancy or to have abortions. The interpretation of cohort studies requires large numbers and multivariate analysis to avoid potential confounding factors.

Prospective studies with non-pregnant HIV-positive controls

Three prospective studies found that HIV progression was greater in women who had been pregnant than in unmatched non-pregnant controls (Delfraissy et al 1989, Deschamps et al 1989, Lindgren et al 1991). In a study of 290 HIV-seropositive women in Paris (Delfraissy et al 1989), progression to CDC group IV within a mean 36 months of follow-up was 15% among women who delivered, versus 3.6% in women who aborted and 5.7% in those who did not become pregnant. As mentioned above, the fall in the CD4 count was significantly greater among the pregnancy group than in controls. In the study from Haiti (Deschamps et al 1989), progression occurred during a mean of 21 months of follow-up in 47% of women who had pregnancies, compared with 26% in those who were not pregnant.

Berrebi and colleagues (1990) performed a prospective study comparing disease progression in three groups: women who were pregnant and delivered, women who had pregnancy terminations and matched non-pregnant controls. All patients were CDC group II or III at inclusion. Nearly all were past or current intravenous drug users. Progression, based on clinical and laboratory criteria, was followed over a mean period of 16 months (range, 3–36 months). Among 35 patients who were pregnant and delivered beyond 28 weeks, four progressed to CDC group IV during the follow-up period; one of these died of neurotoxoplasmosis. Out of 29 controls who miscarried or had first or second trimester terminations of pregnancy, three progressed to CDC group IV; one of these also died of neurotoxoplasmosis. Finally, among 64 matched controls who did not become pregnant during the study period, six progressed to CDC group IV; one of these died of *Pneumocystis carinii* pneumonia. There was no significant difference in the proportion of women developing HIV-related symptoms, according to their pregnancy status. The rate of decrease of CD4 lymphocyte counts, CD4/CD8 ratios and total IgA levels and the prevalence of p24 antigenaemia over the study period did not differ significantly between the three groups. This publication is the largest prospective study with a control group available on the subject.

It offers evidence that pregnancy does not affect disease progression in stage II and III patients. Although the timing of infection was not known in most cases, and possible confounding factors may have been overlooked, an effort was made to match patients for demographics and disease stage. Initial mean CD4 lymphocyte counts were significantly higher among patients who delivered than among those who had terminations or no pregnancy at all, but CD4/CD8 ratios were the same in the three groups. The main weakness of this study, as in most available open observational studies, is the problem of follow-up. The length of follow-up varied widely, nearly one-half of patients being lost to follow-up within a year, some as early as 3 months after inclusion. Life-table analysis would allow for more effective comparison of the groups.

Similarly, a prospective study from Genoa, Italy showed no significant difference in disease progression between women in various stages of disease who had pregnancies and matched non-pregnant controls (Mazzarello et al 1991). Disease progression occurred in 18/35 women who had pregnancies, compared to 15/35 women who had not been pregnant, with a mean follow-up of 41 months.

In a study from the Bronx, USA, Schoenbaum and co-workers (1989), compared disease progression between 56 women who had no live births, 36 with one birth and 49 with two or more live births over a mean of 2.6 years. After controlling for CD4 counts, women who had delivered had no excess disease progression. Other smaller prospective studies including pregnant and non-pregnant HIV-infected women have been presented at international meetings, showing no difference in progression to AIDS (Nachman 1987, DiLenardo et al 1989, Nzila et al 1991). In one small study, the progression rate among pregnant women was actually lower than among non-pregnant women (Bledsoe et al 1990).

In a cross-sectional study of 54 HIV-infected women, we observed that the prevalence of virus excretion in cervico-vaginal secretions was greater among pregnant than among non-pregnant women, when adjusting for disease stage, p24 antigenaemia, CD4 count, sexually transmitted disease and zidovudine therapy (Hénin et al 1993). However, this finding is likely to relate more to local changes than to a decrease in the maternal immune defences.

The design of the non-pregnant control group limits the statistical power of most of the above studies. Since the timing of infection is rarely known, controls cannot be matched for the length of infection. The only criterion for entry is the presence of HIV antibodies. As antibody testing becomes more widespread, less bias towards symptomatic disease would be expected. However, indications for testing vary between countries and between centres. Hence, study patients do not represent a random sample of the overall HIV-infected population. Furthermore, prenatal visits are an occasion for offering routine testing, leading to the possibility that the characteristics of pregnant seropositive women may differ from those of non-pregnant patients. Therefore, non-pregnant controls should be carefully matched for demographics, including risk group and age, as well as for disease stage. Larger prospective studies, including sequential lymphocyte subset counts, would allow for stratifying outcome according to baseline CD4 counts. The time at which pregnant patients are included in the study group must be carefully chosen. Most studies have started follow-up at delivery, which does not account for disease progression during pregnancy itself. However, the major limitation to prospective studies is follow-up. Short-term follow-up would be sufficient to detect rapid disease progression related to pregnancy. However, subclinical pregnancy-related changes would become apparent only upon longer follow-up, which is more difficult to obtain.

NON-SPECIFIC INFECTIOUS MORBIDITY

The data from obstetric cohorts suggest that HIV-infected women are at increased risk of non-AIDS-defining complications, such as upper urinary tract infections, endometritis, cervical papillomavirus infections and intraepithelial neoplasias, syphilis, herpes simplex and pneumopathies (Gloeb et al 1988, Willoughby et al 1989, Selwyn et al 1989, Braddick et al 1990). In the study by Selwyn and associates (1989), 24% of HIV-positive women were hospitalized during pregnancy for non-AIDS-defining infectious diseases, versus 5% for HIV-negative matched controls ($p = 0.04$). Chorioamnionitis has been shown to be more frequent in HIV-seropositive than in seronegative women in some studies (Ryder et al 1989), but not in others (Selwyn et al 1989). Non-specific pregnancy-related infectious complications may represent an immunological burden, which can have an impact on disease progression. In African cohorts, tuberculosis stands out as the major cause of pregnancy-related HIV morbidity and mortality. In a study from Kigali (Msellati et al 1992), 215 HIV-seropositive women and 216 seronegative women matched for age and parity were enrolled at delivery. None fulfilled the definition for AIDS. Among HIV-infected women the incidence of tuberculosis was 1.2 per women-years of follow-up, versus 0.3 in controls (relative risk 4.2; 95% confidence interval 2.8–5.6). The mortality among HIV-infected women in this study was 3.7 per 100 women-years.

Gloeb and colleagues (1992) observed that mothers with herpes genitalis during pregnancy were eight times more likely to develop AIDS. The possibility is open that herpes may have been related to the pregnant state, as well as to latent HIV-induced immunodepression. This example highlights the fact that non-specific infectious morbidity, as well as AIDS-defining opportunistic infections, are relevant to disease progression in HIV infection.

SURVIVAL AND PROGRESSION IN WOMEN WITH ADVANCED DISEASE

Since most of the data on HIV and pregnancy refer to asymptomatic women, little information is available concerning the impact of pregnancy on patients in advanced stages of disease. Early retrospective studies suggested that survival with AIDS may be shortened in pregnant women. The Centers for Disease Control reviewed pregnancy-related deaths in pregnancy and the postpartum period in the USA between 1981 and 1988 (Koonin et al 1989). Six AIDS related deaths had been published and another 20 were identified through the National Pregnancy Mortality Surveillance system. The interval between the termination of pregnancy and death ranged from 1 day to 19 weeks, with a mean of 45 days. The

interval between diagnosis of AIDS and death ranged from 1 day to 15 months, with a mean interval of 113 days. This time interval appeared shorter than those observed at the time for women in general (298 days) or for men (347 days). There was an important bias in that the criterion for inclusion in the study was death within 1 year of delivery. Nevertheless, this review pin-points the fact that the vast majority of HIV-related deaths do not appear in the medical literature. Since 1988, it may be estimated that most HIV-related deaths in pregnancy are not published.

Pneumocystis carinii pneumonia stands out as the most frequent HIV-related infection in pregnancy in the developed countries (Jensen et al 1984, Minkoff et al 1986, Kell et al 1991). Bongain and colleagues (1992) in France reported two cases of fatal *Pneumocystis carinii* pneumonia in the third trimester of pregnancy in patients who were asymptomatic at the beginning of gestation. A large survey covering more than 1000 HIV-infected women who delivered during 1989 in the USA (Stratton et al 1992) confirmed that *Pneumocystis carinii* pneumonia is the most frequent opportunistic infection in seropositive pregnant women in North America, as in France (Fig. 12.3).

Pneumocystis carinii pneumonia was also found to be the leading cause of pregnancy-related deaths from AIDS in the USA (Koonin et al 1989). Outcome for pregnant women with *Pneumocystis carinii* pneumonia appeared worse than those reported at the time for non-pregnant women. Among 16 who died of *Pneumocystis carinii* pneumonia, four died during pregnancy, six within a week after delivery, two within a month and another eight within a year after delivery. The mean interval between diagnosis and death was 59 days (SD ± 42 days), compared to a survival of 187 days (± 208 days) in a CDC reference population of 190 non-pregnant women of reproductive age matched for intravenous drug use. These retrospective data suggest that pregnancy worsens the prognosis of *Pneumocystis carinii* pneumonia. With improvements in prophylaxis, diagnosis and therapy for *Pneumocystis carinii* pneumonia, the outlook for pregnant women with this infection may be improving (Hicks et al 1990).

Nearly all AIDS-defining opportunistic infec-

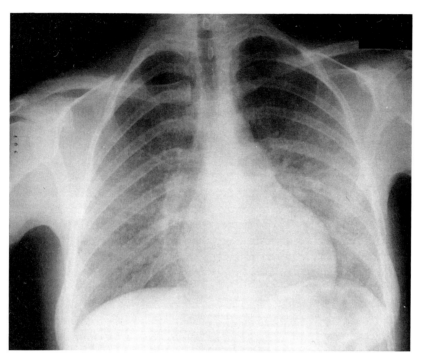

Figure 12.3 *Pneumocystis carinii* pneumonia is the most frequent HIV-related complication in seropositive pregnant women in Europe and North America, as well as the leading cause of death.

tions have been reported in pregnancy, including tuberculosis, oesophageal, bronchial or pulmonary candidiasis, toxoplasmosis, disseminated cytomegalovirus, cryptococcal meningitis and disseminated histioplasmosis (Stratton et al 1992). In addition to *Pneumocystis carinii* pneumonia, the reported causes of death in pregnancy include tuberculosis, *Listeria monocytogenes* and toxoplasmosis (Henrion 1990). However, there exists no information as to whether the course of these diseases is altered in pregnant women. In addition to pregnancy-related immune changes, delays in diagnosis and therapy of opportunistic infections may alter the outcome for HIV infected women during pregnancy.

In the cohort study by Gloeb and co-workers (1992) the median survival of women with AIDS at or following delivery appeared short, compared with survival in men with AIDS. In group IV patients, only $42.9 \pm 18.9\%$ survived 1 year after delivery (Fig. 12.2). Median survival following

diagnosis of AIDS was 189 days. Covariates, such as a history of drug use, sexually transmitted diseases and zidovudine therapy were controlled for; only zidovudine therapy was marginally significant. Unfortunately, the authors did not specify how many of the patients with AIDS at delivery already had symptoms at the beginning of pregnancy, and how many had progressed to AIDS during their pregnancy.

Low CD4 lymphocyte counts are the most well-established prognostic element in HIV-infected persons. Serious infectious morbidity in pregnancy has been shown to be frequent in HIV-infected women with low CD4 counts. In a New York cohort (Minkoff et al 1990), out of 16 women whose CD4 counts dropped below $300/\text{mm}^3$, five experienced serious infections, mostly *Pneumocystis carinii pneumonia*. However, no data have been reported on the rate of decline of CD4 counts in pregnancy following the onset of symptomatic disease.

The potential effects of pregnancy on opportunistic infections are not limited to modifications in immune regulation, but also include local changes. For instance, during parasitemic infections, i.e. toxoplasmosis and crytococcosis, infection of the placenta could theoretically play an aggravating role. Vaginal moniliasis may influence the risk of systemic candidiasis. However, these possibilites have not yet been addressed in the literature.

The only study available comparing survival in AIDS patients according to whether or not they became pregnant is a population-based study by Johnstone and associates (1992b). Survival time after diagnosis of AIDS was compared in five women who were pregnant and 17 women without a pregnancy. Clinical evolution or survival time did not differ between the two groups. However, the number of pregnant women was small. Furthermore, among the five women who had pregnancies, only two went on to term deliveries, and three had terminations. Multicentre studies are under way in France to evaluate the impact of pregnancy on survival in women with symptomatic HIV infections.

Seroconversion in pregnancy

Few cases of documented seroconversion have been reported in pregnant women. Acute primary infection has been shown to be associated with poor outcome in non-pregnant individuals (Isaksson et al 1988). Further studies would be necessary to determine whether the pregnant state exposes to symptomatic seroconversion.

FACTORS INFLUENCING MATERNAL OUTCOME

One of the difficulties in determining the impact of pregnancy on the course of HIV infection is that a number of other factors may influence the rate of progression from an asymptomatic to a symptomatic state, as well as survival rates with AIDS. Comparisons between pregnancy cohorts and published series should be made with utmost caution, if at all. For prospective studies with control groups, given the available population sizes, it would be exceedingly difficult to control

for all putative factors influencing prognosis when performing multivariate analysis. Many of these elements are unknown at present, or are still hypotheses for further research.

These factors are relevant to the extent that they influence the host–virus interaction. The virus itself may be of importance. The vast differences in natural history beween HIV types 1 and 2 offers the most extreme example. Among HIV-1 virus isolates, outcome may differ according to whether they replicate slowly or rapidly, and are syncitia-forming. However, the effects may be confounded by mutations occurring in infected individuals or acquisition of differing strains, through ongoing heterosexual contact or drug injection. The host's susceptibility to HIV disease is thought to be of considerable importance. This topic is under intensive scrutiny in cohorts of long-term survivors with HIV. As mentioned above, age stands out as relating to disease progression. Differences are suspected in the inherent genetic predisposition to HIV infection. The dynamics of the specific immune response, including neutralizing antibodies, may be of importance in disease progression, as well as HIV transmission. Environmental factors, such as malnutrition, smoking, or active drug use, may also be involved. The effect of concomitant drug use on disease progression is dealt with elsewhere in this book. The impact of sexually-transmitted diseases, mentioned above, may be of considerable importance (Phair et al 1992). Host–virus interaction is also thought to be influenced by co-infections with other viruses, such as *Mycoplasma incognitus*, herpes 6, hepatitis C and/or cytomegalovirus (Mandelbrot and Henrion 1991). Mothers who have HIV-infected children have been found to be more likely to develop complications (Scott et al 1989), suggesting that maternal and infant outcome may be related to common prognostic factors. It is thus not surprising to note marked differences in natural history studies from various parts of the world, in particular between Africa, North America and Europe.

An important confounding factor in studies on HIV progression is drug therapy, given either for treatment of complications, or as prophylaxis. Women have been largely underrepresented in clinical trials and pregnant women have been specifically excluded until recently. Pharmacokinetic studies have been conducted in few pregnant women, but have shown results comparable to non-pregnant adults (Watts et al 1991). A US survey reported on the safety of zidovudine use in pregnancy (Sperling et al 1992), but offered no data as to its efficacy on disease progression in a pregnant population. Indications for antiretroviral therapy in pregnant women have tended to be restrictive, because of concern with potential toxicity to the fetus. Currently, zidovudine is recommended in women with symptoms of disease and/or CD4 counts under 200/mm^3 (Sperling & Stratton 1992). There have been anecdotal reports that pregnant women may be more susceptible to side-effects from various medications, such as hepatitis with rifampicin, anaemia with sulphadiazine or hypoglycaemia with pentamidine. Since symptoms such as nausea, rash and anaemia are common in pregnancy, it is often difficult to substantiate maternal drug toxicity. Another area of concern in maternal therapy is the problem of toxicity to the fetus. Most authors agree that aggressive therapy should not be withheld in pregnancy when life-threatening complications occur (Schoenbaum et al 1992). There also appears to be a consensus on the need for secondary prophylaxis, especially following *Pneumocystis carinii* pneumonia or toxoplasmosis. Primary prophylaxis for *Pneumocystis carinii* pneumonia is recommended during pregnancy when CD4 counts fall under 200/mm^3. Aerosolized pentamidine is more widely used in pregnant women than trimethoprim/sulfamethoxazole. There appears to be less consensus concerning primary prophylaxis for toxoplasmosis, tuberculosis, candidiasis and other opportunistic infections. The fact that medications are used with caution in pregnant women could be a confounding element in analysing disease progression and survival.

CONCLUSION

The available evidence does not indicate that pregnancy accelerates progression from asymptomatic HIV infection to AIDS. However, it remains possible that pregnant women are more vulnerable to HIV-related complications, as well as non-AIDS-defining morbidity. It remains to be proven whether pregnancy shortens life expectancy in women with AIDS. Similarly, the impact of pregnancy on CD4 lymphocyte counts appears marginal in the upper ranges, but may be pronounced in patients with low baseline counts. It is not known whether viral load and replication are influenced by pregnancy. The confounding effects of putative cofactors involved in disease progression need to be considered. The key issue in counselling women on reproductive decisions is the danger of mother-to-infant transmission. However, the risk of disease progression must also be emphasized. Patients with advanced disease and/or low CD4 counts are at high risk of complications, whether or not they become pregnant. As more women infected in the 1980s go on to develop symptoms of HIV disease, obstetricians may be confronted with increasing numbers of pregnant women with AIDS. Because maternal deaths have dramatic consequences, women who have advanced-stage disease or poor prognostic markers should clearly be discouraged from becoming pregnant.

REFERENCES

Araneta M R, Lemp G F Cohen J B et al 1991 Survival trends among women with AIDS in San Francisco. Seventh International Conference on AIDS, Florence. Abstract MC3122
Benson C, Sha B, Urbansky P et al 1992 Women and HIV disease: clinical progression and survival in a cohort followed at a university medical center. Eighth International Conference on AIDS, Amsterdam. Abstract MoC0034
Berrebi A, Kobuch W E, Puel J et al 1990 Influence of pregnancy on human immunodeficiency virus disease. Eur J Obstet Gynecol Reprod Biol 37: 211–217
Biedermann K, Rudin C, Irion O et al 1992 Immune parameters in HIV-positive pregnant women. Eighth International Conference on AIDS, Amsterdam. Abstract PoC4725
Biggar R J, Pahwa S, Minkoff H et al 1989 Immunosuppression in pregnant women infected with human immunodeficiency virus. Am J Obstet Gynecol 161: 1239–1244
Blaxhult A, Granath F, Lidman K, Giesecke J 1990 The influence of age on the latency period to AIDS in people infected by HIV through blood transfusion. AIDS 4: 125–129
Bledsoe K, Olopoenia L, Barnes S et al 1990 Effect of pregnancy on progression of HIV infection. Sixth International Conference on AIDS, San Francisco. Abstract ThC652
Bongain A, Fuzibet J G Gillet J Y 1992 Infection à Pneumocystis carinii: deux cas responsables de mort maternelle au cours de la grossesse. Presse Méd 21: 950
Boué F, Dreyfus M, Bridey F et al 1990 Lupus anticoagulant

and HIV infection: a prospective study (letter). AIDS 4: 467–468

Braddick M, Kreiss J K, Embree J E et al 1990 Impact of maternal HIV infection on obstetrical and early neonatal outcome. AIDS 4: 1001–1005

Brettle R P 1992, Pregnancy and its effect on HIV/AIDS. In Johnstone F D (ed) HIV infection in obstetrics and gynaecology. Ballière's Clin Obstet Gynaecol 6: 125–136

Brettle R P, Richardson A M, Burns S M et al 1992 Survival analysis by gender and risk group for HIV in Edinburgh. Eighth International Conference on AIDS, Amsterdam. Abstract MoC0066

Carpenter C C J, Mayer K H, Stein M D et al 1991 Human immunodeficiency virus infection in North American women: experience with 200 cases and review of the literature. Medicine 70: 307–325

Castilla J A, Rueda R, Vargas M L et al 1989 Decreased levels of circulating CD4 + T lymphocytes during normal human pregnancy. J Reprod Immunol 15: 103–111

Chiphangwi J, Nawrocki P, Dallabetta G et al 1991 Post partum T lymphocyte changes in HIV-1 seropositive (SP) and seronegative (SN) Malawian women. Seventh International Conference on AIDS, Florence. Abstract 3233

Ciraru-Vigneron N, Lefèvre-Elbert V, Boval B et al 1992 Evolution and prognostic value of lymphocyte count during pregnancy in healthy women and HIV-infected women. Eighth International Conference on AIDS, Amsterdam. Abstract MoB3048

Creagh T, Thompson M, Morris A, Whyte B 1992 Gender differences in the spectrum of HIV disease. Eighth International Conference on AIDS, Amsterdam. Abstract MoC0032

Delfraissy J F, Pons J C, Séréni D et al 1989 Does pregnancy influence disease progression in HIV-positive women. Fifth International Conference on AIDS, Montreal. Abstract MBP34

Delfraissy J F, Blanche S, Rouzioux C, Mayaux M J 1992 Perinatal HIV transmission: facts and controversies. Immunodefic Rev 3: 305–327

Deschamps N M, Pape J W, Madhauan S et al 1989 Pregnancy and acceleration of HIV-related illness. Fifth International Conference on AIDS, Montreal. Abstract MBP6

DiLenardo L, Truscia D, Gioquinto C, Grella P V 1989 A prospective study of HIV pregnant women. Fifth International Conference on AIDS, Montreal, Abstract MBP14

Dudley D J, Mitchell M D, Creighton K et al 1990 Lymphokine production during term human pregnancy: differences between peripheral leukocytes and decidual cells. Am J Obstet Gynecol 163: 1890–1893

Ellerbrock T V, Bush T J, Chamberland M E, Oxtoby M J 1991 Epidemiology of women with AIDS in the United States, 1981 through 1990. A comparison with heterosexual men with AIDS. JAMA 265: 2971–2975

Ehrnst A, Lindgren S, Dictor M et al 1991 HIV in pregnant women and their offspring: evidence for late transmission. Lancet 2: 203–207

Feinberg B B, Gonik B 1991 General precepts of the immunology of pregnancy. Clin Obstet Gynecol 34: 3–16

Fernandez-Cruz E, Desco M, Garcia Montes M et al 1990 Immunological and serological markers predictive of progression to AIDS in a cohort of HIV-infected drug users. AIDS 4: 987–994

Friedland G H, Saltzman B, Vileno J et al 1991 Survival

differences in patients with AIDS. J Acq Immune Defic Synd 4: 144–153

Gloeb D J, O'Sullivan M J, Efantis J 1988 Human immunodeficiency virus infection in women. I. The effects of human immunodeficiency virus on pregnancy. Am J Obstet Gynecol 159: 756–761

Gloeb D J, Lai S, Efantis J, O'Sullivan M J 1992 Survival and disease progression in human immunodeficiency virus infected women after an index delivery. Am J Obstet Gynecol 167: 152–157

Hénin Y, Mandelbrot L, Henrion R, Pradineaud R, Coulaud J P, Montagnier L 1993 Virus excretion in the cervicovaginal secretions of pregnant and non pregnant HIV-infected women. J Acq Immune Defic Synd 6: 72–75

Henrion R 1990 Virus HIV et périnatalogie. Méd et Hyg 48: 666–672

Hicks M L, Nolan G H, Maxwell S L, Mickle C 1990 Acquired immunodeficiency syndrome and pneumocystis carinii infection in a pregnant woman. Obstet Gynecol 76: 480–481

Isaksson B, Albert J, Chiodi F et al 1988 AIDS two months after primary human immunodeficiency virus infection. J Infect Dis 158: 866–868

Jensen L M, O'Sullivan M J, Gomez del Rio M et al 1984 Acquired immunodeficiency (AIDS) in pregnancy. Am J Obstet Gynecol 148: 1145–1146

Johnstone F D, Kilpatrick D C, Burns S M 1992a Anticardiolipin antibodies and pregnancy outcome in women with human immunodeficiency virus infection. Obstet Gynecol 80: 92–96

Johnstone F D, Willox L, Brettle R P 1992b Survival time after AIDS in pregnancy. Br J Obstet Gynaecol 99: 633–636

Kell P D, Barton S E, Smith D E et al 1991 A maternal death caused by AIDS. Case report. Br J Obstet Gynaecol 98: 725–727

Koonin L M, Ellerbrock T V, Atrash H K et al 1989 Pregnancy-associated deaths due to AIDS in the United States. JAMA 261: 1306–1309

Lapointe N, Boucher M, Samson J, Charest J 1991 Significant markers in the modulation of immunity during pregnancy and post-partum in a paired HIV positive and HIV negative population. Seventh International Conference on AIDS, Florence. Abstract WB2054

Lemp G F, Payne S F, Neal D et al 1990 Survival trends for patients with AIDS. JAMA 263: 402–406

Lindan C P, Allen S, Serufilira A et al 1992 Predictors of mortality among HIV-infected women in Kigali, Rwanda. Ann Int Med 1915: 116

Lindgren S, Anzen S, Bohlin A B et al 1991 HIV and child-bearing: clinical outcome and aspects of mother-to-infant transmission. AIDS 5: 1111–1116

MacCallum L R, Cowan F M, Whitelaw J, Burns S M, Brettle R P 1989 Disease progression following pregnancy in HIV seropositive women. Fifth International Conference on AIDS, Montreal. Abstract MBP3

Mandelbrot L, Henrion R 1991 Human immunodefiency virus and reproduction. Ann NY Acad Sci 626: 484–501

Mazzarello G, Canessa A, Melica F et al 1991 Influence of pregnancy on HIV disease progression. Seventh International Conferrerence on AIDS, Florence. Abstract WC3235

Medley G F, Anderson R M, Cox D R, Billiard L 1987 Incubation period of AIDS in patients infected via blood transfusion. Nature (London) 328: 719–721

Melnick S, Sherer R, Hillman D et al 1992 Gender, HIV-related clinical events, and mortality: preliminary observational data from the community programs for clinical research on AIDS. Eighth International Conference on AIDS, Amsterdam. Abstract MoC0031

Mertz K J, Parker A L, Halpin G J 1992 Pregnancy-related mortality in New Jersey, 1975 to 1989. Am J Pub Health 82: 595–599

Minkoff H, De Ragt R H, Landesman S et al 1986 Pneumocystis carinii pneumonia associated with acquired immunodeficiency syndrome in pregnancy: a report of three maternal deaths. Obstet Gynecol 67: 284–287

Minkoff H, Nanda D, Menez R, Fikrig S 1987 Pregnancies resulting in infants with acquired immunodeficiency syndrome or AIDS-related complex. Obstet Gynecol 69: 285–287

Minkoff H L, Willoughby A, Mendez H et al 1990 Serious infections during pregnancy among women with advanced human immunodeficiency virus infection. Am J Obstet Gynecol 162: 30–34

Minkoff H L, Dehovitz J A 1991 Care of women infected with the human immunodeficiency virus. JAMA 266: 2253–2258

Morlat P, Perneix P, Douard D, Lacoste D, Dupon M, Chêne G, Pellegrin J L, Ragnauc J M, Dabis F 1992 Women and HIV infection: a cohort study of 483 HIV-infected women in Bordeaux, France, 1985–1991. AIDS 6: 1187–1193

Msellati P, Leroy V, Lepage P et al 1992 Natural history of HIV1 infection in pregnant women: a prospective cohort study in Kigali (Rwanda), 1988–1991. Eighth International Conference on AIDS, Amsterdam. Abstract MoC0035

Nachman S 1987 HIV infection during pregnancy: a longitudinal study. Third International Conference on AIDS, Washington. Abstract TP55

Nzila N, Laga M, Brown C, Jingu M, Kivuvu M 1991 Does pregnancy in HIV + women accelerate progression to AIDS? Seventh International Conference on AIDS, Florence. Abstract MC3149

Phair J et al 1992 Acquired immune deficiency syndrome occurring within 5 years of infection with human immunodeficiency virus type 1: the Multicenter AIDS Cohort Study. J Acq Immune Defic Synd 5: 490–496

Ravizza M, Semprini A E, Taglioretti A 1990 CD4 levels in HIV seropositive and HIV seronegative pregnant women. First International Symposium on AIDS and Reproduction, Genoa, p 29

Rawlison K F, Zubrow A B, Harris M A, Jackson V S, Chao S 1984 Disseminated Kaposi's sarcoma in pregnancy: a manifestation of acquired immunodeficiency syndrome. Obstet Gynecol 63: 2S–6S

Reeves G K, Overton S E 1988 Preliminary survival analysis of UK AIDS data. Lancet 1: 880

Reuben J M, Gonik B, Li S et al 1991 Induction of cytokines in normal placental cells by the human immunodeficiency virus. Lymphokine Cytokine Res 10: 195–199

Rothenberg R, Woelfel M, Stoneburner R et al 1987 Survival with the acquired immunodeficiency syndrome. Experience with 5833 cases in New York City. N Engl J Med 317: 1297–1302

Ryder R W, Nsa W, Hassig S E et al 1989 Perinatal transmission of the human immunodeficiency virus type 1 to infants of seropositive women in Zaire. N Engl J Med 320: 1637–1642

Saltzman, R L, Jordan M C 1988 Viral infections. In: Burow G N, Ferris T F, (eds) Medical complications during pregnancy. Saunders, Philadelphia, p 372–388

Schnittmann S M, Greenhouse J J, Psallidopoulos M C et al 1990 Increasing viral burden in CD4-positive T cells from patients with immunodeficiency virus (HIV) infection reflects rapidly progressive immunosuppression and clinical disease. Ann Int Med 438–443

Schoenbaum E E, Davenny K, Selwyn P A, Hartel D, Rogers M 1989 The effect of pregnancy on progression of HIV related disease. Fifth International Conference on AIDS, Montreal. Abstract MBP8

Schoenbaum E E, Davenny K, Holbrook K 1992 Management of HIV disease in pregnancy. In: Johnstone F D (ed) HIV infection in obstetrics and gynaecology. Ballière's Clin Obstet Gynaecol 6:101–124

Scott G B, Fischl M A, Klimas N et al 1985 Mothers of infants with the acquired immunodeficiency syndrome: evidence for both symptomatic and asymptomatic carriers. JAMA 253: 363–366

Scott G B, Hutto C, Makuch R W et al 1989 Survival in children with perinatally acquired human immunodeficiency virus type 1 infection. N Engl J Med 321: 1791–1796

Selwyn P A, Schoenbaum E E, Davenny K et al 1989 Prospective study of human immunodeficiency virus infection and pregnancy outcomes in intravenous drug users. JAMA 261: 1289–1294

Siby T, Thior I, Marlink R et al 1992 Natural history of HIV-2 vs HIV-1: clinical and immunological study in a cohort of female sex workers. Eighth International Conference on AIDS, Amsterdam. Abstract WeC1066

Sperling R S, Stratton P 1992 Treatment options for human immunodeficiency virus-infected pregnant women. Obstet Gynecol 79:443–448

Sperling R S, Stratton P, O'Sullivan M J 1992 A survey of zidovudine use in pregnant women with human immunodeficiency virus infection. N Engl J Med 326:857–861

Sridama V, Pacini F, Yang S L et al 1982 Decreased levels of helper T-cells: a possible cause of immunodeficiency in pregnancy. N Engl J Med 307:352–356

Stratton P, Mofenson L M, Willoughby A D 1992 Human immunodeficiency virus infection in pregnant women under care at AIDS clinical trials centers in the United States. Obstet Gynecol 79:364–368

Szabo S, Miller L H, Sacks H S et al 1992 Gender differences in the natural history of HIV infection. Eighth International Conference on AIDS, Amsterdam. Abstract MoC0030

Watts D H, Brown Z, Tartaglione T et al 1991 Pharmacokinetic disposition of zidovudine during pregnancy. J Infect Dis 163:226–232

Weinberg E D 1984 Pregnancy-associated depression of cell-mediated immunity. Rev Infect Dis 6:814–831

Wetli C V, Roldan E O, Fojaco R M 1983 Listeriosis as a cause of maternal deaths: an obstetric complication of AIDS. Am J Obstet Gynecol 147: 7–9

Willoughby A, Minkoff H, Mendez H et al 1989 Infectious morbidity in pregnant human immunodeficiency virus (HIV) infected women. Pediatr Res 25: A106

Witkin S, McGregor J A 1991 Infection-induced activation of cell-mediated immunity:possible mechanism for preterm birth. Clin Obstet Gynecol 34: 112–121

13. Reproductive decision-making among women with HIV infection

Peter A. Selwyn and Patricia Antoniello

INTRODUCTION

Since early in the AIDS epidemic, one of the more striking and poignant aspects of the epidemic and its consequences has been the issue of mother-to-infant transmission of HIV. This phenomenon has had profound clinical, epidemiological, and social implications, both in industrialized countries and the developing world. Since perinatal transmission continues to be the only significant source of HIV infection in infants throughout the world (Chin 1990, Bennett & Rogers 1990, Gayle et al 1990), there has been considerable interest from a public health perspective in reducing the frequency of this type of transmission. Such interest is understandable and warranted, especially in light of recent projections which anticipate HIV infection emerging as a leading cause of infant mortality and orphanhood in many geographic areas (Chin 1990, Bennett & Rogers 1990).

In parallel to these public health concerns, however, a number of questions have arisen which must be addressed by any strategy aiming to offer appropriate counselling and to prevent perinatal transmission of HIV, including the following:

1. What is the content of counselling which can be given to HIV-infected women concerning their actual risk of transmitting HIV to an infant, in light of given existing uncertainty about prenatal predictors of infection?
2. What, if anything, can be said about the potential adverse effects of pregnancy on HIV infection and vice versa?
3. What is known about the effects, if any, of HIV on reproductive behaviour and pregnancy decision-making among infected women, and how

does this relate to an understanding of reproductive behaviour in general?
4. How does one promote public health objectives without threatening women's autonomy and reproductive freedom (i.e. how does one develop a public health agenda which goes beyond the image of women only as 'vessels' or 'vectors')?

We will review these and related issues with reference both to the existing medical literature and a wider anthropological perspective for examining reproductive behaviour among women with HIV infection. We will also examine the ethical, clinical, and strategic issues involved in developing a framework for HIV-related reproductive counselling.

RISK OF PERINATAL TRANSMISSION

One of the questions most commonly asked by HIV-infected women who are pregnant or considering pregnancy is whether they will or will not transmit HIV to their infants. Unfortunately, as of early 1993, this is not a question that can be answered with certainty in individual cases. Numerous studies of perinatal transmission of HIV have produced estimates of the risk of transmission generally between 13 and 40% (Ryder et al 1988, The European Collaborative Study 1988, 1992; Blanche et al 1989, Goedert et al 1989, Hira et al 1989, Andiman et al 1990, Halsey et al 1990). In the largest such study being conducted in developed countries, the European Collaborative Study (1992), the most recently derived estimate based on 721 children born to 701 HIV-infected mothers was 14.4%. Other studies from industrialized countries have calculated transmission risks of 20–30% (Blanche et al 1989, Goedert et al 1989, Andiman et al 1990). In studies from developing countries, approximately 25% of infants born to 443 HIV-seropositive women in Haiti were estimated to be HIV-infected, as were 39% of infants in separate studies in Zaire and Zambia in a combined sample of nearly 600 infants (Ryder et al 1988, Hira et al 1989, Halsey et al 1990). From studies in developed countries, one would expect that without HIV-specific therapy, between 15 and 30% of infants with perinatal acquired HIV infection would have developed AIDS or died within the first 12–24 months of life (Italian Multicentre Study 1988, Blanche et al 1989, Andiman et al 1990), with higher estimates for the developing world (Ryder et al 1988, Hira et al 1989, Bennett & Rogers 1990, Halsey et al 1990).

Clearly these risks are substantial, and even with conservative estimates of transmission probabilities they would be expected to have a major impact on infant mortality in areas with high levels of HIV infection among women (Chin 1990, Bennett & Rogers 1990). However, it is still possible to examine these probabilities and conclude that the likelihood of an HIV-infected woman having a baby who would be alive and AIDS-free at 2 years of age could exceed 90%. With the advent of HIV-specific therapy and the possibility of improved survival of infected infants (Pizzo et al 1988), the potential risk profile might appear even more favourable. While it has been suggested that a willingness to accept even a 30–50% risk of perinatal HIV transmission might be more common among women accustomed to living with high levels of risk in their daily lives (e.g. active injection drug-users) (Nolan 1989, Selwyn et al 1989a), it has also been observed among non-drug-using middle-class women being screened for genetic disorders that the desire to have a child and carry a pregnancy to term may remain strong even with only a 10% likelihood of a normal outcome (Faden et al 1987). Given these observations, it is perhaps not surprising, as will be discussed in more detail below, that many HIV-infected women have opted to become pregnant or to continue their pregnancies after being informed of the potential risks of perinatal transmission.

Concerning more specific predictors of an individual woman's risk of perinatal HIV transmission, several studies have examined this question; these studies have indeed identified antepartum risk factors, but none which can be used with certainty for individual counselling. These risk factors have included: low maternal CD4+ T lymphocyte count or percentage, maternal HIV disease stage, p24 antigenaemia during pregnancy, prematurity and, possibly, other maternal infections (e.g. syphilis, chorioamnionitis) (Italian Multicentre Study 1988, Ryder et al 1988, The European Collaborative Study 1988, Goedert et al 1989, Andiman 1990, Lindgren et al 1991, Ryder & Temmerman 1991). Early reports suggesting that the absence of maternal antibodies to the gp 120 envelope glyprotein of HIV conferred a higher risk of mother-to-infant transmission have not been substantiated by further studies (Goedert et al 1989, Parekh et al 1991). (The reader is referred to Chapter 15 for an extended discussion of perinatal transmission of HIV.) These observations do permit clinicians to provide somewhat more focused couselling for HIV-infected women (e.g. that the risk of transmission seems to be higher in women who are more symptomatic or in later stages of HIV-related immune suppression), but they still do not permit a precise quantitative estimation of transmission risks for individual women.

Although the diagnostic feasibility has been debated, it may become possible early in pregnancy to determine more precisely the actual risk of a fetus becoming infected with HIV, either through intrauterine diagnostic techniques (Schafer & Koch 1991 or, more likely, the identification of predictive maternal factors. This possibility would no doubt bring a major and welcome change to the content of prenatal counselling of HIV-infected women; however, as discussed below, it will be important in this context to maintain a perspective in which the greater certainty of prediction does not bring with it a greater tendency toward coercion regarding decisions to continue or terminate a pregnancy. The current context of uncertainty, in other words, should not be assumed to be the only basis for a preferred counselling model which is non-directive and non-coercive.

EFFECTS OF HIV INFECTION ON PREGNANCY AND VICE VERSA

A number of studies both in industrialized and developing countries have examined the possible effects of HIV infection on pregnancy complications and outcomes (Gloeb et al 1988, Johnstone et al 1988, Koonin et al 1989, Lallemant et al 1989, Selwyn et al 1989b, Berrebi et al 1990, Braddick et al 1990, Maynard et al 1990, Minkoff et al 1990a, 1990b; Temmerman et al 1990, Brettle & Leen 1991, Lepage et al 1991, Lindgren et al 1991, Ryder & Temmerman 1991, Selwyn et al 1991). Most such studies, and virtually all which have involved HIV-asymptomatic women from industrialized countries, have found little evidence for any direct adverse effect of HIV infection on variables such as spontaneous abortion, obstetrical complications during pregnancy or at delivery, congenital malformations, prematurity, low birth weight, and neonatal mortality. In industrialized countries, where most HIV-infected pregnant women in published reports have had histories of injection drug use (Johnstone et al 1988, Selwyn et al 1989a, Berrebi et al 1990, Maynard et al 1990, Minkoff et al 1990a, Semprini et al 1990, Brettle & Leen 1991) the inference from most such reports has been that drug use and related behaviours are likely to be far more important as risk factors for adverse pregnancy outcomes than HIV infection per se. In several studies from developing countries, however, HIV infection has been associated, though not consistently, with outcomes such as low birth weight, growth retardation, prematurity and fetal wastage (Braddick et al 1990, Miotti et al 1990, Temmerman et al 1990, Lepage et al 1991, Lindgren et al 1991, Ryder & Temmerman 1991). It has been suggested that some of these outcomes may be further related to maternal clinical or nutritional status, or to the presence of other co-occurring conditions in addition to HIV infection (e.g. syphilis). It remains to be determined, especially in developed countries, whether later stages of HIV infection and immune suppression will be more likely to result in adverse pregnancy outcomes, although intuitively one would expect this to be the case. At present, however, in counselling HIV-infected women – particularly those early in the course of HIV disease – one would have little basis to suggest that pregnancy-related complications would be more likely to occur as a direct result of HIV infection itself.

Several analyses have examined the possible risk of the condition of pregnancy on the progression of HIV-related disease (Schoenbaum et al 1989, Selwyn et al 1989b, Berrebi et al 1990, Maynard et al 1990, Brettle & Leen 1991). Concern about this possibility was raised due to the theoretical and known risks of pregnancy on immune function and susceptibility to certain other infections (Weinberg 1984), and to early uncontrolled studies which suggested that HIV-infected women who delivered infants appeared to progress rapidly in their disease course. Subsequent controlled studies from France, the USA and the UK have not found any consistent evidence to suggest that pregnancy has a demonstrable deleterious effect on the natural history of HIV infection in women (MacCallum et al 1989, Schoenbaum et al 1989, Berrebi et al 1990, Brettle & Leen 1991). While one study, without a comparison group, showed a sustained pregnancy-related decline in maternal CD4 + T lymphocyte counts (Biggar et al 1989), this observation was not consistently reproduced in several other studies (Schoenbaum et al 1989, Bisalinkumi et al 1992, Nightingale et al 1992). It must be noted, however, that most of the above-cited studies included women who were mostly at early stages of HIV disease during pregnancy; it remains to be determined whether women in more advanced stages of HIV disease are at risk for more accelerated disease progression as a result of pregnancy.

While pregnancy itself has not appeared as yet to aggravate the clinical course of HIV infection, several studies have documented the occurrence of serious HIV-related infections during pregnancy. These have included bacterial pneumonia (e.g. pneumococcal pneumonia) and other bacterial infections (Selwyn et al 1989b, Berkowitz & La Sala 1990), as well as AIDS-defining opportunistic infections such as *Pneumocystis carinii* pneumonia (PCP) (Minkoff et al 1990b). The risk for PCP and other AIDS-indicator diagnoses during pregnancy has been most pronounced for women with CD4 + counts less than 300 per mm^3 (Minkoff et al 1990b). This observation has important clinical implications for obstetrical management, and also raises additional questions concerning the use of antiretroviral therapy and PCP prophylaxis regimens during pregnancy (Minkoff & Moreno 1990). (A full discussion of these issues is beyond the scope of this chapter; see Chs 14 and 16 in this volume.) Notwithstanding those reports, however, it must be acknowledged that the risk of serious opportunistic infections for immunosuppressed HIV-seropositive women may be no greater in pregnancy than at any other time. While pregnant women with low CD4 + counts should, therefore, be advised that they may be at risk for serious infectious complications during pregnancy, it would be misleading at present to suggest that they would be any less at risk if they were not pregnant.

REPRODUCTIVE BEHAVIOUR AND HIV INFECTION

In examining the literature on HIV and reproductive behaviour, it is helpful to divide this general topic into three more specific areas:

- HIV and it effects on rates of pregnancy or fertility.
- Decisions regarding continuation or termination of pregnancy among HIV-infected women already pregnant
- Occurrence rates and outcomes for subsequent pregnancies among infected women.

We will discuss each of these topics in sequence.

The few published studies in the existing literature suggest that, in general, HIV-infected women as a group do not exhibit lower pregnancy or fertility rates than their HIV-seronegative counterparts (Selwyn et al 1989b, Ryder et al 1991). In one study among drug users in a New York City methadone programme, in which pregnancy rates were monitored by monthly urine pregnancy testing, pregnancy rates for both HIV-seropositive and -seronegative patients were similar, exceeding 10% per year (Selwyn et al 1989b). Since it has been observed that drug users may be less likely to use contraception than some other populations (Ralph & Spigner 1986), and since the relationship between drug use and reproductive behaviour itself may bring certain unique features to this group (Densen-Gerber et al 1972), it may be important

not to over-generalize from these findings. However, studies among other populations have indicated a similar phenomenon. In another small US study, which was not designed as a prospective study of pregnancy, it was noted nevertheless that there was no apparent reluctance among sexual partners of haemophiliacs to become pregnant or carry pregnancies to term (Jason et al 1990). In a larger study in Zaire, which examined fertility rates as an outcome measure of a behavioural intervention to reduce heterosexual transmission of HIV, it was found that fertility rates among HIV-infected women were no lower – and in fact during one time interval were even higher – than rates in HIV-seronegative women (Ryder et al 1991). Here as well, fertility rates were high in both groups.

While it does not seem, therefore, that HIV infection itself has exerted any damping effect on pregnancy or fertility rates among mostly asymptomatic women, it must be noted that with the progression of HIV disease, as with any chronic debilitating illness, the frequency of pregnancy and the rate of live births may indeed diminish. The effects of HIV infection on reproductive endocrinology, especially in women with symptomatic HIV disease, remain largely unexplored; however, the presence of chronic disease, wasting and other associated symptoms would, as with any chronic disease, be expected to result in decreased fertility, whether mediated through behavioural, endocrinological or other changes. Preliminary data from New York suggest that pregnancy and/or live birth rates have indeed been lower among HIV-infected women in advanced stages of disease, when compared to their more asymptomatic counterparts with early HIV infection (Selwyn et al 1991, Sunderland et al 1992). This also raises an additional question which is very germane to the counselling of HIV-infected women considering pregnancy, which is the concern over care and nurturing for the infant in the event of the mother's short-term demise. Ironically, given both this observation (i.e. that late-stage women may be less likely to survive to become mothers to their infants) and the previously noted data concerning an increased risk of HIV transmission with more advanced immune suppression, it is not uncommon for HIV-infected women to choose to bear children earlier than they might otherwise have

Table 13.1 Studies of pregnancy termination decisions among women with HIV infection. Studies include women notified of HIV infection status before or during pregnancy, prior to the local gestational age limit on induced abortion. Most studies excluded women with spontaneous abortions.

City	Population	HIV-seropositive women		HIV-seronegative women (in comparison group)†		Reference
		No. of subjects	No. choosing termination (%)	No. of subjects	No. choosing termination (%)	
Bronx, NY	Methadone program patients	28	14 (50)	36	16 (44)*	Selwyn et al 1989a
Edinburgh, UK	Mixed sample, community-based‡	63	31 (49)	94	33 (35)*	Johnstone et al 1990
Brooklyn, NY	Mixed sample, prenatal clinics‡	32	6 (19)	34	1 (3)**	Sunderland et al 1992
France (multiple sites)	Mixed sample, Ob–Gyn services‡	2023	1008 (50)	—	—	Henrion et al 1991
Brooklyn, NY	Haitian obstetric clinic	9	0	—	—	Holman et al 1989
	Drug users plus Ob–Gyn referrals‡	18	4 (22)	—	—	
Brooklyn, NY New Haven, CT	Mixed sample, Ob–Gyn/paediatric referrals‡	11	3 (27)	—	—	Kurth & Hutchinson 1990
Baltimore, MD	Mixed sample, hospital clinic-based referrals‡	23	3 (13)	—	—	Barbacci et al 1989

* p = not significant; ** $p < 0.05$. † The first three studies had HIV-seronegative comparison groups. ‡ Most studies with mixed population samples had a predominance of injection drug-users among the women studied

contemplated. Though clearly at variance with some existing recommendations that suggest that women 'consider delaying' pregnancy in the setting of HIV infection (CDC 1985), such decisions would in fact be consistent with existing knowledge in this area.

Concerning pregnancy termination rates among women already pregnant, a number of studies have examined this phenomenon (Barbacci et al 1989, Holman et al 1989, Selwyn et al 1989a, Johnstone et al 1990, Kurth & Hutchinson 1990, Henrion et al 1991, Pivnick et al 1991, Sunderland et al 1992). In general, while limited by sampling factors (e.g. enrolling women in prenatal clinics in some cases), these studies have found that fewer than 50% of HIV-infected women who are aware of their HIV antibody status prior to 24 weeks' gestation (or the comparable local limit on induced abortion) have chosen to terminate such pregnancies. This has been observed in several studies from different sites in the USA and Europe (Table 13.1). In two such studies which included HIV-negative comparison groups, in populations of injection drug users there was no statistically significant difference in the frequency of elective termination between HIV-seropositive and -seronegative

women (Selwyn et al 1989a, Johnstone et al 1990). In another study from Brooklyn, HIV-infected women were more likely to terminate, although even among this group the termination rate was only 19% (Sunderland et al 1992). In a large maternity centre-based study in France, which did not include a comparison group, approximately 50% of over 2000 HIV-infected pregnant women chose to terminate and 50% chose to continue their pregnancies (Henrion et al 1991). Taken together, these data suggest that HIV infection has not been strongly associated with decisions to continue or terminate pregnancies within the populations studied to date. However, one must raise the caveat noted earlier for fertility rates, i.e. that women in more advanced stages of disease may choose to terminate more readily than those who are asymptomatic.

In the studies which have examined determinants of HIV-infected women's decisions to terminate or continue pregnancies, a number of predictive factors have been identified (Table 13.2). These have included: previous reproductive history (e.g. women who have previously aborted a pregnancy may be more likely to abort subsequent pregnancies); stage of pregnancy in which HIV

Table 13.2 Factors associated with women's decisions to continue or terminate pregnancies in the setting of HIV infection.

General
Past reproductive history
Social, cultural factors
Demographic factors
Intentionality of pregnancy
Physical and mental health

HIV-specific

Associated with pregnancy termination*	Associated with pregnancy continuation*
Advanced HIV disease	Early asymptomatic HIV infection
Concern for own health	Denial of illness
Completed family size	Desire for child
Unintended pregnancy	Planned pregnancy
Social and moral acceptability of abortion	Religious or moral prohibition on abortion
Family pressure to terminate	Family pressure to continue pregnancy
Fear of having an infected infant	Perceived acceptable risk of transmission
Inability to care for child	Family willingness to care for child
Fear of being unable to parent a child	Desire to leave a legacy after one's own death
HIV infection diagnosed prior to or early in pregnancy	HIV infection diagnosed after first trimester of pregnancy
Availability of abortion services	Lack of access to abortion services
Medical providers' advice to terminate	Social or community value of child-bearing
Fulfilled needs for parenting	Child-bearing as symbol of recovery
Co-residence with previous children	Separation from previous children
Lack of unresolved grief	Grief over prior losses and deaths

* These factors have been found or suggested to be associated with HIV-infected women's decisions to continue or terminate pregnancies, from published reports; factors are often multiple, complex, and are not always consistent predictors of outcome. See text and references

notification takes place (e.g. women informed of their HIV infection status prior to or early in pregnancy may be more likely to terminate than those informed after the first trimester); intentionality of the pregnancy; race, ethnicity or other socio-demographic factors; religious beliefs; family pressures; emotional reaction to the pregnancy; stage of HIV-related disease; level of concern about one's own health or that of an infant; fear of having to abandon an infant due to illness or death; a wish to deny illness and/or leave a legacy in the face of a terminal disease; or the perception of favourable odds of having an uninfected infant (Barbacci et al 1989, Holman et al 1989, Kurth & Hutchinson 1989, 1990; Selwyn et al 1989a, Johnstone et al 1990, Henrion et al 1991, Pivnick et al 1991, Sunderland et al 1992). It must be noted that many of these factors were determined either through retrospective interviews or qualitative analysis of women's pregnancy decisions, and were not always obtained systematically in a way that could allow one to weigh their possible importance. Other important factors, identified in studies among non-HIV-infected women as well, may include: the level and type of familial or social support (some studies have noted that women find greater external support for decisions to continue rather than terminate pregnancies); prior achievement of desired family size and fulfilment of the parenting role; the social or cultural importance of child-bearing in different communities; the symbolic meaning of becoming pregnant and having a child among drug-using women as a sign of regaining control of one's life (including the wish to bear additional children among women whose previous children have been removed by child custody agencies); the desire to please a mate; and the often unconscious desire to bear children as a reaction to grief and loss (Densen-Gerber et al 1972, Bracken et al 1978a, 1978b; Freeman et al 1985; Joyce 1988; Kurth & Hutchinson 1989, 1990; Selwyn et al 1989a; Carovano 1991).

Finally, concerning subsequent pregnancy decisions among women who have already had a pregnancy outcome while aware that they were HIV-infected, published reports amply indicate that there is no consistent pattern to such decisions (Holman et al 1989, Henrion et al 1991, Selwyn et al 1991, Sunderland et al 1992). Women who first chose to terminate one pregnancy have subsequently delivered live births and vice versa, with no apparent predictor of subsequent outcomes (except perhaps, as noted above, the likely effects of more advanced HIV disease resulting in decreased livebirth rates).

Clearly, the factors involved in women's decisions to continue or terminate pregnancy are complex, interconnected and, at best, still poorly understood. Nevertheless, it may be observed that regardless of the circumstances, HIV infection is only one of many variables influencing women's decisions in this area. Counselling must not only attend to the factual information and medical uncertainty regarding transmission and disease risks, but also to the social, cultural and behavioural issues which may be so intimately related to women's pregnancy decisions. The following sections will begin to address these issues from an anthropological perspective.

AN ANTHROPOLOGICAL PERSPECTIVE ON REPRODUCTIVE HEALTH

The provision of medical care to women with HIV disease has been complicated by the need for understanding individual behaviour and the social and cultural factors affecting it. Anthropologists have shown that reproductive choices in general are affected by complex personal issues, family responsibilities and societal expectations and constraints. In addition, reproductive choices can be affected by unintended pregnancy, misinformation about contraception and incompatible conjugal planning. Detailed models of pregnancy decision-making have noted the multiplicity of factors which affect outcomes (Shedlin & Hollerbach 1981).

Reproductive behaviours are often determined in part by birth control technologies and access to health care delivery (Brown 1988, Michaelson 1988). American women, in general, have a high rate of unintended pregnancies which is proportionately higher for women of colour (Williams 1991; however, there are few qualitative data about the practices and beliefs of African-American women and Latinas concerning actual reproductive decision-making (Lazarus 1988, 1990; Mays et al 1989). Since understanding sexual and reproductive behaviours of women affected by HIV disease is essential for the provision of care, ethnographic data which delineate the reproductive behaviours and beliefs of poor women and women of colour would be an important tool for health care practitioners.

Some medical literature assumes that cultural and social factors, such as race, class and ethnicity, are well defined and can be utilized to identify reproductive patterns. However, social scientists themselves have not been able to make accurate generalizations about the relationship among the many variables affecting pregnancy and reproductive practices of women. Moreover, the repro-

ductive behaviours of women in the USA currently most affected by the AIDS epidemic – women of colour – have not been adequately studied as individuals or in groups.

Most women affected by HIV in the USA and other industrialized countries are poor, and consequently their lives are influenced by being economically, socially and politically disadvantaged. Poverty as a factor that crosses race, class and ethnicity has been identified as having a dramatic effect on women's reproductive health and decision-making (Zambrana 1987). Since women affected by HIV are from different social classes and cultural backgrounds than their health care providers, there is a need to focus on the appropriate communication and interpretation of health care information in this context.

There is also a need to go beyond simple stereotypes of behaviour which are often dismissive or oversimplified regarding poor women of colour. If women are not complying with recommended medical therapy procedures, the reason may not be due to apathy or indifference but rather to the inability of the medical care delivery system to reach out to such women in a meaningful and effective way. Mitchell (1988, 1989) asserts that education and information programmes can be successful with women of colour if they are designed creatively and innovatively to address women's needs. More importantly, practitioners should not presume that women are incapable, incompetent or irresponsible if they do not comply with medical advice. Anthropologists have shown that, despite the multiplicity of factors affecting their decisions, most women do deliberate over their reproductive choices. In many cases, however, they may have limited access to appropriate information, and there may be other barriers to receiving appropriate care (Lazarus 1988). Moreover, what has sometimes been considered a lack of decision-making on the part of women may be more accurately described as women making choices with limited information (Lopez 1993) or constrained social options. It is difficult, if not impossible, for women who do not have access to a range of information sources and decision options to make independent judgements and give truly informed consent (Henifin 1989).

The use of cultural categories such as race, class,

ethnicity and gender in the biomedical literature has become problematic when the terminology itself obscures the complexity of human behaviour. In some cases, when these terms are inappropriately applied to those affected by HIV disease, anthropologists have noted the problems of the 'otherization' of groups (Glick Schiller 1992). For example, in the early 1980s the accepted parlance describing HIV transmission emphasized the identification of groups or risk categories rather than the importance of an individual's own behaviour. This served to stigmatize or 'otherize' behaviours attributed to a particular group, often identified by race or sexual preference, rather than assessing practices that placed individuals at risk.

Recently, HIV researchers have begun to assert that the relationship between behaviour and cultural values has been misunderstood (De La Cancela 1989). Since most women affected by HIV are poor, political and economic factors can confound an interpretation of cultural issues. For example, if a woman does not attend a prenatal clinic it may not be that she does not value the service because of cultural norms. Rather, she may be prevented from attending because of pragmatic barriers, such as lack of transportation or child care for older children (Brown 1988). Other authors, for example, have questioned the appropriateness of some frequently cited social science research which reinforces stereotypes of Latinas as submissive or powerless. These authors suggest that using culturally-based gender roles serves to sustain notions of male dominance and female submissiveness (Kline et al 1992). Therefore, while an awareness of cultural factors is important in HIV-related care, this should neither obscure important social and economic factors nor be reduced to a set of inappropriate stereotypes.

An important issue for practitioners working with women at high risk for HIV infection is understanding the conditions surrounding their daily lives. For example, many of these women, especially if they are injection drug-users, face daily crises that threaten the well-being of themselves and their families. Issues of poverty including food, shelter and housing are often more pressing than medical care. Problems surrounding child care may be of paramount concern for many women,

who may express fear of social welfare programmes because of the practice of placing children in foster care. Women who are actively using drugs may be engaged in trying to gain access to drug treatment, obtaining money to maintain their addictions, or simply trying to survive on the street. For women in such circumstances, health and health care issues may be a secondary concern. Many of these problems can not be solved by health or social welfare systems but, at the same time, must be addressed before women can benefit from testing or medical care for HIV disease.

An additional problem for poor women is the lack of trust in the medical care system. In most industrialized countries, medical delivery is hierarchically organized and therefore may not acknowledge the necessity to provide care from a woman-centred perspective. In seeking reproductive health care, poor women must negotiate an alienating and fragmented system, in which there are many implicit and explicit barriers to care (Fee 1982, Michaelson 1988). Studies documenting linguistic barriers and the lack of responsiveness of medical providers to patients' queries serve further to define the impediments to an effective discourse between HIV-infected women and their medical care-givers (Fisher & Todd 1983, West 1984).

EMPOWERMENT

Empowerment may be defined as a process of enabling individuals and groups to participate in action and decision-making. Empowerment involves individuals in a group effort to assess their problems and examines an individual's place within society at a particular place in time. Although empowerment is frequently discussed as a personal attribute, people cannot be empowered; rather, they must enable themselves through a specific process that identifies individual goals within the setting of a community (Freire 1985). Researchers have suggested that empowerment education for women with HIV should be an important aspect of their care, especially for drug-using women who have been alienated from society and often from their own community (Wallerstein & Bernstein 1988). However, one can not assume that empowerment can be achieved without a process that begins with individual self-esteem and results in a comprehension of a place in history and society.

Women with HIV represent a group that has been disenfranchised becasue of their social, economic and political circumstances. The need for empowerment in this group is great, especially with regard to reproductive decision-making, and yet the requisite skills may not be immediately at hand. Consequently, the health provider should evaluate the level of awareness of each client for reproductive decision-making, on an individual basis, while encouraging the process of empowerment for the group as a whole. It is often difficult to make an estimation of this type if the provider does not have a continuing relationship with a client, a situation which argues for the critical need for pregnancy-related counselling of this type to be done in the context of an ongoing therapeutic interaction.

Reproductive counselling for women with HIV infection is a process which requires sensitivity, empathy, thoughtfulness and humility on the part of the care provider, and can best be done effectively in the setting of a primary care relationship. In addition to the necessary trust and mutual respect between patient and provider, it is important for this type of counselling to exist as one part of a comprehensive programme of medical and psychosocial services (Winiarski 1991). The mental health needs of women with HIV infection, which have not been discussed at length in this context, may be especially heightened in pregnancy; feelings of grief, depression and isolation may be aggravated by a decision to terminate a pregnancy, and fear and dependency may become more pronounced after a decision to continue a pregnancy whose outcome may be uncertain (James 1988). Given all of the factors involved in pregnancy-related decision-making, counselling offered outside of the setting of comprehensive primary care services is likely to become paternalistic, hollow and disconnected from the real needs and experience of women.

ETHICAL ISSUES: AUTONOMY, RESPONSIBILITY AND REPRODUCTIVE RIGHTS

It has been suggested that perinatal transmission of HIV may bring into question the principle of a woman's right to autonomy in reproductive decision-making (Bayer 1989, 1990). Others have raised the legitimacy of discussing the issue of whether a woman who is infected with HIV should ever have children (Arras 1990). Embedded in these arguments are questions regarding the limits of individual autonomy in decision-making, the concept of parental responsibility, the possible use of the notion of 'Wrongful life' in the setting of perinatal HIV infection, and the public health imperative of preventing further extension of the AIDS epidemic.

In a thoughtful review of these issues, Nolan (1989) examined the pertinent themes of reproductive autonomy, privacy and public health by comparing HIV disease with genetically transmitted diseases that are similar in rates of transmission, severity of symptoms and prognosis for affected infants. She suggested that children born to HIV-infected women have no greater risk of becoming infected with HIV than the risk of other children acquiring certain transmissible conditions for which they are also born at risk. Further, even if infected with HIV, infants of HIV-infected mothers theoretically pose no greater risk of transmission to others, incur no greater costs for health care services, and are no more likely to reproduce and pass the infection on to their own offspring than is the case for some genetically transmitted diseases (e.g. cystic fibrosis). Nevertheless, it has been noted (Hankins & Handley 1992) that there has been an 'inordinate concentration' on policy debates concerning reproductive decisions and pregnancy termination for HIV-infected women, a focus which is clearly different from what has been the approach to some of these other conditions. Beyond certain unique clinical features of maternal and infant HIV infection (e.g. that mothers and infants share the same illness, from which mothers may die first), Nolan suggested that at least some of the basis for this difference in policy positions may be linked, if unconsciously, to other social factors related to HIV infection in the USA, such as the fact that perinatal HIV transmission over-whelmingly involves poor, often disenfranchised populations, especially women of colour and their children. Unconscious racism, plus the general mood of public fear of HIV infection and AIDS, may lead to a more directive method of repro-ductive counselling among HIV-infected women than might otherwise be the case.

Both concerning HIV infection and more gen-erally, bioethicists have discussed the moral ques-tions raised by decisions to bear children who might be born to a life of illness and suffering, never having been born at all, i.e 'wrongful life' vs 'the value of a life lived under any circumstances' (Asch 1989, Nolan 1989, Purdy 1989, Arras 1990, Kass 1991). While there have been arguments made to support both sides of this issue, with respect to HIV the combined probabilities for a short-term adverse outcome (i.e. serious illness or death) occurring in an infant born to an HIV-infected mother are low enough that, despite its emotional connotations, such a birth would not clearly fit the criteria of wrongful life based on existing discourse. This is likely to become even more the case with the development of additional therapeutic options for paediatric HIV infection. Further, in communities in which women's social roles are often most clearly defined by child-bearing, and in which fertility may be especially important due to high childhood mortality rates, the concept of wrongful life seems even less rel-evant (Mitchell 1988, Carovano 1991).

The structure and method of HIV counselling in the USA has been grounded on the non-directive genetic counselling model, which is based on the premise of ethical neutrality and support for per-sonal choice (Prevention of HIV, ACOG 1987, Nolan 1989, Committee on Ethics 1990, Working Group on HIV Testing 1990, Kass 1991). This perspective was developed against the background of the eugenics controversy and is sensitive to the issues of racism surrounding reproduction (Rapp 1988). Within the context of genetic counselling, it has long been recognized that the very nature and complexity of personal reproductive decisions are such that they cannot be dictated by the larger society. Nolan (1989) cites an early source (Callahan 1979) on genetic counselling from the pre-AIDS era:

Many factors will have to be weighed simultaneously: known objective probabilities interacting with subjective assessements, available family resources, available society resources, effects on sibs and marital relations, commitments to values and worldview, and finally how these would all work together in affecting the welfare of a future child. Since so much of this assessment process is deeply personal, private, and intimately involved with individual differences, prudence has dictated that these decisions be left to the individuals involved.

These considerations have no less relevance in the AIDS era, in which false dichotomies have some-times been erected to oppose the interests of women with those of society or with those of their fetuses or children. Given the complexities of reproductive behaviour, the varied individual and social determinants of personal choice, and the level of existing medical uncertainty regarding peri-natal transmission and the prenatal prediction of HIV disease course in infants – especially with the rapid development of new HIV therapies – it seems presumptuous at best to attempt to dictate women's reproductive decisions based on some purported notion of social good. Clinicians and policy-makers have emphasized that the goal of HIV counselling regarding pregnancy is to provide sufficient information for a woman to make an informed decision about reproductive choice (Minkoff 1987, Prevention of HIV, ACOG 1987, Mitchell 1988, Holman et al 1989, Kurth & Hut-chinson 1989, Selwyn et al 1989a, Committee on Ethics 1990, Kass 1991). Further, it is incumbent upon the health care provider to assess a woman's understanding of information she has received (Kurth & Hutchinson 1989). To do less than this is likely to result in practices which are unjustifiably coercive, discriminating and out of touch with the needs of women with HIV infection.

In this type of environment, one must be especially sensitive both to one's own emotional responses and to the larger context in which the clinical interaction is taking place. Counselling should be done in a way which respects the woman's autonomy and does not impose the prac-titioner's own biases or cultural stereotypes (Hutchinson 1992). Even if one chose explicitly to assert that prevention of prenatal HIV trans-mission were of paramount importance, one would be very unlikely to achieve this result through the active recommendation of pregnancy termination or even systematic pregnancy prevention among infected women (Nolan 1989, Kass 1991). These recommendations may not only be at direct variance with women's own desires and hopes, but they may also, when issued in a directive way, be perceived as yet another expression of paternalism on the part of an alienating and forbidding medical care system. If women began to equate HIV counselling regarding pregnancy with the discouragement of child-bearing, one might predict that such a service would become increasingly irrelevant and distanced from the very population it was intended to engage.

For a non-directive pregnancy counselling model to be successful, the autonomy of the woman must be respected and encouraged. This does not imply that the health care provider should not engage the woman in an open discussion of the implications of the pregnancy (e.g. what effects it might have on her own health, whether she will be able to care for the infant, what her own prognosis is likely to be and so on). Indeed, as in other counselling contexts, the process involved is a mutual and interactive one, and does not consist merely of a one-sided recitation of factual information. The key, however, is to ensure that the provider remains aware not only of the clinical and educational issues, but also of the inherently unequal nature of the provider–patient relationship and the larger social, cultural and economic context within which it unfolds.

To encourage women to make informed decisions about child-bearing and HIV infection, and to help facilitate and support this process of empowerment, does indeed mean at times that one supports a decision to become pregnant or carry a pregnancy to term. However, while this may evoke some deep-seated emotional response in the provider, *not* to proceed in this manner puts one in a position which is at once ethically questionable, clinically compromised, and programmatically ineffective. Ultimately, in fact, the strategy most likely to reduce perinatal transmission of HIV will be based on the empowerment of women to seek greater control over their material, social and reproductive lives, and not on more coercive attempts to impose reproductive decisions from an external source, however well-intentioned.

REFERENCES

Andiman W A, Simpson J, Olson B et al 1990 Rate of transmission of HIV type 1 infection from mother to child and short-term outcome of neonatal infection. AIDS 144: 758–766

Arras J D 1990 AIDS and reproductive decisions: having children in fear and trembling. Milbank Q 68: 353–382

Asch A 1989 Can aborting 'imperfect' children be immoral? In: Arras J, Rhodem J (eds) Ethical issues in modern medicine. Mayfield Publishing, Mountain View Ca, p 317–321

Barbacci M, Chaisson R, Anderson J, Horn J 1989 Knowledge of HIV serostatus and pregnancy decisions. V International Conference AIDS, Montreal. Abstr MBP 10

Bayer R 1989 Perinatal transmission of HIV infection: the ethics of prevention. Clin Obstet Gynecol 32: 497–505

Bayer R 1990 AIDS and the future of reproductive freedom. Milbank Q 68: 179–204

Bennett J V, Rogers M F 1990 Child survival and perinatal infections with HIV. Am J Dis Child 144: 1242–1247

Berkowitz K, LaSala A 1990 Risk factors associated with the increasing prevalence of pneumonia during pregnancy. Am J Obstet Gynecol 163: 981–985

Berrebi A, Kobuch W E, Puel J et al 1990 Influence of pregnancy on HIV disease. Eur J Obstet Gynecol Reprod Biol 37: 211–217

Biggar R J, Pahwa S, Minkoff H L et al 1989 Immunosuppression in pregnant women infected with HIV. Am J Obstet Gynecol 161: 1239–1244

Bisalinkumi E, Nawrocki P, Chao A et al 1992 T-cell subset changes during the after pregnancy in a cohort of HIV-1-seropositive and seronegative African mothers. VIII International Conference on AIDS, Amsterdam, July. (Abstr PoA2086)

Blanche S, Rouzioux C, Moscato M-I G et al 1989 A prospective study of infants born to women seropositive for human immunodeficiency virus type 1. N Engl J Med 320: 1643–1648

Bracken M B, Klerman L V, Bracken M 1978a Coping with pregnancy resolution among never-married women. Am J Orthopsychiatry 48: 320–334

Bracken M B, Klerman L V, Bracken M 1978b Abortion, adoption, or motherhood: an empirical study of decision-making during pregnancy. Am J Obstet Gynecol 130: 251–262

Braddick M R, Kreiss J K, Embree J E, et al 1990 Impact of maternal HIV infection and obstetrical and early neonatal outcome. AIDS 4: 1001–1005

Brettle R P, Leen C L S 1991 The natural history of HIV and AIDS in women. AIDS 5: 1283–1292

Brown S 1988 Prenatal care; reaching mothers, reaching infants. National Academy Press, Washington, DC

Callahan S 1979 An ethical analysis of responsible parenthood. In: Capron A M, Lappe M, Murray R F et al (eds) Genetic counseling: facts, values, and norms. Liss, New York, p 217–238

Carovano K 1991 More than mothers and whores: redefining the AIDS prevention needs of women. Int J Health Services 21: 131–142

Centers for Disease Control 1985 Recommendations for assisting in the prevention of perinatal transmission of human T-lymphotrophic virus type III lymphadenopathy-associated virus and acquired immunodeficiency syndrome. MMWR 34: 721–732

Chin J 1990 Current and future dimensions of the HIV/AIDS pandemic in women and children. Lancet 336: 221–224

Committee on Ethics American College of Obstretricians and Gynecologists 1990 HIV infections: physicians' responsibilities. Obstet Gynecol 75: 1043–1045

De La Cancela V 1989 Minority AIDS prevention: moving beyond cultural perspectives towards sociopolitical empowerment. AIDS Educ Prev 1: 141–153

Densen Gerber J, Wiener M, Hochstedler R 1972 Sexual behavior, abortion, and birth control in heroin addicts: legal and psychiatric considerations. Contemp Drug Probl 1: 783–793

Faden R R, Chwalow A J, Quaid K et al 1987 Prenatal screening and pregnant women's attitudes toward the abortion of defective fetuses. Am J Public Health 77: 288–290

Fee E 1982 Women and health; the politics of sex in medicine. Baywood Publishing, Farmingdale, New York

Fisher S, Todd A D 1983 The social organization of doctor patient communication. Center for Applied Linguistics, Washington, DC

Freeman E, Sondheimer S, Rickels K 1985 Influence of maternal attitudes on urban black teens' decisions about abortion v. delivery. J Reprod Med 30: 731–735

Freire P 1985 Education for critical consciousness. Continuum Press, New York

Gayle J A, Selik R M, Chu S Y 1990 Surveillance for AIDS and HIV infection among black and Hispanic children and women of childbearing age, 1981–1989. MMWR 39 (SS-3): 23–30

Glick Schiller N 1992 What's wrong with this picture? The hegemonic construction of culture: AIDS research in the United States. Med Anthropol 2 (6): 237–254

Gloeb D J, O'Sullivan M J, Efantis J 1988 The effects of human immunodeficiency virus on pregnancy. Am J Obstet Gynecol 159: 756–761

Goedert J J, Mendez H, Drummond J E et al 1989 Mother-to-infant transmission of HIV type 1: association with prematurity or low anti-gp120. Lancet 2: 1351–1354

Halsey N A, Boulos R, Holt E et al 1990 Transmission of HIV-1 infections from mothers to infants in Haiti: impact on childhood mortality and malnutrition. JAMA 264: 2088–2092

Hankins C A, Handley M A 1992 HIV disease and AIDS in women: current knowledge and a research agenda. J Acq Immune Defic Synd 5: 957–971

Henifin M S, Hubbard R, Norsigian J 1989 Position paper: prenatal screening. In: Cohen S, Taub N (eds) Reproductive rights for the 1990's. Humana Press, Clifton, NJ 124–134

Henrion R, Henrion-Geant, Mandelbrot L, Cremieux N 1991 Attitude des femmes enceintes infectees par le VIH. Presse Med 20: 896–898

Hira S K, Kamanga J, Bhat G J et al 1989 Perinatal transmission of HIV-1 in Zambia. Br Med J 299: 1250–1252

Holman S, Berthaud M, Sunderland A et al 1989 Women infected with HIV: counseling and testing during pregnancy. Semin Perinatol 13: 7–15

Hutchinson J 1992 AIDS and racism in America. J Natl Med Assoc 84: 119–124

Italian Multicentre Study 1988 Epidemiology, clinical features and prognostic factors of pediatric HIV infection. Lancet 2: 1043–1045

James M E 1988 HIV seropositivity diagnosed during pregnancy; psychosocial characteristics of patients and their adaptation. Gen Hosp Psychiatry 10: 309–316

Jason J, Evatt B L, and the Hemophilia – AIDS Collaborative Study Group 1990 Pregnancies in HIV-infected sex partners of hemophiliac men. AM J Dis Child 144: 485–490

Johnstone F D, MacCallum I, Brettle R, Inglis J M, Peutherer J F 1988 Does infection with HIV affect the outcome of pregnancy? Br Med J 296: 467

Johnstone F D, Brettle R P, MacCallum L R et al 1990 Women's knowledge of their HIV antibody state: its effect on their decision whether to continue the pregnancy. Br Med J 300: 23–24

Joyce T 1988 The social and economic correlates of pregnancy resolution among adolescents in New York City, by race and ethnicity: a multivariate analysis. Am J Public Health 1988 78: 626–631

Kass, N E 1991 Reproductive decision making in the context of HIV infection; the case for non-directive counseling. In: Faden RR, Geller G, Powers M, (eds) AIDS, women, and the next generation. Oxford University Press, New York, p 308–327

Kline A, Kline E, Oken E 1992 Minority women and sexual choice in the age of AIDS. Soc Sci Med 34: 447–457

Koonin L M, Ellerbrock T V, Atrash H K, et al 1989 Pregnancy-associated deaths due to AIDS in the United States. JAMA 261: 1306–1309

Kurth A, Hutchinson M 1989 A context for HIV testing in pregnancy. J Nurse Midwifery 34: 259–266

Kurth A, Hutchinson M 1990 Reproductive health policy and HIV: where do women fit in? Pediatric AIDS and HIV Infect 1: 121–133

Lallemant M, Lallemant-Le Coeur S, Cheynier E et al 1989 Mother–child transmission of HIV-1 and infant survival in Brazzaville, Congo. AIDS 3: 643–646

Lazarus E 1988 Poor women, poor outcomes: social class and reproductive health. In: Michaelson KL (ed) Childbirth in America: anthropological perspectives. Bergin and Garvey, South Hadley, MA

Lazarus E 1990 Falling through the cracks: contradictions and barriers to care in a prenatal clinic. Med Anthropol 12: 269–287

Lepage P, Dabis F, Hitimana D-G et al 1991 Perinatal transmission of HIV-1: lack of impact of maternal HIV infection on characteristics of livebirths and on neonatal mortality in Kigali, Rwanda. AIDS 5: 295–300

Lindgren S, Anzen B, Bohlin A-B, Lidman K 1991 HIV and childbearing: clinical aspects of mother-to-child transmission. AIDS 5: 1111–1116

Lopez I O 1993 Choices and limited choices: sterilization among Puerto Rican women. Cornell University Press, New York (in press)

MacCallum L R, Cowan F M, Whitelaw J, Burns S M, Brettle R P 1989 Disease progression following pregnancy in HIV-seropositive women. V International Conference on AIDS, Montreal, June. Abstr MBP3

Maynard E C, Indacochea F, Oh W, Peter G 1990 HIV infection and pregnancy outcomes in intravenous drug users (letter). Am J Dis Child 144: 1181–1182

Mays V M, Albee G W, Schneider S S 1989 Primary prevention of AIDS: psychological approaches. Sage Publications, New York

Michaelson K L 1988 Childbirth in America: a brief history and contemporary issues. In: Michaelson KL (ed) Childbirth in America: anthropological perspectives. Bergin and Garvey, South Hadley, MA, 1–24

Minkoff H L 1987 Care of pregnant women infected with human immunodeficiency virus. JAMA 258: 2714–2717

Minkoff H L, Moreno J D 1990 Drug prophylaxis for HIV-infected pregnant women: ethical considerations. Am J Obstet Gynecol 163: 1111–1114

Minkoff H L, Henderson C, Mendez H et al 1990a Pregnancy outcomes among mothers infected with HIV and uninfected control subjects. Am J Obstet Gynecol 163: 1598–1604

Minkoff H L, Willoughby A, Mendez H et al 1990b Serious infections during pregnancy among women with advanced HIV infection. Am J Obstet Gynecol 162: 30–34

Miotti P G, Dallabetta G, Ndovi E, Liomba G, Saah A J, Chiphangwi J 1990 HIV-1 and pregnant women: associated factors, prevalence, estimate of incidence and role in fetal wastage in central Africa. AIDS 4: 733–736

Mitchell, J L 1988 Women, AIDS, and public policy. AIDS Public Pol 3: 50–52

Mitchell J 1989 Drug abuse and AIDS in women and their affected offspring. J Nat Med Assoc 81: 841–842

Nightingale S D, Lawrence J A, Wendell G, Edison R 1992 CD4 count and pregnancy in HIV-seropositive women. VIII International Conference on AIDS, Amsterdam, July. Abstr PoB3056

Nolan K 1989 Ethical issues in caring for pregnant women and newborns at risk for HIV infection. Semin Perinatol 13: 55–65

Parekh B S, Shaffer N, Pau C-P et al 1991 Lack of correlation between maternal antibodies to V3 loop peptides of gp 120 and perinatal HIV-1 transmission. AIDS 5: 1179–1184

Pivnick A, Jacobson A, Eric K et al 1991 Reproductive decisions among HIV-infected, drug-using women: the importance of mother–child coresidence. Med Anthropol Q 5(2(NS)): 153–169

Pizzo P A, Eddy J, Falloon J et al 1988 Effect of continuous infusion of zidovudine (AZT) in children with symptomatic HIV infection. N Engl J Med 319: 889–896

Prevention of human immune deficiency virus infection and acquired immune deficiency syndrome. 1987 American College of Obstetricians and Gynecologists, Washington, DC, p 1–4

Purdy L M 1989 Genetic screening and prenatal diagnosis. In: Arras J, Rhodem J (eds) Ethical issues in modern medicine. Mayfield Publishing, Mountain View, CA, p 311–317

Ralph N, Spigner C 1986 Contraceptive practices among female heroin addicts. Am J Public Health 76: 1016–1017

Rapp R 1988 Chromosomes and communication: the discourse of genetic counseling. Med Anthropol 2: 145–157

Ryder R W, Nsa W, Hassig S E et al 1988 Perinatal transmission of the human immunodeficiency virus type 1 to infants of seropositive women in Zaire. N Engl J Med 320: 1637–1642

Ryder R W, Temmerman M 1991 The effect of HIV-1 infection during pregnancy and the perinatal period on maternal and child health in Africa. AIDS 5 (suppl 1): S75–85

Ryder R W, Batter V L, Nsuami M et al 1991 Fertility rates in 238 HIV-1 seropositive women in Zaire followed for 3 years post-partum. AIDS 5: 1521–1527

Schafer A, Koch M A 1991 Risk factors and diagnostic tools for the detection of maternal fetal HIV-transmission. J Perinat Med 19 (suppl 1): 252–256

Schoenbaum E E, Davenny K, Selwyn P A, Hartel D, Rogers M F 1989 The effect of pregnancy on the progression of HIV-related disease. V International Conference on AIDS, Montreal, June Abstr MBP8

Selwyn P A, Carter R J, Schoenbaum E E, Robertson V J, Klein R S, Rogers M F 1989a Knowledge of HIV antibody status and decisions to continue or terminate pregnancy among intravenous drug users. JAMA 261: 3567–3571

Selwyn P A, Schoenbaum E E, Davenny K et al 1989b Prospective study of human immunodeficiency virus infection and pregnancy outcomes in intravenous drug users. JAMA 261: 1289–1294

Selwyn P A, Davenny K, Buono D, Schoenbaum E E 1991 Continuing study of HIV infection and pregnancies in intravenous drug users (abstr). In: Abstracts of the 119th Annual Meeting of the American Public Health Association. American Public Health Association, Washington, DC p 224

Semprini A E, Ravizza M, Bucceri A, Vucetich A, Pardi G 1990 Perinatal outcome in HIV-infected pregnant women. Gynecol Obstet Invest 30: 15–18

Shedlin M G, Hollerbach P 1981 Modern and traditional fertility regulation in a Mexican community: the process of decision making. Stud Fam Planning 12: 34–42

Sunderland A, Minkoff H L, Handte J, Moroso G, Landesman S 1992 The impact of HIV serostatus on reproductive decisions of women. Obstet Gynecol 79: 1027–1031

Temmerman M, Plummer F A, Mirza N B et al 1990 Infection with HIV as a risk factor for adverse obstetrical outcome. AIDS 4: 1087–1093

The European Collaborative Study 1988 Mother-to-child transmission of HIV infection. Lancet 2: 1039–1042

The European Collaborative Study 1992 Risk factors for mother-to-child transmission of HIV-1. Lancet 339: 1007–1012

Wallerstein N, Bernstein E 1988 Empowerment education: Freire's ideas adapted to health education. Health Educ Q 15: 379–394

Weinberg E D 1984 Pregnancy-associated depression of cell-mediated immunity. Rev Infect Dis 6: 814–831

West C 1984 Medical misfires: mishearings, misgivings, and misunderstandings in physician–patient dialogues. Discourse Proc 7: 107–134

Williams L 1991 Determinants of unintended childbearing among ever-married women in the United States: 1973–1988. Fam Plan Persp 23: 212–221

Winiarski M 1991 AIDS-related psychotherapy. Pergamon Press New York

Working Group on HIV Testing of Pregnant Women and Newborns 1990 HIV infection, pregnant women, and newborns; a policy proposal for information and testing. JAMA 264: 2416–2420

Zambrana R E 1987 A research agenda on issues affecting poor and minority women: a model for understanding their health needs. Women and Health 12 (3/4): 137–155

14. Pregnancy outcome and pregnancy management in HIV-infected women

Frank D. Johnstone

INTRODUCTION

Many HIV-infected women who become pregnant see the main issues of concern for the child as relating to maternal progression of disease and vertical transmission. However, HIV may also impact on infant morbidity and mortality if it has a significant effect on pregnancy outcome.

In theory, pregnancy wastage could result from interference with the fetomaternal immune relationship; early viral infection of the fetus could result in congenital anomaly or reduced fetal growth; maternal immunodeficiency could predispose to chorioamnionitis with the associated risks of preterm labour and stillbirth; the fetus could be damaged by recurrence of other infections, such as cytomegalovirus or toxoplasmosis; and the effect of concurrent infections and poor nutritional status with advancing disease could impair the woman's ability to maintain her pregnancy successfully.

In practice, at least for asymptomatic HIV-infected women in the developed world, such problems do not seem unusually common.

SPONTANEOUS ABORTION

The first report on pregnancy outcome noted an increase in spontaneous abortion in HIV-infected women but concluded that this was probably due to ascertainment bias (Johnstone et al 1988). More recent data from our centre continue to show a higher rate of spontaneous abortion in HIV-seropositive women, but the difference is small and no longer statistically significant. One study on women in the US Army (Lasley-Bibbs et al 1990) compared the reproductive histories of 69 HIV-

positive female soldiers and 276 seronegative women matched for key demographic variables. A significantly greater proportion of pregnancies in the former group ended in spontaneous abortion (risk ratio 4.4, confidence interval 1.5–13.0). However, this study is retrospective and it is not known whether the women were infected at the time of their pregnancies. A small prospective study in New York (Selwyn et al 1989) did not show any increase in spontaneous abortion in the HIV-infected women.

In Africa, studies on very large numbers of HIV-infected women have shown a higher proportion of pregnancies ending in spontaneous abortion. A history of spontaneous abortion was the end-point of studies in Malawi (Miotti et al 1990) and Rwanda (Lepage et al 1991). Such a history was more common in women infected with HIV, but neither HIV status nor syphilis serology was known for the time at which spontaneous abortion occurred. In a large study from Malawi (Miotti et al 1992), 6605 consecutive women were tested for HIV and a history of spontaneous abortion was reported more often by HIV-seropositive than seronegative women (15% vs 7%). In the largest study to date to focus on current abortion, Temmerman and colleagues (1992c) tested 195 women admitted to a hospital in Kenya with abortion. Attempts were made to exclude induced abortion. Controls were selected from antenatal clinic attenders. Spontaneous abortion was independently associated with HIV antibody status (odds ratio 2.2), maternal syphilis seroreactivity (odds ratio 4.3), and vaginal colonization with group B β haemolytic streptococcus (odds ratio 3.2). As with all other studies addressing this issue, there are methodological problems. The abortion and control groups are not strictly comparable, and the selection of the control group has potential for bias. Syphilis correlated with HIV infection and may be responsible for spontaneous abortion, but attempts were made to account for this and other variables and HIV still retained statistical significance.

What theoretical basis might there be for a relationship between HIV infection and spontaneous abortion? Maternal illness itself could be responsible, but direct viral infection is also possible. First trimester trophoblast tissue can be infected with HIV in vitro (Maury et al 1989, Zachar et al 1991), and Lewis and co-workers (1990) claimed that villous trophoblast stained for HIV-1 antigen in pregnancies of 8 weeks gestational age. One plausible mechanism for early spontaneous abortion might be changes in decidual immune cells which could affect implantation and subsequent trophoblast proliferation. There are no published studies on endometrial histochemistry and HIV-infected women in pregnancy, but this is an area which might reward further study.

In conclusion, it is uncertain whether HIV is a direct cause of spontaneous abortion. Most published information suggests a trend in that direction, but the studies are either retrospective or there is doubt about whether the findings could be explained by a correlated variable, such as positive syphilis serology or other infectious disease. On theoretical and observational grounds an increased rate of abortion seems plausible, but the increase is likely to be small.

CONGENITAL ABNORMALITY

A dysmorphic syndrome associated with HIV infection has been reported (Marion et al 1986, 1987). This syndrome included growth failure, microcephaly, flattened nasal bridge, oblique eyes, prominent forehead, triangular philtrum and patulous lips. Subsequent reports have not confirmed this finding (Nicolas 1988, Qazi et al 1988) and HIV dysmorphic syndrome was not seen in the large European collaborative study (1992). At present it seems doubtful that there is a specific syndrome, and the original observations may have been due to confounding from variables such as drug and alcohol use or ethnic group.

Most controlled studies have not specifically reported on structural congenital anomalies. Braddick and co-workers (1990) and Lepage and associates (1991) did not find any association between congenital anomaly and HIV serostatus. Prospective studies (Italian Multicentre Study 1988, Blanche et al 1989, Rogers et al 1989, Andiman et al 1990, European Collaborative Study 1992) are uncontrolled, but have reported on over 1000 babies with more than 18 months follow-up, and have not emphasized unusually high incidences of congenital abnormality.

There seems to be no good evidence that HIV is specifically associated with congenital abnormality. Together with the belief that very early intrauterine infection is uncommon, this makes it unlikely that embryopathy is a major problem with maternal HIV infection.

MATERNAL INFECTIOUS COMPLICATIONS

Whether pregnant women are more susceptible than non-pregnant women to opportunistic infection is unclear. There are theoretical reasons why this might be so, and these have been discussed by Mandelbrot and Henrion (Ch. 12). As would be expected, HIV-infected women are much more likely than seronegative controls to be admitted because of an infectious complication (unpublished data). This includes non-opportunistic infections such as bacterial pneumonia. Several such infections, by affecting maternal well-being, have the potential to impact on pregnancy outcome by causing preterm labour or impairing fetal growth, e.g. severe bacterial pneumonia, tuberculosis, chorioamnionitis and malaria. The prevalence of clinically significant infections during pregnancy has not been studied systematically, but this information should be gathered in large prospective collaborative studies.

Maternal infections could also impact more directly on the fetus or neonate. It is definite that fetal damage may result from reactivation of cytomegalovirus (CMV) infection in pregnancy (Griffiths et al 1991). In most pregnant populations the prevalence of immunity to CMV is 40–60% (Gold & Nankervis 1989) and therefore a high proportion of HIV-infected pregnant women may be at risk. Data from transplant patients have shown that CMV shedding increases with worsening immunosuppression (Gold & Nankervis 1989). There do not appear to be published studies reporting on the prevalence of CMV excretion in newborns in HIV-infected pregnancy, and so far, severe congenital CMV infection does not seem to have been identified as a problem. Several ongoing studies should clarify this.

Transplacental transmission of toxoplasmosis occurs during maternal parasitaemia following primary infection of the mother during pregnancy. Pregnant women with latent infection generally do not transmit toxoplasma to their fetuses (Remington & Desmonts 1990). However, in HIV-infected patients with immune compromise, reactivation of disease occurs in association with parasitaemia. There are very rare cases of transplacental transmission of toxoplasma to the fetus where women were parasitaemic due to reactivated illness (Remington & Desmonts 1990). The frequency of fetal damage from toxoplasmosis where the mother is HIV-infected is unknown.

Reactivation of hepatitis B viraemia does not occur in immune competent individuals but has been reported in an individual with AIDS (Vento et al 1989), and other such cases are known. Because of the serious consequences of neonatal infection (Committee Report 1989) and the high success rate of prevention (Wong et al 1984), hepatitis B status should be checked at booking, and perhaps again in late pregnancy to detect subsequent acquisition of hepatitis B virus or the uncommon situation of reactivation in the previously immune individual.

The major risk with genital herpes is primary infection around the time of delivery (Brown et al 1987). Nevertheless, recurrence of genital herpes does seem to be associated with some risk, and it is theoretically possible that the HIV-infected woman may be more likely to infect her child in this situation because of higher herpes viral load.

At present there are many uncertainties in this area. Fetal damage due to infection with the above agents is very uncommon in the general population, and only the pregnancies of severely immunocompromised HIV-infected women – a small proportion of the total – may be at increased risk.

It will therefore require large collaborative studies and data collection over a long period before the situation is clear.

PREGNANCY COMPLICATIONS

Early reports referred to a high incidence of preterm labour, Caesarean section, syphilis and low birth weight in the pregnancies of HIV-infected women (Minkoff et al 1989 Gloeb et al 1988). These studies were uncontrolled and illicit drug use and poverty are known to be associated with both HIV infection and poor pregnancy outcome.

The first controlled study showed both case and control groups to have a high incidence of preterm labour, intrauterine growth retardation and low birth weight. However, there were no differences according to HIV serostatus (Johnstone et al 1988). Further data from this centre, on larger numbers, have shown HIV-infected pregnancies to have no increase in pregnancy or delivery complications, except for infection (unpublished). A prospective study of methadone clinic attenders did not show differences in pregnancy complications or outcome (Selwyn et al 1989). Similar findings were reported from New York (Minkoff et al 1990), Milan (Semprini et al 1990) and Toulouse (Berrebi et al 1991). However, because of small numbers, all these studies lack statistical power.

These data from the USA and Europe contrast with the information from Africa, where several large studies from Zaire (Ryder et al 1989, Kamenga et al 1991), Congo (Lallemant et al 1989), Zambia (Hira et al 1989), Kenya (Braddick et al 1990, Temmerman et al 1992b), Uganda (Guay et al 1990) and Rwanda (LePage et al 1991, Bulterys et al 1991) compare pregnancy outcome in women who were infected with HIV with women who were not. These studies include 2249 infected mothers and 4308 HIV-seronegative controls. HIV seropositivity was associated with preterm delivery in some studies (Ryder et al 1989, Guay et al 1990, Temmerman et al 1992b) but not others (Kamenga et al 1991, Braddick et al 1990, LePage et al 1991, Bulterys et al 1991); increased perinatal deaths in some studies (Ryder et al 1989, Guay et al 1990, Bulterys et al 1991) but no difference in others (Braddick et al 1990, LePage et al 1991).

An increase in chorioamnionitis in HIV-positive pregnancies was reported in one study (Ryder et al 1989), bleeding in the third trimester in another (Braddick et al 1990) and twinning in another (Lallemant et al 1989).

A large and important case-control study in Nairobi (Temmerman et al 1990) focused on adverse pregnancy outcome: 373 women who delivered a preterm baby, 324 who delivered a baby small for gestational age, 120 who had an intrauterine death and 69 with an intrapartum death were compared for HIV status with 711 controls. HIV seropositivity was more common in the case groups but so were other, potentially confounding, features such as primiparity, lack of antenatal clinic attendance and maternal syphilis infection. However, linear logistic regression retained HIV status as a statistically significant associated outcome with modestly increased odds ratios of 2.1 (preterm birth), 2.3 (small for gestational age), 2.7 (intrauterine death) and 2.9 (intrapartum death).

There are several reasons why HIV infection might influence pregnancy complications. One important pathway could be via an increased rate of chorioamnionitis. This was certainly reported in one large controlled study (Ryder et al 1989) where pregnancies from 475 seropositive women were compared with those from 615 seronegative women matched for age and parity. Not only was chorioamnionitis more common in the former group, but babies were more frequently premature and the neonatal death rate was increased. Pathological changes have been described with greater frequency in placentas from HIV-seropositive women compared with those from seronegative controls. For example, Bulfamante and colleagues (1991) described a higher incidence of chorioamnionitis and omphalitis, villous immaturity and plasma cell infiltrates in 91 placentas from HIV-seropositive women. In a further study highlighting chorioamnionitis, Nyongo and co-workers (1992) reported from Kenya on 638 mothers delivering preterm and 862 term controls. Maternal HIV seropositivity was associated with prematurity (odds ratio 1.9). In a subset where the placenta was examined, moderate/severe chorioamnionitis was found in 23% of preterm and in 8% of term placentas (odds ratio 3.4). Within preterm deliveries the placentas showed chorioamnionitis in 37% of cases where the woman was HIV-seropositive, and 18% of matched HIV-seronegative cases. In addition to preterm delivery, chorioamnionitis in association with amniotic fluid infection could account for a higher rate of stillbirth.

HIV infection could also operate on pregnancy complications through other systemic infections, maternal debility and weight loss. Possible reasons for the discrepancy between different studies, particularly those from Africa and Europe and the United States, will be discussed below.

BIRTH WEIGHT

In published controlled studies in Europe and the USA, HIV infection has not been associated with a difference in birth weight (Johnstone et al 1988, Selwyn et al 1989, Minkoff et al 1990, Semprini et al 1990, Berrebi et al 1991). One study using multivariate analysis suggested there might be a small, but statistically significant, decrease in birth weight associated with maternal HIV infection (Johnstone et al 1991).

In contrast to most reports from the developed world, all studies from Africa seem to show decreased birth weight in pregnancies where the mother is HIV-infected (Table 14.1). There is some evidence that the decrease in fetal size is related to the stage of maternal disease (Ryder et al 1989, Guay et al 1990). An important and consistent observation is that birth weight seems unrelated to the infant's eventual HIV status (Italian Multicentre Study 1988, Blanche et al 1989, Ryder et al 1989, European Collaborative Study 1991).

If HIV is associated with decreased birth weight (and this is discussed below) there are a number of possible explanatory mechanisms. One is that this could be an effect of antiphospholipid antibodies. Raised levels of circulating antibodies to the divalent phospholipid, cardiolipin (anticardiolipin antibodies) are found in a substantial minority of patients infected with HIV, independent of clinical status (Boue et al 1990, MacLean et al 1990). Raised levels of anticardiolipin antibodies have also been shown in low risk obstetric populations to be associated with

Table 14.1   Controlled studies from Africa with data on birth weight (NS, not significant; NND, neonatal death)

First author	Year of publica-tion	Country	Number of sero-positive preg-nancies	Number of sero-negative preg-nancies	Rate of prematurity (usually < 38 weeks)	Perinatal death	Birth weight	Difference from sero-negative controls	Statistical signifi-cance (p value)
Ryder	1989	Zaire	466	606	Increased (p < 0.01)	Increased NND (p < 0.0001)	Decreased	− 409 g (AIDS) − 176 g (non-AIDS)	< 0.01
Lallemant	1989	Congo	64	130	Increased (NS)	Increased (NS)	Decreased	− 266 g	< 0.01
Hira	1989	Zambia	227	1727	Increased (NS)	Increased (NS)	Decreased	Not stated More low birth weight	< 0.001
Braddick	1990	Kenya	177	326	Increased (NS)	Increased (NS)	Decreased	− 130 g	< 0.005
Guay	1990	Uganda	206	444	Increased (p < 0.0001)	Increased (p < 0.01)	Decreased	− 190 g	< 0.001
Kamenga	1991	Zaire	350	280	No difference	No difference	Decreased	− 160 g	< 0.001
Bulterys	1991	Rwanda	166	209	No difference	No difference	Decreased	− 135 g	0.06
Lepage	1991	Rwanda	215	216	Increased (NS)	Increased (NS)	Decreased	− 130 g	< 0.01
Temmerman	1992	Kenya	378	370	Increased (p < 0.001)	Increased (NS)	Decreased	− 155 g	< 0.001

adverse pregnancy outcome, including preterm delivery and intrauterine growth retardation (Lockwood et al 1989, Perez et al 1991). In the only study to examine this in HIV-infected pregnancy (Johnstone et al 1992a), one-quarter of the 55 such women had raised anticardiolipin antibodies (greater than four standard deviations above the mean for a reference population). There was, however, no relationship with clinical features, gestational age at delivery or birth weight. It seems most likely that anticardiolipin antibodies provoked by HIV have a narrow specificity for cardiolipin, and unlike those provoked by auto-immunity are unrelated to phospholipid antibody syndrome.

DELIVERY

There is little information about labour and delivery complications in HIV-infected women. Nevertheless, labour ward management is likely to become more of a focus for critical review and interest, particularly as the birth process may be a significant time for transmission of HIV to the

baby (Goedert et al 1991, Krivine et al 1992, Ch. 15). Other important issues are support to the mother around delivery, and the prevention of spread of HIV to health care workers.

Caesarean section rates have been reported in two large studies of vertical transmission (Italian Multicentre Trial 1988, European Collaborative Study 1992). Both studies reported a high Caesarean section rate, 23% in the Italian Multicentre Trial and 26% in the European Collaborative Study. Both studies were uncontrolled and the reasons for Caesarean section were not given. In controlled studies, Selwyn and colleagues (1989) found 36% of 25 HIV-infected women had Caesarean section as opposed to 14% of seronegative women, a result, despite the very small numbers, which approached statistical significance (p = 0.06). In contradistinction, Minkoff and co-workers (1990) found no excess in Caesarean sections in their larger prospective study (12% compared with 18% for seronegative controls). In the Edinburgh cohort of women exposed to the risk of HIV infection, meconium staining of the liquor was more common compared with neighbourhood controls, but was equally common in HIV-ser-opositive and risk-exposed seronegative women. The rates of induction of labour, use of epidural anaesthesia or oxytocin, assisted vaginal delivery, episiotomy and Caesarean section were not related to serostatus and were similar to neighbourhood controls and the general hospital population. None of the large studies from Africa seem to have pub-lished on fetal distress in labour, labour com-plications or operative delivery.

It seems likely that there are no major differences attributable to HIV infection in labour and delivery outcome. In immunocompromised women, it is plausible that premature rupture of the mem-branes may occur more frequently, and in such women the risk of chorioamnionitis may be increased. Similarly, the risk of postoperative wound infection or postpartum endometritis may be greater. Reluctance to do fetal scalp sampling or to apply scalp electrodes (because of the theoretical risk that a wound on the fetal head, exposed directly to infected maternal fluids, could increase the risk of HIV transmission to the baby) could possibly result in additional Caesarean sections. Drug use is consistently reported to be associated with persistent breech presentation, and this mal-presentation could contribute to an increase in use of Caesarean section. However, the major factor which could result in a big change in practice would be convincing evidence that most vertical transmission occurs around delivery, that this could be significantly reduced by elective Cae-sarean section, and that other interventions were not effective. None of these three possibilities has yet been proven, but this is an area of intense interest and further data should accumulate rapidly.

DISCREPANCIES BETWEEN STUDIES

There are obvious differences in the results of studies on pregnancy outcome from Africa com-pared with those from Europe and the USA. One reason may simply be that published work from the developed world has included only very small numbers of pregnancies. Each of these studies lacks statistical power to detect a true difference in birth weight or pregnancy complications. This is particularly so if an adverse effect is found only in

symptomatic, immunocompromised individuals, who comprise a small proportion of HIV-infected women.

Whether the data from African studies can be assumed causally to relate HIV infection with preg-nancy outcome is neither straightforward nor clear-cut: nor is the assumption that these findings apply equally in Europe and America.

In the African studies, control subjects are often loosely matched (because they delivered the same day, were matched for age and parity alone, or were simply matched with all other pregnancies), and this makes it difficult to attribute differences only to HIV status. It is clear that seropositive women differ from controls in other (though related) characteristics apart from HIV status. These vary in different geographical areas. However, statistically significant differences which might be relevant include age (Hira et al 1989, LePage et al 1991), unmarried status (Hira et al 1989, Braddick et al 1990, LePage et al 1991), primiparity (LePage et al 1991), more sexual part-ners (Hira et al 1989, Braddick et al 1990), pros-titution (Braddick et al 1990), alcohol consumption during pregnancy (Braddick et al 1990), travel to other African countries (Hira et al 1989, Braddick et al 1990), gonorrhoeal and chlamydial infections (Braddick et al 1990), and positive syphilis serology (Miotti et al 1990, Temmerman et al 1992b). It is thus clear that control groups in these studies differ from cases, not only in HIV status but also in ways which are classically recognized as likely to affect birth weight or pregnancy outcome. In several studies, attempts have been made using linear logistic regression to allow for these differences, but not all potential confounders can be included, and residual features distinguishing HIV-infected women are likely to remain to confound the analysis.

Even if the reports from Africa can be accepted as true direct effects of HIV infection (and the consistency of reports on reduced birth weight from many different countries with studies using different designs is particularly impressive), the findings may not apply equally in the developed world. It would be expected that women with symptoms would have less favourable pregnancy outcomes and there is some evidence that this is so (Ryder et al 1989, Guay et al 1990). Whereas the great majority of pregnant women studied in the developed world were asymptomatic, HIV clinical disease may have been more common in the African studies. Thus 18% of women in one study had AIDS (Ryder et al 1989), while women who reported symptoms, a non-specific guide to illness, comprised 53% and 17% of other studies (Hira et al 1989, Braddick et al 1990). Differences in African populations may also be due to the load of other infectious diseases, which do not appear to have been examined in any of the published studies. Reactivation of tuberculosis appears very common in HIV-positive individuals and maternal ill health due to this or other endemic parasitic infections could account for the observed differences in pregnancy outcome. Malaria is endemic in several of the countries where HIV has been studied. If HIV infection resulted in a higher malarial parasite load this could explain some of the association with adverse pregnancy outcome, as this organism is known to be associated with increased rates of prematurity, low birth weight and neonatal death (Blacklock & Gordon 1925, Archibald 1958, Jelliffe 1968). Finally, differences in African populations may relate to initial and continuing nutritional status. African women may have entered pregnancy in a more vulnerable nutritional state, so that any effect of HIV is more apparent, and HIV disease in Africa may be more likely to have a weight-losing pattern. Data on prepregnancy maternal weight or weight gain during pregnancy have not been reported.

In conclusion, it seems most likely that when women are asymptomatic and not significantly immunocompromised, HIV infection per se does not have a major effect on pregnancy outcome. It is possible, from the African studies, that even early disease may have a slight effect on birth weight, spontaneous abortion and preterm labour. However, the major effect is likely to be due to advancing HIV disease, with the accompaniment of other infections (including chorioamnionitis) and deteriorating nutritional status. It seems inevitable that there will then be a detrimental effect on pregnancy, and there are data suggesting that this is so.

TREATMENT AND PREGNANCY OUTCOME

Most published studies reflect natural history, but increasingly reports on pregnancy outcome will also reflect medical intervention. This is a relatively unexplored area. Use of zidovudine in 43 pregnancies (Sperling et al 1992) was not associated with major side-effects in mothers or babies, and whether vertical transmission may be reduced by zidovudine prophylaxis is the subject of an ongoing trial (Sperling, Ch. 16).

It is possible that *Pneumocystis carinii* pneumonia prophylaxis with co-trimoxazole could be protective for other infections, apart from *Pneumocystis*, perhaps even chorioamnionitis, and as data from large collaborative studies accumulate, more insight into the effect of this intervention on gestation and birth weight should be obtained.

Trials examining several other strategies to reduce perinatal transmission are being discussed, including speculation about giving HIV hyperimmune globulin to the mother in later pregnancy (Mofenson & Burns 1991). A trial of an AIDS vaccine ran into problems, because manufacturers were reluctant to collaborate (McBride 1991). Some of the potential risks of vaccination for pregnant women were raised by Nixon (1991), who suggested that active immunization could accelerate cytotoxic T lymphocytes and antibody-driven HIV escape mutants, while passive immunization could result in viral mutation to highly virulent strains. All trials, particularly those using drugs with no established safety record in pregnancy, should pay careful attention to recording pregnancy outcome, as well as the risk of the baby being infected.

MANAGEMENT OF PREGNANCY

It can be seen that there are few purely obstetrical issues, and that pregnancy management is dominated by effective communication, up to date knowledge, and expertise in the care of HIV disease. Many of the issues in pregnancy care have been discussed more comprehensively elsewhere in this book and this short section aims simply to draw together these different threads. There have been several reviews dealing with management in pregnancy (Henrion 1988, Dinsmoor 1989, Minkoff 1989, Minkoff & Dehovitz 1991, Johnstone 1992b).

One important principle of care is that it has to be supportive, and this often involves a multiagency approach. The general practitioner, the community midwife, a physician with a special interest in HIV disease and the paediatrician who will follow up the baby may all be involved as well as hospital obstetrical staff. Social, drug and support group workers may also make a valuable contribution to the care of some patients. While this skill mix offers many advantages and opportunities to the pregnant woman, it also carries the risk of conveying different, partially confusing messages, and can involve duplication of effort. There is therefore an obligation on such a team to maintain effective communication among its members as well as with the woman.

Table 14.2 Investigations which may be appropriate depending on local laboratory facilities and local levels of disease

Assessment of HIV disease
  CD4 + lymphocyte count
  p24 antigen
  p24 antibody titre
  β_2 microglobulin
Baseline titres of conditions which may affect the fetus
  hepatitis B
  cytomegalovirus
  toxoplasmosis
Screening for other related maternal disease
  Mantoux test
  other sexually transmitted diseases
  colposcopy

Investigations which might be done at first contact in pregnancy, additional to routine antenatal tests, are shown in Table 14.2. CD4 lymphocyte count decreases by about 100/mm^3 in the first few weeks of normal non-HIV-infected pregnancy (unpublished data). Thereafter the count remains lower, but there may be an increase towards non-pregnant values by term (Castilla et al 1989). This count is affected by marked diurnal variation with a nadir in the late morning. The rate of loss of CD4 cells within cohorts is of the order of 60–100 cells/mm^3 per year (Bird 1992). It is probably the most useful single assessment of disease progression, and forms an important part of the framework for discussion about pregnancy, termination and prophylaxis. Nevertheless, few

studies have examined the power of single CD4 counts to predict prognosis in individual patients (Bird 1992). In general terms, opportunistic infection is very unlikely with a CD4 count > 300/mm^3 and *P. carinii* pneumonia prophylaxis is appropriate at a CD4 count $\leq$ 200/mm^3. Most clinicians would stick to these same figures for pregnancy even though CD4 count is reduced during this time.

Tuberculosis is a major problem in some parts of America and Africa. In the United States, Schoenbaum and colleagues (1992) recommended that determination of latent tuberculous infection should be part of the initial evaluation of pregnant HIV-infected women, and stressed the importance of prophylaxis against active tuberculosis in all ppd-reactive HIV-infected pregnant women. Depending on local prevalence of other sexually transmitted diseases, these may also be screened (Minkoff & Dehovitz 1991). As discussed in Chapter 19, cervical intraepithelial neoplasia is more common in HIV-infected women and there are anecdotal reports of very rapid progression to invasive carcinoma. Many HIV-infected women are reluctant to attend clinics and the opportunity may be taken during pregnancy to carry out colposcopy in the woman who has not been screened.

When termination of pregnancy is an available option this should be discussed. Assessment of risks of disease progression and vertical transmission can to a certain extent be individualized for each patient. The framework for discussion has been discussed in Chapter 13.

Where the woman decides to continue the pregnancy, the plan of assessment and management should be discussed with her and related issues such as maintenance drug use, plans for reduction, *P. carinii* pneumonia prophylaxis and antiretroviral therapy can be explored. As Mitchell et al (1990) has pointed out, 'in discussing potential therapies with most pregnant women, the usual maternal response is concern for the fetus. It is important that the woman with a CD4 count < 200/mm^3 understands that the risks from these therapies to the fetus remain theoretical, while the risks to herself of delayed treatment are better documented'.

It is helpful if the woman understands the symptoms of infection which may be significant during pregnancy and is encouraged to report these early. Other than infection, there do not appear to be major obstetrical problems specifically associated with HIV. However, there are often associated factors, such as drug use, heavy cigarette smoking, and adverse living conditions which may predispose to intrauterine growth retardation. For this reason careful attention should be paid to fetal growth.

Antenatal procedures which potentially could micro-innoculate maternal blood into the fetal compartment, and hence infect the baby, include:

- Chorion villus sampling
- Amniocentesis
- Cordocentesis
- Placental biopsy.

How real a risk they pose is unknown, but in one study of HIV transmission in the second trimester the only fetus in which maternal cells were demonstrated was the only one in which fetocopy had been done (Mano & Cherman 1991).

Attention has recently focused on the possibility that a high proportion of infection may occur around delivery (Ch. 15), and this in turn has raised the question of whether transmission may be reduced by performing elective Caesarean section. At present, evidence is inconclusive, and the general belief is that mode of delivery should continue to be indicated by standard obstetrical factors. However, this opinion may have to be revised as more evidence accumulates. The issue is not only transmission rate. As Fuith and associates (1992) have pointed out, anaesthesia and surgery are known to induce important changes of the immune system (Slade et al 1975), and it is conceivable that surgery could have some effect on maternal disease. There is also likely to be a higher risk of postoperative infectious morbidity for HIV-infected women.

Interventions which could theoretically have an effect on risk of vertical transmission include:

- Elective Caesarean section
- Application of fetal scalp electrode
- Fetal scalp blood sampling
- Early artificial rupture of membranes
- Vacuum/forceps delivery

- Episiotomy
- Early cord clamping
- Early bathing of baby

There is no conclusive evidence about application of scalp electrodes and fetal scalp sampling, but the European Collaborative Study (1992) found HIV infection to be more common in babies in whom these procedures were done, though only in units where these procedures were not routine. Early artificial rupture of the membranes has not been shown to have clear advantages obstetrically, and could allow more contact of maternal cervical secretion and blood from cervical dilatation with the baby. Similarly, vacuum extraction may carry a higher risk of causing abrasions to the fetal skull than forceps delivery. Early cord clamping might reduce the risk of maternal cells gaining access to the fetal blood stream as the placenta detaches, and early bathing of the baby minimizes the time of contact of maternal blood with the baby's body surface. These procedures do have potential disadvantages. Early cord clamping reduces the baby's blood volume, can predispose to anaemia, and in preterm babies, perhaps to respiratory distress syndrome. Early bathing of the baby in a relatively cool labour ward can predispose to hypothermia. Therefore, judgement about the management of each baby has to be made on an individual basis, and in the knowledge that evidence of the value of these minor changes in practice is unlikely to emerge.

Women in developed countries where bottle feeding is relatively safe should be advised against breast-feeding (Dunn et al 1992). The balance of risk may be different in situations where formula milk is not readily available and where poor standards of hygiene are used in constituting milk powder. In such situations breast feeding should continue to be promoted, as offering infants the optimum chances for survival. The postnatal period is a useful time to review arrangements for follow-up of mother and baby, to answer questions about the baby and risk of HIV infection and to discuss contraception.

The risk of nosocomial transmission is very small but remains real, and has attracted great attention. Operating practices need to change in obstetrics to minimize current rates of needle-stick injury and blood contamination. This is discussed in Chapter 22. An excellent recent review of precautions recommended in surgical practice has been published by the Joint Working Party (1992).

Progress is being made in elucidating several aspects of the interaction between HIV and pregnancy. Optimal management may well change as more information becomes available. It is important for those involved in looking after HIV-infected women in pregnancy to encourage participation in multicentre trials where efficacy of treatment is not established, and to remain receptive to new, proven advances so that their patients can have maximum benefit.

REFERENCES

Andiman W A, Simpson B J, Olson B, Dember L, Silva T J, Miller G 1990 Rate of transmission of human immunodeficiency virus type 1 infection from mother to child and short-term outcome of neonatal infection. Results of a prospective cohort study. Am J Dis Child 144: 758–766

Archibald H M 1958 Influence of maternal malaria on newborn infants. Br Med J 2: 1512–1514

Berrebi A, Lahlov M, Puel J et al 1991 Effects of HIV infection on pregnancy. VII International Conference on AIDS, Florence, June. Abstract WV2042

Bird A G 1992 Monitoring of disease progression of HIV infection. In: Bird AG (ed) Immunology of HIV infection. Kluwer Academic Publications, London, p 91–111

Blacklock B, Gordon R M 1925 Malarial parasites in the placental blood. Ann Trop Med Parasitol 19: 37–45

Blanche S, Rouzioux C, Moscato M-L et al 1989 A prospective study of infants born to women seropositive for human immunodeficiency virus type 1. N Engl J Med 320: 1643–1648

Boue F, Dreyfus M, Bridey F, Delfraissy J G, Dormont J, Tchernia G 1990 Lupus anticoagulant and HIV infection: a prospective study. AIDS 4: 467–468

Braddick M R, Kreiss J K, Embree J E et al 1990 Impact of maternal HIV infection on obstetrical and early neonatal outcome. AIDS 4: 1001–1005

Brown Z A, Vontver L A, Benedetti J et al 1987 Effects on infants of a first episode of genital herpes during pregnancy. N Engl J Med 317: 1246–1251

Bulfamante G, Muggiasca L, Conti M et al 1991 Placental morphological findings in HIV positive pregnancies: frequency and correlation to the clinical status of mothers and their babies. Abstracts of the VII International Conference on AIDS, Florence, June. Abstract WC3249

Bulterys M, Chao A, Kurawige J B et al 1991 Maternal HIV infection and intrauterine growth: a prospective cohort study in Butare, Rwanda. VII International Conference on AIDS, Florence, June. Abstract WC3224

Castilla J A, Rueda R, Vargas M L, Gonzalez-Gomez F, Garcia-Olivares E 1989 Decreased levels of circulating CD4 + T lymphocytes during normal human pregnancy. J Reprod Immunol 15: 103–111

Committee Report 1989 Prevention of perinatal transmission of hepatitis B virus: prenatal screening of all pregnant women for hepatitis B surface antigen. NY State J Med 89: 352–354

Cook G S 1990 Toxoplasma gondii infection: a potential danger to the unborn fetus and AIDS sufferer. Q J Med 273: 3–19

Dinsmoor M J 1989 HIV infection and pregnancy. Med Clin N Am 73: 701–711

Dunn D T, Newell M L, Ades A E, Peckham C S 1992 Risk of human immunodeficiency virus type 1 transmission through breast feeding. Lancet 340: 585–588

European Collaborative Study 1991 Children born to women with HIV-1 infection: natural history and risk of transmission. Lancet 337: 253–260

European Collaborative Study 1992 Risk factors for mother-to-child transmission of HIV-1. Lancet 339: 1007–1012

Fuith L C, Czarnecki M, Wachter H, Fuchs D 1992 Mode of delivery in HIV-1 infected women (letter). Lancet 339: 1603

Gloeb D J, O'Sullivan M J, Efantis J 1988 Human immunodeficiency virus infection in women 1. The effects of human immunodeficiency virus on pregnancy. Am J Obstet Gynecol 159: 756–761

Goedert J J, Duliege A M, Amos C I, Felton S, Biggar R J 1991 High risk of HIV-1 infection for first-born twins. Lancet 338: 1471–1475

Gold E, Nankervis G A 1989 Cytomegalovirus. In: Evans A S (ed) Viral infections in humans. Plenum Medical Book Company; New York, p 175–189

Griffiths P D, Baboonian C, Rutter D, Peckham C 1991 Congenital and maternal cytomegalovirus infections in a London population. B J Obstet Gynecol 98: 135–140

Guay L, Mmiro F, Ndugwa et al 1990 Perinatal outcome in HIV-infected women in Uganda. VI International Conference on AIDS, San Francisco, June. Abstract ThC42

Henrion R 1988 Pregnancy and AIDS. Hum Reprod 3: 257–262

Hira S K, Kamanga J, Bhat G J et al 1989 Perinatal transmission of HIV-1 in Zambia. Br Med J 299: 1250–1252

Italian Multicentre Study 1988 Epidemiology, clinical features and prognostic factors of paediatric HIV infection. Lancet 2: 1043–1045

Jelliffe E F P 1968 Low birth weight and malarial infection of the placenta. Bull WHO 38: 69–78

Johnstone F D, Kilpatrick D C, Burns S M 1992a Anticardiolipin antibodies and pregnancy outcome in women with human immunodeficiency virus infection. Obstet Gynecol 80: 92–96

Johnstone F D 1992b Management of pregnancy in women with HIV infection. Br J Hosp Med 48: 664–670

Johnstone F D, MacCallum L, Brettle R et al 1988 Does infection with HIV affect the outcome of pregnancy? Br Med J 296: 467

Johnstone F D, MacCallum L R, Brettle R P et al 1991 Population based, controlled study; effects of HIV infection on pregnancy. VII International Conference on AIDS, Florence, June. Abstract no WC3239

Joint Working Party of the Hospital Infection Society and the Surgical Infection Study Group 1992 Risks to surgeons and patients from HIV and hepatitis: guidelines on precautions and management of exposure to blood or body fluids. Br Med J 305: 1337–1343

Kamenga M, Manzila T, Behets F et al 1991 Maternal HIV infection and other sexually transmitted diseases and low birth weight in Zairian children. VII International

Conference on AIDS, Florence, June. Abstract WC3244

Krivine A, Firtion G, Cao L, Francoual C, Henrion R, Lebon P 1992 HIV replication during the first weeks of life. Lancet 339: 1187–1189

Lallemant M, Lallemant-LeCoeur S, Cheynier D et al 1989 Mother–child transmission of HIV-1 and infant survival in Brazzaville, Congo. AIDS 3: 643–646

Lasley-Bibbs V, Renzullo P, Goldenbaum M et al 1990 Patterns of pregnancy and reproductive morbidity among HIV infected women in the US Army: a retrospective study. VI International Conference on AIDS, San Francisco, June. Abstract ThC655

Lepage P, Dabis F, Hitimana D-G et al 1991 Perinatal transmission of HIV-1: lack of impact of maternal HIV infection on characteristics of live births and on neonatal mortality in Kigali, Rwanda. AIDS 5: 295–300

Lewis S H, Reynolds-Kohler C, Fox H E, Nelson J A 1990 HIV-1 in trophoblastic and villous Hofbauer cells, and haematological precursors in eight week fetuses. Lancet 335: 565–568

Lockwood C J, Romero R, Feinberg R G, Clyne L P, Coster B, Hobbins J C 1989 The prevalence and biologic significance of lupus anticoagulant and anticardiolipin antibodies in a general obstetric population. Am J Obstet Gynecol 161: 369–373

McBride G 1991 Vaccines for HIV infected pregnant women? Br Med J 303: 665

MacLean C, Flegg P J, Kilpatrick D C 1990 Anticardiolipin antibodies and HIV infection. Clin Exp Immunol 81: 263–266

Mano H, Cherman J-J 1991 Fetal human immunodeficiency virus Type 1 infection of different organs in the second trimester. AIDS Res Hum Retroviruses 7: 83–88

Marion R W, Wiznia A A, Hutcheon G, Rubinstein A 1986 Human T-cell lymphotrophic virus III (HTLV-III) embryopathy: a new dysmorphic syndrome associated with intrauterine HTLV-III infection. Am J Dis Child 140: 638–640

Marion R W, Wiznia A A, Hutcheon R G, Rubinstein A 1987 Fetal AIDS syndrome score correlation between severity of dysmorphism and age at diagnosis of immunodeficiency. Am J Dis Child 141: 429

Maury W, Potts B J, Rabson A B 1989 HIV-1 infection of first trimester and term human placental tissue: a possible mode of maternal–fetal transmission. J Infect Dis 160: 583–588

Minkoff H L 1989 AIDS in pregnancy. Curr Probl Obstet Gynecol Fertil 12: 206–228

Minkoff H L, Dehovitz J A 1991 Care of women infected with the human immunodeficiency virus. JAMA 266: 2253–2257

Minkoff H, Nanda D, Menez R, Fikrig S 1989 Pregnancies resulting in infants with acquired immunodeficiency syndrome of AIDS related complex. Obstet Gynaecol 69: 285–287

Minkoff H L Henderson C, Mendez H et al 1990 Pregnancy outcomes among mothers infected with human immunodeficiency virus and uninfected control subjects. Am J Obstet Gynecol 163: 1598–1604

Miotti P G, Dallabetta G, Ndovi E et al 1990 HIV-1 and pregnant women: associated factors, prevalence, estimate of incidence and role in fetal wastage in central Africa. AIDS 4: 733–736

Miotti P G, Dallabetta G A, Chiphangwi J D et al 1992 A retrospective study of childhood mortality and spontaneous abortion in HIV-1 infected women in urban Malawi. Int J Epidemiol 21: 792–799

Mitchell J L, Brown G M, Loftman P, Williams S B 1990 HIV infection in pregnancy: detection, counselling and care. Pediatric AIDS and HIV Infection: Fetus to Adolescent 1: 78–82

Mofenson L M, Burns D N 1991 Passive immunisation to prevent mother–infant transmission of human immunodeficiency virus: current issues and future directions. Pediatr Infect Dis J 10: 456–462

Nicolas S 1988 Is there an HIV associated facial dysmorphism? Pediatr Ann 5: 353

Nixon D 1991 Vaccines for HIV infected pregnant women? (letter). Br Med J 303: 1061

Nyongo A, Gichangi P, Temmerman M, Ndinya-Achola J, Piot P 1992 HIV infection as a risk factor for chorioamnionitis in preterm birth. VIII International Conference on AIDS, Amsterdam, July. Abstract POB3469, P3165

Perez M C, Wilson W A, Brown M L, Scopelitis E 1991 Anticardiolipin antibodies in unselected pregnant women: relationship to fetal outcome. J Perinatol 11: 33–36

Qazi Q H, Sheikh T M, Fikrig S 1988 Lack of evidence for craniofacial dysmorphism in perinatal HIV infection. J Pediatr, 112: 7–11

Remington J S, Desmonts G 1990 Toxoplasmosis. In: Remington J S, Klein J D (eds) Infections for the fetus and newborn infant. W B Saunders, Philadelphia; p 89–105

Rogers M F, Ou C Y, Rayfield M et al 1989 Use of the polymerase chain reaction for early detection of the proviral sequences of human immunodeficiency virus in infants born to seropositive mothers. New York City Collaborative Study of Maternal HIV Transmission and Montefiore Medical Center HIV Perinatal Transmission Study Group. N Engl J Med 320: 1649–1654

Ryder R W, Nsa W, Hassig S E et al 1989 Perinatal transmission of the human immunodeficiency virus type 1 to infants of seropositive women in Zaire. N Engl J Med 320: 1637–1642

Schoenbaum E E, Davenny K, Holbrook K 1992 The management of HIV disease in pregnancy. Baillieres Clin Obstet Gynaecol 6: 101–124

Selwyn P A, Schoenbaum E E, Davenny K et al 1989 Prospective study of human immunodeficiency virus infection and pregnancy outcomes in intravenous drug users. JAMA 261: 1289–1294

Semprini A E, Ravizza M, Bucceri A et al 1990 Perinatal outcome in HIV-infected pregnant women. Gynecol Obstet Invest 30: 15–18

Slade M S, Simmons R L, Yunis E et al 1975 Immunodepression after major surgery in normal patients. Surgery 78: 363–372

Sperling R S, Stratton P, O'Sullivan M J et al 1992 A survey of zidovudine use in pregnant women with human immunodeficiency virus infection. N Engl J Med 326: 857–861

Temmerman M, Plummer F A, Mirza N B et al 1990 Infection with HIV as a risk factor for adverse obstetrical outcome. AIDS 4: 1087–1093

Temmerman M, Ali F M, Ndinya-Achola et al 1992a Rapid increase of both HIV-1 infection and syphilis among pregnant women in Nairobi, Kenya. AIDS 6: 1181–1185

Temmerman M, Kodvoi T, Plummer F A, Ndinya-Achola J O, Piot P 1992b Maternal HIV infection as a risk factor for adverse obstetric outcome. VIII International Conference on AIDS, July. Abstract Poc 4232

Temmerman M, Lopita M I, Sanghui H C G et al 1992c. The role of maternal syphylis, gonorrhoea and HIV-1 infection in spontaneous abortion. Int J Std AIDS 3: 418–422

Vento S, Perri G D, Luzzati R et al 1989 Clinical reactivation of hepatitis B in anti-Hbs positive patients with AIDS. Lancet 1: 332–333

Wong V C, Reesink H W and Ip H M M et al 1984 Prevention of the HB$_s$Ag carrier state in newborn infants of mothers who are chronic carriers of HB$_s$Ag and HB$_e$Ag by administration of hepatitis B vaccine and hepatitis B immunoglobulin. Lancet 1: 921–926

Zachar V, Noskov-Lauritsen H, Juhl C et al. 1991 Susceptibility of cultured human trophoblast to infection with human immunodeficiency virus type 1. J Gen Virol 72: 1253–1260

15. Vertical transmission

Jacqueline Y. Q. Mok

The human immunodeficiency virus (HIV) infects children by mother-to-child transmission; through contaminated blood or blood products; through the use of inadequately sterilized equipment; or rarely, because of child sexual abuse. On a global scale, the majority of paediatric HIV infections are attributable to transmission from mother to child (vertical transmission). Table 15.1 summarizes the ways in which children can be infected with HIV.

Table 15.1 Routes of infection in children

Mother to child
  intrauterine
  intrapartum
  breast milk
Blood and blood products
Child sexual abuse
Multiple injections with inadequately sterilized equipment

ROUTES OF VERTICAL TRANSMISSION

The basic routes by which HIV can pass from mother to child are:

1. Intrauterine (transplacental)
2. Intrapartum (at the time of delivery)
3. Postpartum (mainly through breast milk).

The relative risks associated with each mode of transmission have not been quantified, and important questions regarding the mechanism, timing and route of transmission remain unanswered. For effective intervention to occur, it is important to know the exact time when infection from mother to child takes place.

Intrauterine transmission

The placental cells which are likely to be susceptible to infection by the virus are the trophoblasts and the macrophages (Hofbauer cells). Potential routes whereby HIV gains access to the fetal circulation include direct infection of the syncytiotrophoblast layer; infection of the Hofbauer cells; or invasion through the villous stroma into the fetal circulation. It is possible that free virus or HIV-laden maternal lymphocytes could be transferred to the fetus. In vitro studies suggest that the placenta could become infected with HIV by the interaction of virus-infected maternal lymphocytes with syncytiotrophoblast in direct contact with maternal blood in the intervillous space, while trophoblast cells exposed to cell-free HIV for up to 24 hours showed no evidence of virus uptake or replication (Douglas et al 1991).

In an attempt to localize HIV-positive cells in the placenta, immunoperoxidase techniques were used. HIV p24 antigen was detected in villous Hofbauer cells, decidual macrophages, intermediate trophoblast and villous endothelium in four of nine placentas from HIV-infected women (Martin et al 1992). Another group of workers found p24/55 antigen to be located exclusively in the cytoplasm of stromal macrophages located within chorionic villi, but specifically not within the trophoblastic layer (Mattern et al 1992). While virological and histological evidence of HIV replication was found in about 25% of placentas obtained at term from HIV-infected women, the presence of infection in the placentas did not correlate with infant infection status.

The role of placental macrophages in mother-to-child transmission of HIV therefore remains unclear. The macrophage could protect the fetus from HIV infection; or could serve to breach the placenta barrier, at times acting as an effective reservoir of HIV infection.

HIV antigen has been demonstrated in fetal and amniotic cells at 15 weeks' gestation (Sprecher et al 1986), in the organs of a 20-week-old fetus (Jovaisas et al 1985) and also in an infant born at 28 weeks' gestation by Caesarean section (Lapointe et al 1985). Studies of aborted fetal material suggest that infection is established by the first trimester, as early as the 8th week of gestation (Lewis et al 1990).

Isolated case reports of early HIV disease in neonates also support intrauterine infection. Rudin and co-workers (1992) presented a case of severe congenital symptomatic HIV infection detected at 21 weeks' gestation. At birth, the infant had petechiae with hepatosplenomegaly with anaemia, thrombocytopenia, leukopenia and lymphopenia. Ultrasonography revealed a pericardial effusion. HIV was cultured from plasma, while pericardial fluid was positive for p24 antigen. There was no evidence of other congenital infections. In another case report, *Pneumocystis carinii* pneumonia was diagnosed in a 19-day-old infant, again implicating intrauterine infection causing immune compromise in the newborn (Beach et al 1991). Finally, evidence for early intrauterine infection comes from reports of the 'fetal AIDS syndrome' (Marion et al 1986, 1987) where dysmorphic features observed in newborns were attributed to congenital infection with HIV. The presence of embryopathy has not been confirmed in larger prospective studies (European Collaborative Study 1988), and its existence remains in question.

Intrapartum transmission

The large quantities of infectious blood and amniotic fluid present during delivery raise the possibility that, like hepatitis B, infection with HIV could occur around the time of delivery. HIV has been isolated from vaginal and cervical secretions from HIV-positive women (Wofsy et al 1986, Vogt et al 1987). Although no case has been documented where intrapartum infection occurred, circumstantial evidence presented recently suggests

that some infection could occur during birth.

The International Registry of HIV-exposed twins (Goedert et al 1991) showed a higher risk of HIV infection in first-born twins. Where there was HIV discordance, 25% of firstborns were infected compared to 8% of second-born twins. The data suggested that a substantial portion of HIV infection occurred during the passage of the first twin through the birth canal. However, no attempt was made by the authors to examine the effects of parity, or to differentiate emergency from elective Caesarean section. Also, no comment was made on the state of the membranes or the length of membrane rupture. The data, however, provide exciting insights into the timing of infection from mother to child, as well as possible ways of preventing infection in the newborn by passive and active immunization at birth.

Ehrnst and co-workers from Sweden also presented evidence for late transmission (1991). In a study of 44 pregnant women during 47 pregnancies (19 of which were terminated), HIV was detected during pregnancy in 83%, from either peripheral blood mononuclear cells or plasma. Despite the high frequency of viraemia during pregnancy, the isolation rate of HIV from newborns at birth was low. By 6 months of age, five of 19 infants (26%) were shown to be infected by positive virus cultures. The detection of HIV was attempted in 12 abortuses, by virus isolation, in situ hybridization or polymerase chain reaction, and was not regarded as 'definitely present' in any fetus. The authors' conclusion was that most cases of transmission occurred close to or at delivery. Although their laboratory had a high frequency of positive isolations from asymptomatic HIV-infected adults, the decreased sensitivity of the test when small volumes of blood are used from newborns could account for some of the negative cultures at birth. An alternative explanation is that intrauterine infection could remain latent at birth, and requires 'trigger events' in the early newborn period for HIV replication to occur.

Postpartum transmission

After delivery, the infant could become infected through close contact with maternal secretions. Most cases of infection acquired in the postpartum period have been as a result of breast feeding. Other retroviruses (e.g. HTLV-1) can be transmitted via breast milk (Hino et al 1985, Ando et al 1987). HIV has been detected in cell-free human milk (Thiry et al 1985), and early reports of paediatric AIDS cases which implicated breast milk as a source of infection have come from children whose mothers were infected from postpartum transfusions of infected blood, and probably infected their children prior to seroconversion while being highly infectious (Ziegler et al 1985, Lepage et al 1987, Weinbreck et al 1988).

The additional risk of breast-feeding in established HIV infection had been poorly quantified due to the failure of prospective studies to recruit sufficiently large numbers of exclusively breast- or bottle-fed infants. Recently, the European Collaborative Study (1992) analysed the rate of vertical transmission, based on 721 children born to 701 mothers. In a multivariate analysis, the odds ratio of transmission was twofold higher in breast-fed versus never-breast-fed children, despite the short (4 weeks) median duration of breast-feeding. The balance of evidence was in favour of HIV transmission through breast milk, even in mothers with established infection.

The relative importance of breast milk as a source of HIV infection remains unquantified. In developing countries, the primary causes of infant deaths are malnutrition and infectious diseases, which would increase if breast milk was withdrawn. It is therefore important to assess the baby's risk of dying if not breast-fed. In each country and locality, specific guidelines should be developed to help practitioners to examine the circumstances for each individual woman. The World Health Organization (1992) recommends that in all populations, breast-feeding should continue to be protected, promoted and supported.

Bimodal distribution of paediatric HIV infection

While several mechanisms and various timings for HIV infection in children have been postulated, the exact proportion of vertical transmission attributed to each route remains unknown. Large retrospective and prospective studies of HIV-infected children suggest that early and late infection can

occur, and that the timing of infection is likely to influence the clinical presentation in the child. In the European Collaborative Study (1991), survival methods were used to estimate that 83% of 64 infected children showed signs of HIV infection within the first 6 months of age. Of these children, 26% developed AIDS by 12 months and 17% died of HIV-related causes. After the 1st year, the rate of progression of HIV disease slowed down considerably with most children remaining stable over the study period. The French prospective study (Blanche et al 1990) also estimated the early onset of AIDS in approximately 30% of infected children. Early infection, in the first trimester, could have devastating effects on the fetal immune system and lead to the severe infantile form of paediatric HIV disease. On the other hand, infection around the time of delivery, when the immune system is more mature, could result in the more slowly progressive form of HIV disease seen in some children who survive into adolescence without therapy.

RATE OF MOTHER-TO-CHILD TRANSMISSION

The efficiency of mother-to-child transmission of HIV has been estimated to vary from 13 to 32% in developed countries, and from 28 to 52% in developing countries. This wide variation is due to differences in study design, definition of infection in the child, and methods of calculation of transmission. Earlier reports were biased in that they were retrospective in design, identifying women only after they had given birth to a child with AIDS (Scott et al 1985, Minkoff et al 1987). In the last 8 years, numerous cohorts have been established to evaluate the rate of mother-to-child transmission, but differences in recruitment procedures, diagnostic criteria and measurement of transmission rate have made it impossible to compare results.

An earlier report from the European Collaborative Study (1988) which quoted a transmission rate of 24%, included children who were antibody-negative, but culture-positive. The phenomenon of 'antibody-negative culture-positive children' is hard to quantify, and some instances must be explained by laboratory error.

The revised transmission rate from the European Collaborative Study (1991) was 12.9% (95% confidence interval 9.5–16.3%), based on 372 children of at least 18 months of age with known infection status. Interestingly, 2.5% of children who remained healthy, seronegative and had no immune dysfunction were found to have positive virus cultures. The long-term outlook for these children remains uncertain. With newer, more sensitive techniques for detecting proviral sequences, reports are emerging of HIV antibody-negative-polymerase chain reaction-positive children (Laure et al 1988, De Rossi et al 1988, Rogers et al 1989). Extreme caution must be exercised when interpreting these results, as the diagnostic methods are still under evaluation and the numbers of children reported are small.

Standard laboratory tests include detection of HIV antibody or antigen, or culture methods. Most workers accept the definition proposed by the Centers for Disease Control (1987), using HIV antibody testing and the age limit of 15 months as a cut-off for 'indeterminate' children. However, the European Study used 18 months as an upper limit because survival curve estimations showed that 10.2% of children who lost maternal antibody did so after 15 months, and 2.5% after 18 months. Where authors have used 1 year as the cut-off age to define infection (Ryder et al 1989), the transmission rate could well be overestimated.

Where a combination of tests are used, the sensitivity is increased. The addition of newer, highly sensitive techniques such as the polymerase chain reaction will further increase the transmission rate. Furthermore, earlier reports which included children with symptoms and signs suggestive of HIV infection, in the absence of abnormal laboratory results, resulted in higher rates of transmission.

The Working Group on Mother-to-Child transmission of HIV (Dabis 1992) evaluated all the cohort studies, and recommended a standardized methodological approach as follows:

1. Enrolment and follow-up procedures: the cohort should include all children born to all known HIV-infected women, to avoid selection bias. Follow-up should be prospective, from birth, so that infected children are not enrolled when symptoms are identified.

Table 15.2   Diagnostic criteria and case definitions (adapted from Dabis 1992)

HIV-related signs and symptoms
  diarrhoea persisting for > 15 days
  oral candidiasis beyond the neonatal period
  generalized lymphadenopathy
  failure to thrive
  recurrent parotitis > 1 month
  herpes zoster infection
  recurrent pneumonia > two occasions

Probable HIV death
  AIDS
  at least one HIV-related sign and/or symptom when last seen, and dying from severe infection or persistent diarrhoea beyond the age of 4 weeks

2. Diagnostic criteria and case definitions: HIV-related signs and symptoms, as well as HIV-related deaths were defined (Table 15.2). A classification system of children born to HIV-infected mothers was proposed (Fig 15.1) according to their probable HIV infection status during the first 15 months of life.

3. Measurement and comparison of mother-to-child transmission rates: completeness of follow-up was clearly desired but rarely achieved. Details of loss to follow-up, including the age at which the infant was last seen, should be documented. Losses to follow-up might bias a reported transmission rate in either direction. A comparison of mortality rates in the first 15 months, seen in the infants of HIV-infected vs non-infected mothers would allow an estimation of excess mortality.

One proposed indirect measurement of transmission rate used antibody results combined with an estimate of excess mortality, viz:

$$TR = \frac{m1 - m0 + [p \times (1 - m1)]}{1 - m0}$$

where TR = transmission rate, $m1$ = probability of dying before 15 months for children born to HIV-infected women, $m0$ = probability of dying before 15 months for children born to HIV-negative women, and p = proportion of surviving children who are HIV antibody-positive at 15 months.

While most calculations of transmission rate exclude children of indeterminate and unknown

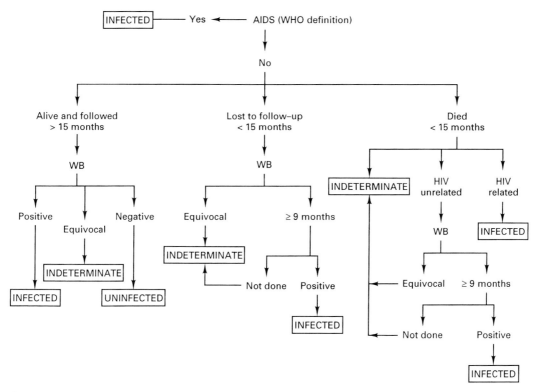

Figure 15.1 Classification system for children born to HIV-infected mothers (Dabis 1992); WB = Western blot

infection status, the information provided by children of indeterminate status allows calculation of lower and upper estimates of transmission rate. The Working Group proposed the following:

1. Assuming that all indeterminate children are uninfected,

$$TR \text{ (lower estimate)} = \frac{\text{no. of infected children}}{\text{no. in cohort}}$$

2. Assuming that all indeterminate children are infected,

$$TR \text{ (upper estimate)} =$$
$$\frac{\text{no. of infected children} + \text{no. of indeterminate children}}{\text{no. in cohort}}$$

3. Assuming that indeterminate children provide no information on infection status,

$$TR \text{ (intermediate estimate)} =$$
$$\frac{\text{no. of infected children}}{\text{no. of infected children} + \text{no. of uninfected children}}$$

From the above, it can be seen that properly conducted studies to estimate transmission rate require evaluations of the correct numerator as well as denominator. They are therefore difficult to organize, for methodological reasons and in the climate of new tests for early diagnosis. It is important, however, that results on mother-to-child transmission rates can be compared between cohorts from different geographical areas.

FACTORS INFLUENCING VERTICAL TRANSMISSION

The risk of transmission of HIV from an infected woman to her child depends on multiple factors which have yet to be unravelled. The stage of maternal disease could influence her infectivity, and hence the efficiency of transmission. It would appear, from studies of heterosexual transmission, that the rate of transmission was greater for men with full-blown AIDS (53%) than for those without symptoms (18%). The risk was also significantly increased when CD4 + lymphocyte counts were below 150 cells/mm³, with an odds ratio of 4.1 (European Study Group, 1989). The reason could be due to an increased virus load with advanced disease, leading to more efficient transmission. It has also been suggested that virus mutation with time could lead to more virulent and infectious strains of HIV (Cheng-Meyer et al 1988).

One study from Zaire (Ryder et al 1989) examined maternal health and related this to infant outcome. Of 466 HIV-infected women, 85 met the WHO definition of AIDS, and a subset of 37 women had CD4 + counts monitored. Those who were immunologically compromised (CD4 < 400 cells/mm³) were more likely to transmit HIV to their infants. In the European Collaborative Study (1992) selected risk factors for vertical transmission were examined using multivariate analysis, while controlling for other factors. A low CD4 count (< 700 cells/mm³) and p24 antigenaemia were predictive of vertical transmission, whereas non-specific clinical manifestations of HIV infection were not. Risk of vertical transmission increased threefold when the CD4 count fell below 700 cells/mm³, a level which is higher than currently recommended for initiating prophylactic therapy in HIV-infected adults.

The passage of maternal antibodies to the infant constitutes a natural model for the study of epitope-specific antibodies and their role in preventing or predicting infection in the infant. In a small study where 55 mother–infant pairs were evaluated, 16 infants were infected (Goedert et al 1989). Transmitting mothers were found to lack a gp120 band while non-transmitting mothers were postulated to confer immunological protection to their offspring by a high-affinity antibody to a gp120 epitope. These findings were corroborated by those of Rossi et al (1989) in a retrospective analysis of sera from 33 children born to HIV-infected women. Sera from uninfected children were found selectively to contain maternal antibodies to certain epitopes of gp120, and this was further substantiated in a prospective analysis where again, antibodies to the same envelope protein were detected almost exclusively in sera from mothers of uninfected infants. This promising work was refined by Devash and co-workers

(1990) who identified the region (principal neutralizing domain) within the envelope glycoprotein which in turn contains a highly conserved tetramer of amino acids, with variable sequences on either side. A retrospective analysis of 15 mother–infant pairs demonstrated that all 11 infected infants, as well as their mothers, had low levels of maternal antibodies to the gp120 principal neutralizing domain. The protective effect of gp-120 antibodies in mother-to-child transmission was not supported by results from the New York Collaborative Study (Parekh et al 1991). Clearly, further work is needed to determine whether specific maternal humoral responses influence HIV transmission from mother to child.

Although only 33 children were born before 34 weeks' gestation in the European Collaborative Study (1992), the infection rate of 33% was more than double that for children born thereafter. HIV infection per se might be expected to lead to preterm delivery, but the infected children were not observed to be small for dates. Infants born preterm could be more susceptible to infection because of low levels of passively transferred maternal antibodies (Goedert et al 1989). The data from the European Collaborative Study showed the transmission rate to level off after 34 weeks' gestation, suggesting that some infection occurred around the time of delivery, rendering preterm infants susceptible because they were born before transfer of protective maternal antibodies.

Obstetrical procedures have also been postulated to influence HIV transmission to the child. Data from the International Registry of HIV-exposed twins (Goedert et al 1991) suggested that a substantial portion of HIV transmission could occur as the first twin passed through the birth canal, and the benefits of Caesarean delivery prior to membrane rupture should be reconsidered. The Italian Multicentre Study (1988) had highlighted vaginal delivery as an added risk to the child, but only when considered together with breastfeeding.

Although transmission at delivery could occur, some prospective studies have shown no differences in infection rate in children delivered vaginally or by Caesarean section (Goedert et al 1991, Hutto et al 1991). Results from the European Collaborative Study (1992) showed some protective effect of Caesarean section which was not of statistical significance. Until randomized controlled trials are conducted, available evidence does not justify routine Caesarean section for HIV-infected women. Procedures or interventions during vaginal delivery did not affect the rate of transmission, but it would seem prudent to avoid such instrumentation which could result in the introduction of potentially infectious blood from mother to an otherwise uninfected child.

Other maternal factors which might influence HIV transmission have not been studied as intensively. Maternal intravenous drug use, parity or age at the time of delivery was not associated with increased risk of transmission (European Collaborative Study 1992). Preliminary results from Edinburgh (Hague et al 1991) suggest that delivery of the infant within a year of maternal seroconversion increased the risk of transmission, again highlighting infectiousness of the mother during primary infection.

Host genotypes might also influence the infant's susceptibility to infection, but these have not been studied in detail, as they have been in other cohorts, e.g. in haemophiliacs, in whom infection was associated with the HLA haplotype A1, B8, DR3 (Steel et al 1988). In a small study from Edinburgh (Kilpatrick et al 1991), the HLA frequencies were obtained from 47 infants born to HIV-positive women. Comparing the HLA antigen frequencies between infected and uninfected infants, HLA-DR3 was threefold higher in the infected infants. The combination A1, B8, DR3 was weakly associated with susceptibility to infection, while A3, B7, DR2 might confer some measure of protection. Table 15.3 summarizes factors which have been postulated to influence transmission of HIV from mother to child. Until more data are available, it is impossible to quantify the relative risks associated with each factor, and it is likely that several factors will combine to identify the woman at high risk of vertical transmission. Until then, it is still pertinent to offer individually tailored advice to the HIV-positive pregnant woman, taking into account her clinical and immunological status.

DIAGNOSIS OF THE INFECTED INFANT

Successful interventions to stop perinatal transmission depend on the ability to diagnose the infected infant in the first few months of life. Signs and symptoms which occur in the 1st year of life are neither specific nor sensitive. The presence of maternal HIV antibody at birth, and its persistence to 18 months, limits the usefulness of antibody testing in young infants. Also, some HIV-infected infants may be antibody-negative due to immune dysfunction, making the interpretation of results from antibody testing very difficult. A number of techniques designed to detect the virus, or to assess the infant's immune response to HIV, are discussed below.

Detection of HIV antibody produced by the infant

When serial samples of the infant's serum are tested, using enzyme-linked immunosorbent assay (ELISA) or Western blot methods, a rising titre in ELISA or an increasing number of bands on Western blot provide evidence that the response indicates de novo antibody production by the infant rather than passively transferred maternal antibodies.

A specific immune response in the infant which

Table 15.3 Risk factors for mother-to-child transmission

Maternal factors
    advanced disease, as measured by:
        clinical staging
        low CD4 + lymphocyte counts
        p24 antigenaemia
        elevated serum levels of $\beta2$ microglobulin, neopterin or
          IgA
    increased infectivity during primary infection
    presence of other sexually transmitted diseases
    protective antibodies against:
        gp120
        principal neutralizing domain
        V3 loop

Viral factors
    virulent mutant strain of HIV

Host factors
    preterm delivery
    HLA specificities

Obstetrical factors
    vaginal delivery
    invasive procedures during labour

Breast milk

would indicate infection is the presence of IgA or IgM HIV-specific antibodies, which do not cross the placenta. After removal of IgG with recombinant protein G, Weiblen and co-workers (1990) studied 64 samples from 38 infected infants, and found IgA HIV antibodies in 66% of the infants, with IgM HIV antibodies detected in 33%. The correlation with clinical information suggested that detection of HIV-specific IgA was an effective method for early diagnosis. These findings concurred with those reported earlier by a Swiss group (Schupbach et al 1989) who found that 62% of 21 infected children had either HIV-specific IgM or IgA present in cord blood sera, with 19% testing positive for both. Other workers have found a lack of correlation between IgM levels and infection status of the infant (Johnson et al 1989), due most likely to the short duration of IgM production, and to the interference of the IgM assay by the presence of IgG.

A simple modification of IgA detection was applied to a group of African children with AIDS, or who were at risk of HIV infection. Local immunity against HIV was examined, using tears (Renom et al 1990). The presence of lacrimal IgA antibodies directed against gp120, gp160, p18 and p24 core proteins was detected in 90% of children hospitalized for AIDS, and in 15% of children born to seropositive mothers. No IgA antibodies were detected in tears from control children. Although the minimal age for appearance of IgA-secreting cells was not examined, a 3-month-old child possessed anti-HIV IgA in tears.

HIV-specific IgA has been detected in saliva (Archibald et al 1990). Using Western blotting methods, the presence of anti-gp 160 IgA was found in the saliva of 10 out of 11 infected infants aged 6–46 months. Since IgA antibodies to other antigens can be elicited as early as birth, the presence of salivary HIV-specific IgA could prove a useful diagnostic test. There are obvious advantages in using saliva or urine for the detection of HIV infection in children, as venesection can be difficult in very young children. Saliva and urine samples are also safer to handle than blood specimens, and there is no risk of needle-stick injury. Robertson et al (1992) used an IgG capture enzyme immunoassay (GACELISA) and accurately identified all eight infected children with saliva and urine testing. The standard ELISA gave positive results with 7/8 saliva and 2/8 urine specimens. No false-positive results were seen from seven control children.

In a study of the pattern of HIV-specific IgG responses in infants born to HIV-infected women, the presence of antibodies to certain gag peptides (p17/9 and p24/59) was suggested as an early marker of infection (Broliden et al 1989). In a single case report, specific anti-HIV IgG1 and IgG3 subclass antibodies were detected between the 8th and 12th weeks of life, with no IgG2 or IgG4 detected. This would suggest neonatal synthesis of specific antibodies and thus HIV infection (Pyun et al 1987).

The presence of antibody-producing B lymphocytes indicates previous stimulation of the infant's immune system by HIV. The in vitro production of HIV-specific antibodies (IVAP) method was evaluated in 141 children born to HIV-positive mothers (Amadori et al 1990). The sensitivity was 90–95%, at least as sensitive as virus culture, after the first 2 months of life when the possibility of contamination by maternal cells has ceased.

HIV culture

Virus culture, either from peripheral blood mononuclear cells or plasma, remains the diagnostic standard against which newer techniques are measured. The amount of virus present can be quantified, and the frequency of positive isolations increases as HIV infection progresses (Ehrnst et al 1988, Ho et al 1989, Coombs et al 1989). Although highly specific, virus culture requires relatively large blood volumes and during asymptomatic HIV infection, false-negative results may occur. Cultures usually take 7–28 days to complete, and require specially designated equipment and skilled personnel.

By co-culturing patient cells with peripheral blood mononuclear cells from healthy donors, viral replication properties have been studied (De Rossi et al 1991). Three different phenotypes of HIV were identified according to their capacity to replicate in vitro – rapid, intermediate and slow strains. A significant association was observed between the in vitro growth pattern, proviral copy number in vivo and the clinical outcome.

HIV antigen

The presence of HIV antigen in the serum or plasma reflects viral replication. Enzyme-linked immunosorbent assays for detection of p24 core antigen are commercially available, and a positive result provides clear evidence of HIV infection. Its usefulness as a diagnostic test was assessed in 77 HIV-infected children. Antigenaemia was detected in six of 15 (40%) asymptomatic children, 33 of 47 (70%) children with AIDS-related illnesses and in all 27 of those with AIDS. Half the plasma specimens from children less than 6 months old contained antigen, but none in 10 samples taken during the 1st week of life. About 70% of specimens from infants aged 7–12 months, without symptoms, were positive for HIV antigen (Borkowsky et al 1989). Antigen testing was found to be an early predictor of HIV infection, with a single positive test having a positive predictive value of 89% (95% confidence interval, 67–99%). For 36 children tested in the 1st month of life, the specificity of antigen testing was 100%, but the sensitivity was only 20%. In the first 6 months of life, the overall sensitivity was less than 50% (Andiman et al 1992). Although specific, the transient nature of antigenaemia during early infection leads to false-negative results and limits its usefulness. Using acid to dissociate antigen from immune complexes, positive results were obtained in 145 of 162 samples from 47 infected children older than 1 month of age (Quinn et al 1992). This sensitivity of 89.5% compares with 18% when the assay was performed without acid dissociation.

HIV genomic material

Specific nucleic acid sequences can be amplified and detected using the polymerase chain reaction (PCR). This technique requires 1–3 ml of blood, and results can be obtained within a day. Laure and co-workers (1988) used primers directed against the gag and pol regions, and were able to detect HIV infection in infants 2–3 days after birth. No clinical follow-up was provided in this study. Rogers et al (1989) reported on the use of PCR for early detection of proviral sequences. Using two primer pairs, PCR was positive on blood obtained in the neonatal period in five of seven infants in whom AIDS subsequently developed, at a mean of 9.8 months after the positive PCR result. No infant, including those who developed AIDS, tested positive for HIV antigen during this time. Further analyses were done during the postneonatal period, at a median age of 5 months, and the PCR was positive in all six infants who later had AIDS, and in four of 14 infants with non-specific evidence of HIV infection. False-positives could arise, due to the extreme sensitivity of the test. The long-term outlook for children with proviral sequences detected by PCR but who become seronegative remains unknown (Laure et al 1988).

The urgent need for rapid and sensitive methods for early diagnosis has led to the search for HIV-RNA in plasma samples. Using the self-sustained sequence replication reaction (3SR) to amplify HIV-RNA, Bush et al (1992) found concordance between 3SR amplification and plasma virus culture in 14 of 19 high-risk paediatric patients. In five discordant samples, four were positive by 3SR and negative by culture. Unfortunately, no clinical information was provided on the children, limiting the usefulness of the data.

De Rossi et al (1988) compared the use of PCR with IVAP to diagnose HIV infection in infants, and concluded that a combination of tests was likely to yield the best results. The usefulness of an HIV diagnostic panel was reiterated by Petru and co-workers (1992). Using p24 antigen detection, HIV culture, and PCR, specificities were all 100%. The sensitivities, however, were 65%, 92%, and 97%, respectively. Until new techniques have been evaluated and correlated with clinical follow-up of the infants, extreme caution should be used in interpreting single results.

Surrogate markers of infection

In the absence of a sensitive, definitive test for the early diagnosis of HIV infection, monitoring immunoglobulins has proved valuable. A small study from Edinburgh (Mok et al 1989) found that in children with proved HIV infection, hypergammaglobulinaemia (especially IgG) was noted as early as 6 months, and often predated clinical signs. In the European Collaborative Study (1991) hypergammaglobulinaemia identified 77% of infected children at 6 months with 97% specificity, with a positive predictive value of 80%.

Non-specific markers of lymphocyte and macrophage activation, such as serum $\beta2$ microglobulin and neopterin levels, have been used to attempt early diagnosis. Serial determinations may be useful to detect changes, but it is not known how early in life these markers of infection are elevated. Optimal interpretation of results requires correlation with the natural history of HIV disease, as well as comparison with other methods. At present, no single test has been standardized or evaluated which can reliably identify all HIV-infected infants in the first few months of life. Table 15.4 lists some commonly used tests for early diagnosis.

Table 15.4   Tests used in early diagnosis of HIV infection in infants

Detection of infant HIV antibody
  HIV-specific IgA or IgM
  IgG capture enzyme immunoassay
  IgG subclasses
  in vitro antibody production by B lymphocytes

Detection of HIV
  virus culture from peripheral blood mononuclear cells or plasma
  HIV antigen, after acid dissociation
  HIV-DNA or RNA detected by polymerase chain reaction

Surrogate markers of infection
  hypergammaglobulinaemia
  elevated serum $\beta2$ microglobulin
  elevated serum neopterin

ANTENATAL DIAGNOSIS

In modern obstetrical practice, the prenatal diagnosis of genetic disorders is routine. Varying degrees of success have been achieved for the prenatal diagnosis of congenital infections, and attention has focused on the applicability of diagnostic techniques to the antenatal diagnosis of HIV infection.

Although HIV has been identified from amniotic cells and fluid (Sprecher et al 1986), the presence of HIV does not necessarily imply infection in the fetus, unless fetal cells are examined. Chorionic villous sampling carries a high risk of exposing fetal tissue to infected maternal blood, and the procedure is usually performed so early in ges-

tation that HIV infection might not have occurred in the fetus. Percutaneous umbilical blood sampling was performed by Daffos and co-workers (1989) on two HIV-seropositive women just prior to pregnancy termination at 24 and 27 weeks gestation. No virus was detected in either fetal blood specimen, but no postmortem virological studies were performed to establish the infection status of the abortuses.

The major concern surrounding antenatal diagnosis of HIV infection is that the procedure itself will inoculate an otherwise uninfected infant. False-positive results may be obtained from fetal samples contaminated with maternal blood. Before antenatal diagnosis can be offered routinely, it will be necessary to study seropositive women who have already elected to terminate their pregnancy, and fetal samples should be correlated with examinations of autopsy material.

With recent debate on the timing of mother-to-child infection, it is important to consider the implications of negative tests obtained during the antenatal period. The inability to detect HIV in fetuses or at birth favours the hypothesis that transmission of the virus takes place at the end of pregnancy or during delivery. Krivine et al (1992) were unable to detect the presence of HIV at birth in almost 70% of babies subsequently found to be infected.

INTERRUPTION OF VERTICAL TRANSMISSION

The prevention of vertical transmission of HIV depends on knowing when transmission is most likely to occur. If transmission occurred in utero, antiretroviral treatment of the mother during pregnancy could be administered. Even so, the teratogenic effects of drugs must be weighed against the benefits. The use of zidovudine during pregnancy was reported by two groups of Italian workers recently. Ferrazin et al (1991) treated seven HIV-infected pregnant women from 16 to 30 weeks' gestation till delivery. No side-effects were noted in the women, and although the newborns had macrocytosis, this was reversible by 2 months of age. Nine pregnant HIV-infected women treated with zidovudine were reported by Carcassi and co-workers (1991). Five women had continuous therapy, while four were only treated for the first 2 months. No teratogenic effects or haematological toxicity were observed in the infants. Only one of nine infants appeared to be infected with HIV and the authors speculated that this was due to irregular therapy in the mother. A single case report has documented the failure of zidovudine to prevent vertical transmission, despite therapy throughout pregnancy and cord concentrations of the drug equivalent to maternal levels (Crane et al 1991). The efficacy of zidovudine in preventing transmission of HIV from mother to child is best assessed in a large randomized placebo trial.

If transmission occurred around the time of delivery, therapeutic options include administration of hyperimmune immunoglobulin and vaccine to the newborn, similar to strategies to prevent hepatitis B infection. Twin studies could provide some insight into the mechanism of infection. Proximity to the cervix would put the first twin at risk from infected maternal secretion, from fetal scalp blood sampling or scalp electrodes. The second delivered twin could, in theory, be at greater risk of infection from maternal blood by remaining attached to the placenta for longer. The International Registry of HIV-exposed twins (Goedert et al 1991) provided data to suggest that proximity and passage through the birth canal were major contributors to intrapartum transmission of HIV. It was postulated that the first-born twin was in more intimate contact with infectious blood and secretions compared to the second twin. The authors suggested that a trial be undertaken to study the efficacy of using antiretroviral agents to irrigate the birth canal, as well as a reconsideration of elective Caesarean section prior to membrane rupture.

Experience with antiretroviral therapy in infants with asymptomatic HIV infection is still limited. In theory, treatment may be more effective if given as soon after infection as possible. However, difficulties surround the early diagnosis of the infected infant; and it would be unethical to use potentially toxic drugs on all infants born to HIV-infected women without identifying the truly infected ones. The approaches to the interruption of vertical transmission of HIV infection will be challenging, requiring studies into the complex physiological interactions between mother, placenta and fetus, to unravel the precise mechanism and timing of infection.

SUMMARY

Since AIDS was first described in children, much has been learnt about the epidemiology, clinical presentations and natural history of perinatally-acquired HIV disease. As yet, several questions remain unanswered about the timing and mechanisms of vertical transmission, the relative risks associated with each mode of transmission, the rate of transmission from mother to child and the factors which might contribute to the efficiency of transmission. Data presented in the early 1980s suggest that intrauterine exposure posed the greatest risk; but more recent reports have speculated that infection could occur at or around the time of delivery. The infectivity of breast milk is also emerging as an important factor in HIV transmission from mother to child.

The prospects for intervention to stop transmission from mother to child rest on the ability to identify HIV-infected women; the knowledge of how and when the virus infects the fetus; and how to identify, as early as possible, those truly infected infants. Resources should therefore be set aside for routine screening for HIV in antenatal women. There is also a need to quantify the contribution made by intrauterine vs intrapartum events. Lastly, promising new techniques designed to detect neonatal HIV infection must be properly evaluated against standard methods, and correlated with clinical outcome. Only then can there be the scientific basis for the optimal design and choice of therapies to interrupt the transmission of HIV from a mother to her offspring.

REFERENCES

Amadori A, De Rossi A, Chieco Bianchi L, Giaquinto C, De Maria A, Ades A E 1990 Diagnosis of human immunodeficiency virus 1 infection in infants: in vitro production of virus-specific antibody in lymphocytes. Pediatr Infect Dis J 9: 26–30

Andiman W A, Silva T J, Shapiro E D, O'Connor T, Olson B 1992 Predictive value of the HIV-1 antigen test in children born to infected mothers. Pediatr Infect Dis J 11: 436–440

Ando Y, Nakano S, Saito K et al 1987 Transmission of adult T cell leukemia retrovirus (HTLV-1) from mother to child:

comparison of bottle with breast-fed babies. Jpn J Cancer Res 78: 322–324

Archibald D W, Johnson J P, Nair P et al 1990 Detection of salivary immunoglobulin A antibodies to HIV-1 in infants and children. AIDS 4: 417–420

Beach R S, Garcia E R, Sosa R, Good R A 1991 Pneumocystis carinii pneumonia in a HIV-1 infected neonate with meconium aspiration. Pediatr Infect Dis J 10: 953–954

Blanche S, Tardieu M, Duliege A et al 1990 Longitudinal study of 94 symptomatic infants with perinatally acquired human immunodeficiency virus infection. Evidence for a bimodal expression of clinical and biological symptoms. Am J Dis Child 144: 1210–1215

Borkowsky W, Krasinski K, Paul D et al 1989 Human immunodeficiency virus type 1 antigenemia in children. J Pediatr 114: 940–945

Broliden P A, Moschese V, Ljunggren K et al 1989 Diagnostic implication of specific immunoglobulin G patterns of children born to HIV-infected mothers. AIDS 3: 577–582

Bush C E, Donovan R M, Peterson W R 1992 Detection of HIV type 1 RNA in plasma samples from high-risk pediatric patients by using the self-sustained sequence replication reaction. J Clin Microbiol 30: 281–286

Carcassi C, Chiappe F, Lecca U et al 1991 A study of nine infants born from HIV-1 positive mothers who continued treatment with AZT during pregnancy. Abstracts of the Seventh International Conference on AIDS, Florence. WC 3228

Centers for Disease Control 1987 Classification system for human immunodeficiency virus (HIV) infection in children under 13 years of age MMWR 36: 225–30, 235–6

Cheng-Meyer C, Seto D, Tateno M, Levy J A 1988 Biological features of HIV-1 that correlate with virulence in the host. Science 240: 80–82

Coombs R W, Collier A C, Allain J-P et al 1989 Plasma viremia in human immunodeficiency virus infections. N Engl J Med 321: 1626–1631

Crane L, Schuman P, Cohen F, Moore E, Kauffman R 1991 Failure of zidovudine to prevent vertical transmission of HIV. Abstracts from the Seventh International Conference on AIDS, Florence. MC 3182

Dabis F 1992 Methodological issues in mother-to-child transmission of HIV. Abstracts of the VIII International Conference on AIDS, Amsterdam. PoC 4218

Daffos F, Forestier F, Mandelbrot L, Pialoux G, Rey M A, Brun Vezinet F 1989 Prenatal diagnosis of HIV infection: two attempts using fetal blood sampling. J Acq Immune Defic Synd 2: 205–207

De Rossi A, Amadori A, Chieco Bianchi L et al 1988 Polymerase chain reaction and in-vitro antibody production for early diagnosis of paediatric HIV infection. Lancet 2: 278

De Rossi A, Pasti M, Mammano F, Ometto L, Giaquinto C, Chieco-Bianchi L 1991 Perinatal infection by HIV-1: relationship between proviral copy number in vivo, viral properties in vitro and clinical outcome. J Med Virol 35: 283–289

Devash Y, Calvelli T A, Wood D G, Reagan K J, Rubinstein A 1990 Vertical transmission of human immunodeficiency virus is correlated with the absence of high-affinity/avidity maternal antibodies to the gp 120 principal neutralizing domain Proc Natl Acad Sci USA 87: 3445–3449

Douglas G C, Fry G N, Thirkill T et al 1991 Cell mediated infection of human placental trophoblast with HIV in vitro. AIDS Research and Human Retroviruses 7: 735–740

Ehrnst A, Sonnerborg A, Bergdahl S, Strannegard O 1988 Efficient isolation of HIV from plasma during different stages of HIV infection. J Med Virol 26: 23–32

Ehrnst A, Lindgren S, Dictor M, Johansson B et al 1991 HIV in pregnant women and their offspring: evidence for late transmission. Lancet 338: 203–207

European Collaborative Study 1988 Mother-to-child transmission of HIV infection. Lancet 2: 1039–1043

European Study Group 1989 Risk factors for male to female transmission of HIV. Br Med J 2998: 411–415

European Collaborative Study 1991 Children born to women with HIV-1 infection: natural history and risk of transmission. Lancet 337: 253–258

European Collaborative Study 1992 Risk factors for mother-to-child transmission of HIV-1. Lancet 339: 1007–1012

Ferrazin A, Terragna A, Loy A et al 1991 Zidovudine therapy of HIV infection during pregnancy: assessment of the effect on the newborns. Abstracts from the Seventh International Conference on AIDS, Florence. MC 3023

Goedert J J, Mendez H, Drummond J E et al 1989 Mother-to-infant transmission of human immunodeficiency virus type 1: association with prematurity or low anti-gp120. Lancet 2: 1351–1354

Goedert J J, Duliege A M, Amos C I, Felton S, Biggar R J 1991 High risk of HIV-1 infection for first-born twins. The international registry of HIV-exposed twins. Lancet 338: 1471–1475

Hague R A, Mok J Y Q, MacCallum L, Burns S, Yap P L 1991 Do maternal factors influence the risk of vertical transmission of HIV? Abstracts from the Seventh International Conference on AIDS, Florence. WC 3237

Hino S, Yamaguchi K, Katamine S et al 1985 Mother-to-child transmission of human T cell leukemia virus type 1. Jpn J Cancer Res 78: 474–480

Ho DD, Moudgil T, Alam M 1989 Quantitation of human immunodeficiency virus type 1 in the blood of infected persons. N Engl J Med 321: 1621–1625

Hutto C, Parks W P, Lai S et al 1991 A hospital-based prospective study of perinatal infection with HIV type 1. J Pediatr 118: 347–353

Italian Multicentre Study 1988 Epidemiology, clinical features, and prognostic factors of paediatric HIV infection. Lancet 2: 1043–1046

Johnson J P, Nair P, Hines S E et al 1989 Natural history and serologic diagnosis of infants born to human immunodeficiency virus-infected women. Am J Dis Child 143: 1147–1153

Jovaisas E, Koch M A, Schafer A, Stauber M, Lowenthal D 1985 LAV/HTLV-III in 20-week fetus. Lancet 2: 1129

Kilpatrick D C, Hague R A, Yap P L, Mok J Y Q 1991 HLA antigen frequencies in children born to HIV-infected mothers. Disease Markers 8: 1–6

Krivine A, Firtion G, Cao L et al 1992 HIV replication during the first weeks of life. Lancet 339: 1187–1189

Lapointe N, Michaud J, Pekovic D, Chausseau J P, Dupuy JM 1985 Transplacental transmission of HTLV-III virus. N Engl J Med 312: 1325–1326

Laure F, Courgnaud V, Rouzioux C et al 1988 Detection of HIV1 DNA in infants and children by means of the polymerase chain reaction. Lancet 2: 538–541

Lepage P, Van de Perre P, Carael M et al 1987 Postnatal transmission of HIV from mother to child. Lancet 2: 400

Lewis S H, Reynolds Kohler C, Fox H E, Nelson J A 1990 HIV-1 in trophoblastic and villous Hofbauer cells, and haematological precursors in eight-week fetuses. Lancet 335: 565–568

Marion R W, Wiznia A A, Hutcheon G, Rubinstein A 1986 Human T-cell lymphotropic virus type III (HTLV-III) embryopathy. A new dysmorphic syndrome associated with intrauterine HTLV-III infection. Am J Dis Child 140: 638–640

Marion R W, Wiznia A A, Hutcheon R G, Rubinstein A 1987 Fetal AIDS syndrome score. Correlation between severity of dysmorphism and age at diagnosis of immunodeficiency. Am J Dis Child 141: 429–431

Martin A W, Brady K, Smith S I et al 1992 Immunohistochemical localization of HIV p24 antigen in placental tissue. Hum Pathol 23: 411–414

Mattern C F T, Murray K, Jensen A, Farzadegan H, Pang J, Modlin J F 1992 Localization of HIV core antigen in term human placentas. Pediatrics 89: 207–209

Minkoff H, Nanda D, Menez R, Fikrig S 1987 Pregnancies resulting in infants with acquired immunodeficiency syndrome or AIDS-related complex: follow-up of mothers, children, and subsequently born siblings. Obstet Gynecol 69: 288–91

Mok J Y, Hague R A, Yap P L et al 1989 Vertical transmission of HIV: a prospective study. Arch Dis Child 64: 1140–1145

Parekh B S, Shaffer N, Pau C P et al 1991 Lack of correlation between maternal antibodies to V3 loop peptides of gp120 and perinatal HIV-1 transmission. AIDS 5: 1179–1184

Petru A, Dunphy M G, Azimi P et al 1992 Reliability of polymerase chain reaction in the detection of HIV infection in children. Pediatr Infect Dis J 11: 30–33

Pyun K H, Ochs H D, Dufford M T, Wedgwood R J 1987 Perinatal infection with human immunodeficiency virus. Specific antibody responses by the neonate. N Engl J Med 317: 611–614

Quinn T C, Kline R, Moss M, Livingston R A, Hutton N 1992 Acid dissociation of immune complexes improves the diagnostic utility of p24 antigen detection in perinatally acquired HIV-1 infection. VIII International Conference on AIDS, Amsterdam, Abstr ThC 1579

Renom G, Bouquety J C, Lanckriet C, Georges A J, Siopathis M R, Martin P M 1990 Detection of anti-HIV IgA in tears of children born to seropositive mothers is highly specific. Res Virol 141: 557–562

Robertson P, Burns S M, Yap P L, Mok J Y Q, Parry J V 1992 The use of saliva and urine for the detection of HIV infection in children: preliminary report. Pediatr AIDS and HIV Infect 3: 12–14

Rogers M F, Ou C Y, Rayfield M et al 1989 Use of the polymerase chain reaction for early detection of the proviral sequences of human immunodeficiency virus in infants born to seropositive mothers. New York City Collaborative Study of Maternal HIV Transmission and Montefiore Medical Center HIV Perinatal Transmission Study Group. N Engl J Med 320: 1649–1654

Rossi P, Moschese V, Broliden P A et al 1989 Presence of maternal antibodies to human immunodeficiency virus 1 envelope glycoprotein gp 120 epitopes correlates with the uninfected status of children born to seropositive mothers. Proc Natl Acad Sci USA 86: 8055–8058

Rudin C, Meier D, Pavic N et al 1992 Intrauterine onset of symptomatic HIV disease. Abstracts of the VIII International Conference on AIDS, Amsterdam. PoC 4734

Ryder R W, Nsa W, Hassig S E et al 1989 Perinatal transmission of the human immunodeficiency virus type 1 to infants of seropositive women in Zaire. N Engl J Med 320: 1637–1642

Schupbach J, Wunderli W, Kind C, Kernen R, Baumgartner A, Tomasik Z 1989 Frequent detection of HIV- and IgG-specific IgM and IgA antibodies in HIV-positive cord-blood sera: fine analysis by western blot. AIDS 3: 583–589

Scott G B, Fischl M A, Klimas N et al 1985 Mothers of infants with the acquired immunodeficiency syndrome. Evidence for both symptomatic and asymptomatic carriers. JAMA 253: 363–366

Sprecher S, Soumenkoff G, Puissant F, Degueldre M 1986 Vertical transmission of HIV in 15-week fetus. Lancet 2: 288–289

Steel C M, Ludlam C A, Beatson P, Peutherer J F 1988 HLA haplotype A1 B8 DR3 as a risk factor for HIV-related disease. Lancet 1: 1155–1158

Thiry L, Sprecher Goldberger S, Jonckheer T et al 1985 Isolation of AIDS virus from cell-free breast milk of three healthy virus carriers. Lancet 2: 891–892

Vogt M W, Witt D J, Craven D E, Byington R et al 1987 Isolation patterns of the human immunodeficiency virus from cervical secretions during the menstrual cycle of women at risk for the acquired immunodeficiency syndrome. Ann Intern Med 106: 380–382

Weiblen B J, Lee F K, Cooper E R et al 1990 Early diagnosis of HIV infection in infants by detection of IgA HIV antibodies. Lancet 335: 988–990

Weinbreck P, Loustaud V, Denis F et al 1988 Postnatal transmission of HIV infection. Lancet 1: 482

Wofsy C B, Cohen J B, Haver L B, Padian N S et al 1986 Isolation of AIDS-associated retrovirus from genital secretions of women with antibodies to the virus. Lancet 1: 527–529

World Health Organization Global Programme on AIDS 1992 Consensus statement from the WHO/UNICEF consultation on HIV transmission and breast feeding. Geneva 30 April–1 May 1992

Ziegler J B, Cooper D A, Johnson R O, Gold J 1985 Postnatal transmission of AIDS-associated retrovirus from mother to infant. Lancet 1: 896–898

16. Prophylaxis and treatment during pregnancy

Rhoda Sperling

BACKGROUND

Infection with the human immunodeficiency virus (HIV) remains a global pandemic (Chin 1990). World-wide, the large increases in the number of infected women reflect a steady increase in HIV-1 infections among heterosexual populations.

In the USA, blinded seroprevalence surveys among child-bearing women are being conducted and provide data on patterns and trends of HIV infection among women and newborns (Ellerbrock & Rogers 1990); similar studies are being conducted in other parts of the world. As the number of HIV-infected pregnant women has grown, obstetricians have been faced with the challenge of developing appropriate management protocols. Antepartum management should include: assessing maternal immunological function; initiating or continuing HIV-1-related prophylactic and therapeutic treatments of proven efficacy; recognizing and treating frequently seen concomitant infections; monitoring the fetus; and participating (when available) in trials designed to interrupt perinatal HIV-1 transmission.

The treatment of a medical problem as complex as HIV-1 during pregnancy requires a consideration of maternal risks, maternal benefits, fetal risks, and fetal benefits. Although optimal therapeutic regimens for a pregnancy complicated by HIV-1 infection have yet to be defined, disclosure and consideration of the range of therapeutic options are essential components of appropriate prenatal care. The pregnant woman should make decisions regarding an acceptable level of maternal and fetal neonatal risks after risk–benefit discussions with her physicians. The ethical complexity of this decision-making process has been eloquently discussed in a recent article by Minkoff and Moreno (1990).

IMMUNOLOGICAL EVALUATION AND MONITORING

Non-pregnant adults

T cell lymphocyte levels remain the primary laboratory determinant for initiating both anti-retroviral treatment and prophylaxis against *Pneumocystis carinii* pneumonia. Individuals who have absolute T helper (CD4+ lymphocyte) cell counts less than 200 cells/mm^3 or less than 20% of total lymphocytes have significant immune suppression and are at high risk for the development of opportunistic infections (Masur et al 1989).

At a state-of-the-art conference at the National Institutes of Health (NIH) in March 1990 it was recommended that a baseline CD4+ cell count be obtained at diagnosis of HIV infection. For infected individuals with a cell count greater than 600 cells/mm^3, testing should be repeated in 6 months. CD4+ cell counts were recommended every 3 months for those with baseline counts below 600 cells/mm^3. A count less than 200 cells/mm^3 should be reconfirmed 1 week later. After the count falls below 200 cells/mm^3 and the patient has been placed on *P. carinii* pneumonia prophylaxis and zidovudine therapy, further CD4+ counts are not required (NIAID/NIH 1990).

Pregnant women

The recommendations described above are probably appropriate for HIV-infected pregnant women. Although some obstetric experts recommend obtaining a CD4 + cell count each trimester, that approach would be expensive and its benefit has not yet been demonstrated. Although there are theoretical concerns that pregnancy could result in an acceleration of HIV-related disease progression (Brabin 1985), and modest decreases in maternal CD4 + cell counts have been reported in HIV-infected pregnant women (Biggar et al 1989), preliminary studies have not demonstrated accelerated HIV disease progression related to pregnancy (Berrebi et al 1990).

P. CARINII PNEUMONIA PROPHYLAXIS

Non-pregnant adults

P. Carinii pneumonia remains the most common opportunistic infection in HIV infection, and mortality for the first episode is 5–20% (Centers for Disease Control 1989). The recurrence risk for those not receiving prophylaxis is high (CDC 1989). Therapies aimed at the prevention of the first episode of P. carinii pneumonia are referred to as primary prophylaxis and those targeted at preventing subsequent episodes are referred to as secondary prophylaxis.

Certain immunological and clinical indices are helpful in predicting which HIV-infected individuals should receive primary prophylaxis. Although data on women are unavailable, the Multicenter AIDS Cohort Study of homosexual men found that 8.4% and 18.4% of individuals with CD4 + cell counts less than 200 cells/mm^3 develop P. carinii pneumonia by 6 and 12 months, respectively (Phair et al 1990). For individuals with counts of 201–350 cells/mm^3, the risk of developing pneumonia within 6 months has been estimated to be 0.5% (Phair et al 1990). Therefore, prophylaxis should be reserved for individuals whose CD4 + cell counts are below 200 cells/mm^3. After an episode of pneumonia, relapse occurs in 50% of zidovudine treated patients by 8 months and in 70–80% by 18 months. (Fischl et al 1988, CDC 1989). Therefore, secondary prophylaxis is indicated for all individuals with a prior history of P. carinii pneumonia regardless of CD4 + cell count.

The treatments used most commonly for prophylaxis have been oral trimethoprim–sulfamethoxazole and aerosolized pentamidine. A recent National Institutes of Health-funded AIDS Clinical Trial Group study of secondary prophylaxis found that in zidovudine-treated patients, trimethoprim–sulfamethoxazole (one double-strength tablet every day) was superior to aerosolized pentamidine (300 mg every 4 weeks) (Hardy et al 1992). The most efficacious regimen for primary prophylaxis is not yet known. There is an ongoing multicentred study comparing trimethoprim–sulfamethoxazole, aerosolized pentamidine, and a third oral agent, dapsone.

Trimethoprim–sulfamethoxazole, one double-strength tablet twice daily, given with folinic acid, 5 mg once daily, was the first reported effective regimen for primary prophylaxis in HIV-1-infected individuals (Fischl et al 1988), but was poorly tolerated. Fevers, rash, neutropenia and elevated transaminase levels have often required a change in therapy (Kobrinsky & Ramsay 1981, Gordin et al 1984, Kovacs et al 1984, Fisch et al 1988). Because toxicities appear to be dose-dependent, low-dose trimethoprim–sulfamethoxazole, once daily or three times per week, has been used. A retrospective series of low-dose, intermittent administration (one double-strength tablet every Monday, Wednesday, and Friday) given without folinic acid rescue strongly supports the efficacy and tolerance of this approach (Ruskin & La-Riviere 1991).

Aerosolized pentamidine provides effective prophylaxis when given at a dose of 300 mg once a month (Hirschel et al 1991). Aerosolized administration offers the theoretical advantage of targeting drug distribution to the alveoli. Although this route reduces systemic toxicity associated with parenteral administration, it has been associated with local treatment failure and systemic pneumocystosis (Abd et al 1988, Jules-Elysee et al 1990). Administration of aerosolized pentamidine is expensive and requires a system that will deliver the appropriate size particles intra-alveolarly while protecting other patients and health care workers from environmental contamination (CDC 1989, 1990). Of particular concern is environmental contamination with tuberculosis from aerosolized pulmonary secretions. Because the incidence of tuberculosis among HIV-infected patients in the USA is high, it is recommended that all patients be screened for active tuberculosis before aerosolized pentamidine therapy is initiated (CDC 1990). Screening should include a medical history, a tuberculin skin test, and a baseline chest radiograph.

The most common toxicities caused by aerosolized pentamidine are cough (38%) and bronchospasm (15%) (Diagnostic and therapeutic technology assessment 1990), both of which may be mitigated or eliminated by the use of inhaled bronchodilators. Chemical conjunctivitis and pneumothorax have been reported in patients receiving aerosolized therapy. Other side-effects include neutropenia, anaemia, liver function abnormalities, renal insufficiency, and hyper- and hypoglycaemia; however, these adverse reactions are less marked in aerosol administration compared to parenteral.

Because of the high incidence of rash and side-effects associated with oral trimethoprim–sulfamethoxazole, dapsone has been advocated for oral maintenance therapy. There are few published data on its effectiveness for primary prophylaxis and dapsone has yet to be approved by the Food and Drug Administration in the USA for this indication.

Pregnant women

Because *P. carinii* pneumonia is an important cause of AIDS-related maternal mortality (Minkoff et al 1986, Koonin et al 1989), HIV-infected pregnant women with a history of this opportunistic infection or with a CD4 + cell count less than 200 cells/mm³ should receive prophylaxis. In the absence of pregnancy-specific pharmacokinetic information, a regimen approved for non-pregnant adults outlined previously should be considered.

Pentamidine, when delivered via aerosol for prophylaxis, has little systemic absorption and may have little effect on the fetus, making it the first choice of some obstetricians for primary prophylaxis.

The fetal and newborn safety of trimethoprim–sulfamethoxazole in human pregnancy is of concern as both trimethoprim and sulfamethoxazole readily cross the placenta. In some animal models, these agents have been reported to cause congenital malformations (Helm et al 1976). Sulfamethoxazole alone, in corresponding doses, was not embryotoxic. To date, human teratogenicity with either drug, singularly or in combination, has never been reported (Williams et al 1969, Heinonen et al 1977).

Experience with trimethoprim–sulfamethoxazole in human pregnancy has been limited by the theoretical concern of maternal treatment precipitating newborn kernicterus. Sulfonamides displace bilirubin from its albumin binding site, resulting in increases in circulating unconjugated bilirubin. In premature newborns who have received sulfonamide therapy *after* birth, high levels of unconjugated bilirubin have been associated with kernicterus (Silverman et al 1956). During pregnancy, unconjugated bilirubin will cross the placental barrier but it is effectively cleared from the fetus by the placenta (Palmisano & Palhill 1979). A recent review of the English language literature failed to reveal any cases of newborn kernicterus following *maternal* sulfamethoxazole therapy. Newborns also have a relative deficiency of glucose-6-phosphate dehydrogenase and glutathione, and, therefore, may be at increased risk of haemolysis precipitated by the ingestion of sulfonamides (Brown & Cevik 1965). Cases of newborn haemolysis have been reported following maternal ingestion of long-acting sulfonamides (Brown & Cevik 1965), but cases of newborn haemolysis precipitated by maternal sulfamethoxazole therapy have not been reported in the literature.

Since the morbidity and mortality of *P. carinii* pneumonia remain high, and fetal or newborn morbidity after maternal receipt of prophylaxis has not been clearly demonstrated, withholding therapy is unjustified. When considering trimethoprim–sulfamethoxazole therapy either in the first trimester or at term, the theoretical risks of teratogenicity or newborn kernicterus should be reviewed with the patient. In addition, newborns of mothers who have received sulfonamide therapy should have appropriate haematological monitoring.

Maternal safety of trimethoprim–sulfamethoxazole therapy is also of concern because the combination commonly causes neutropenia

(Gordin et al 1984, Fischl et al 1988) and may also cause megaloblastic anaemia due to an anti-folate effect (Kobrinsky & Ramsay 1981). Although concurrent administration of folinic acid prevents megaloblastic anaemia without inter-fering with antibacterial activity (Zinner & Mayer 1990) recent data demonstrating efficacy of low-dose, three times weekly prophylaxis suggest the use of folinic acid may not be necessary (Ruskin & LaRiviere 1991). During pregnancy, a complete blood count (CBC) is recommended every 2 weeks to monitor maternal haematological toxicity.

There is no reported clinical experience with the use of dapsone in HIV-infected pregnant women. As dapsone significantly affects the glucose-6-phosphate dehydrogenase system its use in preg-nancy is of concern. Dapsone has been used in pregnancy for the treatment of both leprosy and dermatitis herpetiformis and in uncontrolled studies fetal abnormalities have not been reported (UPSC 1990). Animal reproduction studies have yet to be conducted with dapsone. The drug has been shown to be carcinogenic in mice and rats (UPSC 1990). Until controlled trials of dapsone vs trimethoprim–sulfamethoxazole for primary prophylaxis are completed, trimethoprim–sul-famethoxazole remains the oral treatment of choice in pregnant women.

ZIDOVUDINE AND OTHER ANTIRETROVIRAL THERAPY

Non-pregnant adults

The dideoxynucleoside analogues are a family of antiretroviral agents with activity against the human immunodeficiency virus (Yarchoan et al 1989). Therapy with zidovudine, the first member of this family to be approved for the treatment of HIV disease, has become a routine part of the care of HIV-infected individuals. Zidovudine therapy is not curative. Zidovudine inhibits viral reverse transcriptase and when the drug achieves adequate intracellular concentrations in an uninfected cell, it can prevent the HIV-1 virus from reproducing.

For individuals with AIDS or AIDS-related complex and/or CD4+ cell counts less than 200 cells/mm^3, zidovudine therapy has been shown to decrease mortality, frequency and severity of opportunistic infections and to delay progression of immune deterioration (Fischl et al 1987). Zido-vudine therapy has also been shown to delay the onset of AIDS in asymptomatic HIV infected sub-jects with fewer than 500 CD4+ cells/mm^3 (Volberding et al 1990). Early treatment with zido-vudine remains controversial. Questions of long-term benefit, toxicity and emerging drug resistance are unanswered. The minimum effective dose of zidovudine has not been established. Earlier studies utilized 1500 mg daily, but more recent studies have found 500 mg daily to be effective. The currently recommended oral dose in adults is 500 mg daily (100 mg five times daily).

Adverse haematological effects, including mac-rocytosis, anaemia, and neutropenia have been reported (Richman et al 1987). Clinically sig-nificant anaemia has been a problem in both pae-diatric and adult treatment trials. Lower doses have been associated with diminished toxicity. Dose interruption or reduction is recommended for a haemoglobin less than 8.0 g/dl and gran-ulocytopenia less than 750 cells/mm^3. During treatment, a complete blood count with differential should be done monthly for the first 3 months and then every 3 months. Chronic zidovudine use has also been associated with both a peripheral myop-athy and a polymyositis-like-syndrome.

Late-appearing, non-metastasizing vaginal tumours have been seen in a small number of mice and rats exposed to high doses of zidovudine throughout their life span; toxicology experts believe that species differences make it unlikely that this observation is predictive of human car-cinogenicity (NIAID 1990).

Other nucleoside analogues, didanosine (ddI) and dideoxycytidine (ddC), have recently been added to the clinical armamentarium. Didanosine was originally approved for salvage therapy for patients who either failed or who had become intol-erant of zidovudine. However, a recent report of patients on long-term zidovudine suppression found that patients switched from zidovudine to low-dose didanosine therapy had a lower rate of AIDS-defining illnesses (Kahn et al 1992). The minimal effective dose of didanosine and the best time to begin treatment with this agent have not yet been determined. There are as yet no data to support the use of didanosine alone as the initial therapy in patients with advanced HIV-1 infection.

In early studies, didanosine therapy did not result in bone marrow suppression, a major adverse effect of zidovudine, but instead had the limiting toxic effects of pancreatitis and sensory peripheral neuropathy (Yarchoan et al 1990). In a recently published trial, low-dose didanosine had a toxicity profile that was more favourable than that of zidovudine (Kahn et al 1992).

Pregnant women

Most obstetrical experts offer zidovudine therapy to pregnant women with AIDS, AIDS-related complex, or CD4 + cell counts below 200 cells/mm^3. Delaying treatment until the postpartum period in women at high risk for clinical deterioration may adversely affect both short-term and long-term maternal outcome. In the absence of pharmacokinetic data in pregnant women, the dose recommended for non-pregnant adults (100 mg five times daily) should be administered. The maternal benefits of zidovudine therapy during pregnancy for women with CD4 + cell counts between 200 and 500 cells/mm^3, as well as the risks of delaying treatment until the postpartum period, are unclear.

The effects of zidovudine on the fetus or on the pregnancy are unknown. Of particular concern with zidovudine use during pregnancy is the possibility of teratogenicity, fetal haematological toxicity, and/or any unanticipated long-term toxicities.

Teratology studies in animals have been reported. Earlier studies failed to demonstrate impaired fertility or fetal harm; however, a recent study of zidovudine in pregnant rats found developmental malformations and skeleton variations in dams treated with 3000 mg/kg per day from gestational days 6–15 (Burroughs–Wellcome 1992). Twelve percent of the fetuses were malformed; the most frequently observed malformations were absent tail, anal atresia, fetal oedema, situs inversus, diaphragmatic hernia, bent limbs, and bone and rib abnormalities. The clinical relevance of this data is unknown as the doses used far exceeded the estimated human exposure with currently recommended oral doses. In another study, a direct toxic effect on developing mouse embryos was reported resulting in early pregnancy resorptions (Toltzis et al 1991). Another recent study utilizing an in vitro rat embryo model compared zidovudine to four other nucleoside analogues (vidarabine phosphate, dideoxyadenosine (ddA), dideoxycytidine (ddC), and ganciclovir) and found that zidovudine was the least embryotoxic (Klug et al 1991). In vivo experiments by the same investigators found no teratogenic abnormalities with zidovudine after in utero exposure (Klug et al 1991).

There is increasing experience with zidovudine use in human pregnancy. Pharmacokinetic studies have confirmed transplacental passage of the drug with concentrations in the fetal compartment similar to those found in the maternal circulation. (Watts et al 1991). A retrospective series of 43 women who had received zidovudine during pregnancy has been published (Sperling et al 1992). In this reported series, zidovudine was well tolerated by the pregnant women and was not associated with malformations in the newborns, premature births or fetal distress. There was no pattern of haematological toxicity observed in the newborns. Of the 12 infants with first trimester exposure, no teratogenic abnormalities occurred. However, this small number of first trimester exposures cannot be used to predict the potential human teratogenic risk of zidovudine. Ongoing surveillance of zidovudine safety in pregnancy is being conducted by the manufacturer, Burroughs-Wellcome, through their pregnancy registry and also in ongoing clinical trials. Until more data are available, first trimester use of this agent should be considered carefully in the context of maternal benefits compared to unknown fetal teratogenic risks.

The possibility of clinically significant fetal marrow suppression after transplacental passage of zidovudine requires close antepartum assessment. Serial sonographic assessment is currently the only practical method for monitoring fetuses for the development of in utero anaemia. In general, fetuses will not develop hydrops unless severely anaemic with haemoglobin concentrations 7–10 g/dl below the normal mean for gestational age (Nicolaides et al 1988).

Since haematological toxicities have been observed in non-pregnant adults, pregnant women taking zidovudine should be monitored for anaemia and granulocytopenia by complete blood counts with differentials every month. In the absence of standards for pregnancy, the guidelines for non-pregnant adults should be followed; indications of toxicity that require dose interruption or reduction include a haemoglobin less than 8 g/dl and absolute granulocyte count (polymorphonuclear cells and bands) less than 750 cells/mm^3. In addition, newborns born to pregnant women who have taken zidovudine should be screened for haematological toxicity, with close follow-up of any abnormalities. Serum chemistries should also be obtained in all pregnant women as a baseline, with any abnormalities followed closely. Of particular concern are hepatic enzyme abnormalities since zidovudine is cleared by hepatic glucuronidation.

The effect of zidovudine treatment on mother-to-child transmission of HIV is unknown and is the subject of an ongoing National Institutes of Health-funded trial.

Less is known about the effects of other nucleoside analogues on pregnancy. Based on toxicities reported in early trials of didanosine, there is concern about the possibility of fetal and/or maternal pancreatitis complicating maternal therapy. As with the use of any drug in pregnancy, there are also concerns about teratogenicity and unanticipated long-term toxicities. There is a lack of reported experience with the safety of didanosine in human pregnancy. Limited pharmacokinetic studies have reported that didanosine crosses the placental barrier and the concentrations achieved in amniotic fluid and fetal blood are lower than that in maternal blood (Pons et al 1991).

From information provided by the manufacturer of didanosine (Bristol-Myers Squibb Company), animal reproduction studies in rats and rabbits with doses up to 12 and 14 times the estimated human exposure, found no evidence of impaired fertility or harm to the fetus. However, until further information is available about didanosine, recommendations for its use in pregnancy cannot be made.

RECOGNITION AND TREATMENT OF FREQUENTLY SEEN CO-INFECTIONS

Infections that are frequently seen in HIV-1-infected pregnant women that require therapy include sexually transmitted pathogens (*Chlamydia trachomatis* and *Neisseria gonorrhoea*, *Treponema pallidum*, and herpes simplex virus), mucocutaneous fungal infections, as well as tuberculosis (both skin conversions and active pulmonary disease).

STRATEGIES TO REDUCE PERINATAL TRANSMISSION

The risk of vertical transmission from mother-to-child has been difficult to determine, the reported transmission rates have varied widely in different geographic areas from 13% in Western Europe (European Collaborative Study 1991) to rates as high as 40% in Africa. (Hira et al 1987, Ryder et al 1989).

Limitations in the understanding of the pathogenesis of maternal–child transmission have hampered the development of trials to interrupt perinatal HIV-1 transmission. Trial design would be improved if the factors contributing to the timing and to the mechanism of maternal-child infection were better elucidated including:

- When during gestation infection occurs
- Whether infection occurs because of transplacental passage of virus or newborn or mucocutaneous exposure
- The nature of the protective maternal immunologic response
- The contribution of suspected maternal cofactors associated with transmission, including maternal viral burden, maternal immunological status and co-infections associated with placental inflammation.

The therapeutic strategies that have been proposed to prevent maternal–child transmission include antiretroviral therapy, passive immunotherapy, active immunotherapy, and combination therapy.

The first large-scale trial of an antiretroviral agent to prevent perinatal HIV-1 transmission is the National Institutes of Health (NIH)-funded AIDS Clinical Trial Group (ACTG) 076 study.

ACTG 076 is a phase III trial to evaluate the efficacy, safety and tolerance of oral zidovudine for the prevention of maternal–child transmission. Protocol 076 is a randomized, double-blind placebo-controlled trial. According to the protocol, maternal therapy is administered antepartum after the first trimester (after organogenesis), is continued intrapartum, and is also given to the newborn for 6 weeks post-delivery. The scientific rationale for this study is twofold: that zidovudine will reduce the maternal viral burden to which the fetus/newborn is exposed, and that zidovudine will provide to both the fetus and newborn post-exposure prophylaxis prior to and during viral exposure. The study began in May 1991 and is being closely monitored for both safety and efficacy; the first interim efficacy analysis should be available at the end of 1993.

A trial of passive immunotherapy is also being planned with a HIV hyperimmune gammaglobulin preparation (HIVIG). HIVIG is a preparation of highly purified human immunoglobulin containing high titres of antibody to HIV structural proteins with considerable functional activity in virus neutralization and antibody-dependent cytotoxicity assays. This product is prepared from the plasma of HIV-1-seropositive donors. Donors are clinically asymptomatic, with a CD4 + cell count equal to or above 400 cells/mm^3. The donor plasma contains high titres of antibodies to p24 antigen (an index of strong immune response to HIV); high virus neutralizing activity; high reactivity with MN strain V3 loop peptide; is negative for HIV p24 antigen; and is unable to infect phytohaemagluttinin-stimulated normal lymphocytes in the presence of interleukin-2. The preparation of HIVIG includes multiple steps to inactivate HIV.

Initial studies in chimpanzees have found that HIVIG protected against a low viral challenge but not against a higher dose challenge (Eichberg 1991). In the cynomolgus monkey model, hyperimmune serum to HIV-2 and simian immunodeficiency virus (SIV sm) obtained from vaccine-immunized monkeys was protective when administered 6 hours prior to a viral challenge (Putkonen et al 1991).

Another strategy that is also being explored to prevent perinatal transmission is active immunization of pregnant women and their newborns.

The proposed immunizing antigen is a recombinant glycoprotein from the HIV envelope (gp 120). Several lines of evidence suggest that gp 120 is the HIV-1 protein with the greatest potential as a vaccine against HIV-1:

- gp 120 is the major protein on the surface of the virus and mediates the attachment of HIV-1 to its cellular receptor, CD4
- Antibodies to gp 120 are known to neutralize HIV-1 infectivity in vitro
- Recent studies have shown that immunization with recombinant gp 120 can elicit an immune response able to protect chimpanzees from intravenous infection by a homologous isolate of HIV-1.

However, the amino acid sequence of the gp 120 region can vary as much as 40% from isolate to isolate. Thus, the identification of an immunogen that can elicit broadly neutralizing antibodies to different HIV-1 isolates is a major challenge in vaccine development.

Ongoing and future treatment trials to interrupt perinatal HIV-transmission will likely result in a better understanding of the clinical, virological and immunological factors influencing transmission.

REFERENCES

Abd A G, Nierman D M, Ilowite J S, Pierson R N, Bell A L 1988 Bilateral upper lobe Pneumocystis carinii pneumonia in a patient receiving inhaled pentamidine prophylaxis. Chest 94: 329–331

Berrebi A, Kobuch W E, Puel J et al 1990 Influence of pregnancy on human immunodeficiency virus disease. Eur J Obstet Gynecol Reprod Biol 37: 211–217

Biggar R J, Pahwa S, Minkoff H et al 1989 Immunosuppression in pregnant women infected with human immunodeficiency virus. Am J Obstet Gynecol 161: 1239–1244

Brabin B J 1985 Epidemiology of infection in pregnancy. Rev Infect Dis 7: 579–603

Brown A K, Cevik N 1965 Hemolysis and jaundice in the newborn following maternal treatment with sulfamethoxypyridozine. Pediatrics 36: 742–744

Burroughs–Wellcome 1992 Letter to investigators, June 1992. Burroughs–Wellcome Co., Triangle Park, North Carolina

Centers for Disease Control 1989 Guidelines for prophylaxis against Pneumocystis carinii pneumonia for persons infected with human immunodeficiency virus. MMWR 38 (S-5): 1–9

Centers for Disease Control 1990 Guidelines for preventing the transmission of tuberculosis in health care settings, with special focus on HIV-related issues. MMWR 39 (RR-17): 1–27

Chin J 1990 Current and future dimensions of the HIV/AIDS pandemic in women and children. Lancet 336: 221–224

Diagnostic and therapeutic technology assessment (DATTA) 1990 Prophylactic treatment for opportunistic infections in HIV-positive patients: aerosolized pentamidine. JAMA 263: 2510–2514

Eichberg J W 1991 Experience with seventeen HIV vaccine efficacy trials in chimpanzees. VII International Conference on AIDS, Florence, Italy, June 1991. Abstract FA2

Ellerbrock T V, Rogers M F 1990 Epidemiology of human immunodeficiency virus infection in women in the United States. Obstet Gynecol Clin N Am 17: 523–544

European Collaborative Study 1991 Children born to women with HIV-infection: natural history and risk of transmission. Lancet 337: 253–259

Fischl M A, Richman D D, Grieco M H et al 1987 The efficacy of azidothymidine (AZT) in the treatment of patients with AIDS and AIDS-related complex. A double-blind, placebo-controlled trial. N Engl J Med 317: 185–191

Fischl M A, Dickinson G M, La Voie L 1988 Safety and efficacy of sulfamethoxazole and trimethoprim chemoprophylaxis for Pneumocystis carinii pneumonia in AIDS. JAMA 259: 1185–1189

Gordin F M, Simon G L, Wofsy C B, Mills J 1984 Adverse reactions to trimethoprim/sulfamethoxazole in patients with AIDS. Ann Intern Med 100: 495–499

Hardy D W, Feinberg J, Finkelstein D M et al 1992 A controlled trial of trimethoprim-sulfamethoxazole or aerosolized pentamidine for secondary prophylaxis of Pneumocystis carinii pneumonia in patients with the acquired immunodeficiency syndrome. N Engl J Med 327: 1842–1848

Heinonen O P, Slone D, Shapiro S 1977 Birth defects and drugs in pregnancy. Publishing Sciences Group, Littleton, Massachusetts

Helm J, Kretzschmar R, Leuschner F, Neumann W 1976 Untersuchungen uber den Einfluss der Kombination Sulfamoxol Trimethoprim and Fertilitat und Embryonalentwicklung an Ratten und Kaninchen. Arzneimittel Fnorsch 26: 643–651

Hira S K, Kamanga J, Bhat G J et al 1987 Perinatal transmission of HIV-1 in Zambia. Br Med J 229: 1250–1253

Hirschel B, Lazzarin A, Chopard P et al 1991 A controlled study of inhaled pentamidine for primary prevention of Pneumocystis carinii pneumonia. N Engl J Med 324: 1079–1083

Jules-Elysee K M, Stover D E, Zaman M B, Bernard E M, White D A 1990 Aerosolized pentamidine: effect on diagnosis and presentation of Pneumocystis carinii pneumonia. Ann Intern Med 112: 750–757

Kahn J O, Lagakos S W, Richman D D et al 1992 A controlled trial comparing continued zidovudine with didanosine in human immunodeficiency virus infection. N Engl J Med 327: 581–587

Klug S, Lewandowski C, Merker H J et al 1991 In vitro and in vivo studies on the prenatal toxicity of the five virustatic nucleoside analogues in comparison to aciclovir. Arch-Toxicol 65(4): 283–291

Kobrinsky N L, Ramsay N K 1981 Acute megaloblastic anemia induced by high-dose trimethoprim-sulfamethoxazole. Ann Intern Med 94: 780–781

Koonin L M, Ellerbrock T V, Atrash H K et al 1989 Pregnancy-associated deaths due to AIDS in the United States. JAMA 261: 1306–1309

Kovacs J A, Hiemenz J M, Macher A M et al 1984 Pneumocystis carinii pneumonia: a comparison between patients with the acquired immunodeficiency syndrome and patients with other immunodeficiencies. Ann Intern Med 100: 663–671

Masur H, Ognibene F P, Yarchoan R et al 1989 CD4 counts as predictors of opportunistic pneumonias in human immunodeficiency virus infected individuals. Ann Intern Med 111: 223–231

Minkoff H, deRegt R H, Landsman S, Schwartz R 1986 PCP pneumonia associated with AIDS in pregnancy: a report of three maternal deaths. Obstet Gynecol 67: 284–287

Minkoff H L, Moreno J D, 1990 Drug prophylaxis for human-immunodeficiency virus-infected pregnant women: ethical considerations. Am J Obstet Gynecol 163: 1111–1114

NIAID 1990 Expert panel clears AZT neonate trials after reviewing data on carcinogenicity. AIDS Research Exchange, Summer: 1–3

NIAID/NIH State-of-the Art Conference 1990 AZT therapy for early HIV infection. Clin Courier 8: 1–8

Nicolaides K H, Soothill W, Clewell W H et al 1988 Fetal hemoglobin measurement in the assessment of red cell immunization. Lancet 1: 1073–1075

Palmisano P A, Palhill R B 1979 Fetal pharmacology. Pediatr Clin N Am 19: 3–20

Phair J, Muno A, Detels R et al 1990 The risk of Pneumocystis carinii pneumonia among men infected with human immunodeficiency virus type 1. N Engl J Med 322: 1607–1608

Pons J C, Boudon M C et al 1991 Fetoplacental passage of 2',3' dideoxyinosine (letter). Lancet 337: 732

Putkonen P, Thorstensson R, Ghayamizadeh L et al 1991 Prevention of HIV-2 and SIV(sm) infection by passive immunization in cynomolgus monkeys. Nature (London) 320: 1637–1642

Richman D D, Fischl M A, Grieco M H et al 1987 The toxicity of azidothymidine (AZT) in the treatment of patients with AIDS and AIDS-related complex: a double-blind, placebo-controlled trial. N Engl J Med 317: 192–197

Ruskin J, LaRiviere M 1991 Low-dose co-trimoxazole for prevention of Pneumocystis carinii pneumonia in human immunodeficiency virus disease. Lancet 337: 468–471

Ryder R W, Nsa W, Hassig S E et al 1989 Perinatal transmission of the human immunodeficiency virus type 1 to infants of seropositive women in Zaire. N Engl J Med 320: 1637–1642

Silverman W A, Anderson D H, Blanc W A, Crozier D N 1956 A difference in mortality rate and incidence of kernicterus among premature infants allotted to two prophylactic antibacterial regimens. Pediatrics 18: 614–625

Sperling R S, Stratton P, O'Sullivan M J et al 1992 A survey of zidovudine use in pregnant women with human immunodeficiency virus infection. N Engl J Med 326: 857–861

Sullivan L Public health service press release

Toltzis P, Marx C M, Kleinman N, Levine E M, Schmidt E V 1991 Zidovudine-associated embryonic toxicity in mice. J Infect Dis 163: 1212–1218

UPSC 1990 Dapsone. In: USP DI, Drug information for the health care professional, USPC, Rockville, MD, vol IA, p 1106–1108

Volberding P A, Lagakos S W, Koch M A et al 1990 Zidovudine in asymptomatic human immunodeficiency virus infection: a controlled trial in persons with fewer than 500 CD4-positive cells per cubic millimeter. N Engl J Med 322: 941–949

Watts D H, Brown Z A, Tartaglione T et al 1991
    Pharmacokinetic disposition of zidovudine during
    pregnancy. J Infect Dis 163: 226–232
Williams J D, Brumfitt W, Condie A P, Reeves D 1969 The
    treatment of bacteriuria in pregnant women with
    sulfamethoxazole and trimethoprim. Postgrad Med J 45
    (Suppl): 71–76
Yarchoan R, Mitsuya H, Myers C E, Broder S 1989 Clinical
    pharmacology of 3'azido-2'3'-dideoxythymidine

(zidovudine) and related deideoxynucleoside. N Engl J Med
    321: 726–728
Yarchoan R, Pluda J M, Thomas R V et al 1990 Long-term
    toxicity/activity profile of 2',3'-dideoxyinosine in AIDS or
    AIDS-related complex. Lancet 336: 526–529
Zinner S, Mayer K 1990 Sulfonamides and trimethoprim. In:
    Mandel G L, Douglas R G, Bennett J E (eds) Principles
    and practice of infectious diseases. Churchill Livingstone,
    New York, p 325–333

17. Clinical manifestations, management and therapy of HIV infection in children

Frederick Mambwe Kaoma and Gwendolyn B. Scott

INTRODUCTION

The human immunodeficiency virus (HIV) infection has been documented in children for over a decade (CDC 1982: Oleske et al 1983, Rubenstein et al 1983, Scott et al 1984). Reports from the World Health Organization estimate more than 10 million HIV-infected persons world-wide, and of these more than 500 000 represent women with AIDS-defining conditions. More than 750 000 are infants and children, the majority of whom are in Africa (Chin 1990). As the number of infected women has increased, consequently so has the problem of paediatric AIDS. Based on 1989 estimates, more than 6000 HIV-positive women will deliver in the USA within the next year (Gwinn et al 1991). With an estimated perinatal transmission rate of 30%, at least 2000 HIV-infected infants will be born annually in the USA alone. About 80% of the HIV infection in children seen in the USA and in Europe is a result of perinatal transmission of HIV from mother to infant (Oxtoby 1990). Europe, France, Italy and Spain currently have the highest numbers of perinatally HIV-infected children. Since the routine screening of blood products, transmission of HIV through blood transfusion is rare. However, recent outbreaks of AIDS in children in Russia and Romania related to transfusion of unscreened blood and use of poorly sterilized needles raise the concern that these modes of transmission of HIV may still be a risk for children in some areas of the world.

Epidemiologically, HIV in children has been a disease confined to large inner city neighbourhoods involving substance-abusing women or partners of HIV-infected men. The disease is now apt to be seen even in the suburbs and in middle income-group families, and continues to rise in all sectors of the population. The large metropolitan centres on the eastern coast of the continental USA including New Jersey, New York, Washington DC and Florida, represent 54% of the total number of paediatric AIDS cases seen in the USA. Recently there is a greater proportion of cases occurring in rural areas as seen in surveys among women delivering in smaller cities and rural areas and in the large migrant worker community (CDC 1992a, 1992b).

Paediatric HIV infection is a chronic multisystemic disease with a high morbidity and mortality. Significant progress has been made in the past decade in the diagnosis, treatment and management of the HIV-infected child. Ideally, the at-risk infant should be identified at birth so close medical follow-up with appropriate diagnostic tests and early initiation of prophylaxis and therapy can be instituted. To accomplish this, maternal knowledge of HIV status is essential. The paediatrician should co-ordinate the care for both at-risk infants and infected infants in consultation with a specialist in HIV care. HIV/AIDS was the first and second leading cause of death in Hispanic and black children 1–4 years of age in New York State in 1991 and the seventh leading cause of death in the state for all children. It is expected to become one of the ten leading causes of death in all ages of children by the end of 1992 in the USA (Novello et al 1989, Oxtoby 1990). The following sections review the management and treatment of infants at risk for perinatal HIV infection as well as for those children with diagnosed HIV infection.

MANAGEMENT OF THE INFANT BORN TO AN HIV-SEROPOSITIVE MOTHER

The management of the at-risk infant begins at birth. Between 13 and 39% of infants born to HIV-seropositive mothers will be infected with HIV. The goals of close medical follow-up are to establish a diagnosis of infection as soon as possible, to initiate appropriate therapies and to monitor for clinical signs of HIV disease and disease progression. The mother should be counselled about the risk of her infant having HIV infection, the anticipated visit schedule, the importance of maintaining good health and nutrition for her newborn, and a discussion of signs and symptoms that should prompt a medical visit. In countries where alternatives to breast milk are available and can be given safely, breast-feeding should be discouraged because of the slight incremental risk of HIV transmission to the infant via breast milk (Van de Perre et al 1991, de Martino et al 1992). In developing countries, WHO recommends that mothers with HIV infection breast-feed their infants, because the advantages of breast-feeding far outweight the slightly increased risk of HIV transmission in these settings.

At birth, infants born to HIV-infected mothers are HIV-seropositive as a result of passive transfer of maternal antibody across the placenta. Clinically they usually show no signs of HIV infection. Management includes routine well-child care including immunizations as well as immunological monitoring and tests specific for diagnosis of HIV infection. Table 17.1 outlines a schedule of visits and the recommended testing at each visit. Physi-cal examination includes vital signs, evaluation of each organ system, an assessment of nutritional status and developmental and neurological assessment. Baseline laboratory studies should include a complete blood count, tests of renal and hepatic function, quantitative immunoglobulins, and lymphocyte count with subset analysis. Monitoring of the CD4 count is critical for initiation of *Pneumocystis carinii* pneumonia (PCP) prophylaxis as well as antiretroviral therapy.

DIAGNOSIS

Early diagnosis of HIV infection is important so children can receive appropriate medical care, be assessed for antiretroviral therapy and prophylaxis and have access to clinical drug trials. In the neonate, maternal antibody is transferred across the placenta and may persist for up to 15–18 months of age. Thus, the routinely performed enzyme-linked immunosorbent assay (ELISA) antibody test for detection of IgG antibody and the Western blot are not reliable for diagnosis of infection in the child less than 18 months of age. Virus culture is the most reliable laboratory test for diagnosis of HIV infection in the young infant. P24 antigen testing, if positive, is diagnostic, but this test has a low sensitivity in the 1st year of life. The polymerase chain reaction detects viral HIV-DNA in cells and has a high sensitivity and specificity. Using these techniques, nearly 50% of all infected infants can be diagnosed within the first few days of life, 90% by 3 months of age and nearly 100% by 6 months of age (Report on the

Table 17.1 Follow-up schedule for children at risk for HIV infection

Age (months)	Physical examination	Complete blood count	Absolute CD4 + count	Quantitative immunoglobulins	ELISA/WB	P24Ag/PCR/Viral culture
1	+	+	+	+	+	+
2	+		+			+
4	+	+	+			
6	+	+	+	+		+
9	+	+	+			
12	+	+	+	+	+	
15	+	+	+		+	
18	+	+	+	+	+*	
21	+	+	+		+	
24	+	+	+	+	+	

* Child is considered not infected if two consecutive antibody tests are negative; ELISA, enzyme-linked immunosorbent assay; WB, Western blot; PCR, polymerase chain reaction

Consensus Workshop 1992). Thus, one or more of these diagnostic tests should be done as soon as possible after birth. If the tests are negative then they should be repeated at 3 and 6 months of age (see Table 17.1). If one of the virus-specific tests is positive, a presumptive diagnosis of HIV infection may be made, but a second blood specimen should be obtained for testing to confirm the first positive test. Other tests currently under investigation for early diagnosis of HIV infection in infants include the detection of HIV-specific IgA antibody and in vitro production of HIV antibody (Landesman et al 1991, Quinn et al 1991). Increase in the IgG and IgA classes of immunoglobulins is one of the earliest detectable immune abnormalities in HIV infection (Hutto et al 1991). Children with a persistent antibody response to HIV after 18 months of age are considered infected. Most uninfected children will have lost maternal antibodies by 10 months of age (European Collaborative Study 1991). The 'at risk' child is considered not infected if after 18 months of age there are no clinical signs of infection, no immunological abnormalities and the HIV antibody test has been negative on two consecutive determinations done at least 1 month apart.

CHILDHOOD IMMUNIZATIONS

Immunization against common childhood infectious diseases in HIV-infected children has to be considered in light of the possible vaccine reactions and the risk of disease. The safety profile of live vaccines in HIV-infected children versus the availability of inactivated preparations are other important considerations. HIV-infected children have a higher incidence of most vaccine-preventable diseases. Table 17.2 outlines the immunizations for children with HIV infection as recommended by The American Academy of Pediatrics (1988) and the World Health Organization (1987).

There are limited data on the use of live viral and bacterial vaccines in children with HIV. Measles vaccine is recommended for children with HIV infection because of the reports of severe measles in symptomatic children with HIV (CDC 1988a). The World Health Organization has recommended the use of oral polio vaccine in all children in developing countries. In the USA and Europe, inactivated polio vaccine is recommended in place of oral polio vaccine for immunocompromised hosts, including children with HIV infection. Inactivated polio vaccine is recommended also for normal children living in households with immunocompromised family members since the virus can be excreted and transmitted to others. Rarely, cases of polio vaccine-associated poliomyelitis related to the use of the oral vaccine have been reported. Diphtheria, tetanus toxoid, pertussis vaccine and measles, mumps, rubella (MMR) vaccinations are given to both symptomatic and asymptomatic children. Other vaccines recommended include the *Haemophilus influenza* conjugate vaccine, hepatitis B vaccine, pneumococcal vaccine, and influenza vaccine.

Asymptomatic HIV-infected children living in areas with a high prevalence of tuberculosis can receive BCG vaccine, since the possible com-

Table 17.2 Recommendations for immunization of HIV-infected infants and children (adapted from WHO 1987 and AAP 1991)

Type of vaccine	World Health Organization (WHO)		American Academy of Pediatrics (AAP)	
	Asymptomatic	Symptomatic	Asymptomatic	Symptomatic
Diptheria-pertussis-tetanus (DPT)	yes	yes	yes	yes
Oral polio	yes	yes	no	no
Inactivated polio	—	—	yes	yes
Measles-mumps-rubella (MMR)	yes	yes	yes	yes
Influenza	yes	no	Should be considered	yes
Bacillus Calmette-Guérin (BCG)*	yes	no	no	no
Pneumococcal	—	—	yes	yes
Haemophilus B conjugate	—	—	yes	yes
Hepatitis B vaccine	—	—	yes	yes

*WHO recommends use of BCG in areas of high tuberculosis prevalence

plications of the vaccination are less than the risk of acquiring active tuberculosis (CDC 1988b, WHO 1987). However, symptomatic HIV-infected children are not candidates for this vaccine. In the USA and many parts of Europe, BCG is not routinely used.

Since immunization may not produce protective antibody titres in all HIV-infected children, especially those with B cell dysfunction and impaired antibody formation, tetanus-prone wounds, and exposure to measles and varicella should receive passive prophylaxis using the appropriate immune globulin preparations.

DEFINITION AND CLASSIFICATION

Clinical studies conducted in various centres around the world have given us a better understanding of the natural history and evolution of HIV infection in infants and children. The Centers for Disease Control and Prevention (CDCP) has defined AIDS in infants and children as a disease with an underlying immunodeficiency that is not explained by other causes; laboratory evidence of HIV infection; and the presence of at least one of the following: opportunistic infection, lymphoid interstitial pneumonitis, recurrent invasive bacterial infection (two or more episodes in a 2-year period), encephalopathy, wasting syndrome, and/or malignancy (CDC 1987a). The CDCP classification of paediatric HIV infection outlined in Table 17.3 describes the spectrum of disease and was designed for epidemiological and surveillance purposes (CDC 1987b). This classification is currently being reviewed and redesigned to better reflect the clinical stages of infection. The WHO clinical case definition of AIDS in children is in use in most developing nations. It is based on both clinical and epidemiological information. Weight loss, failure to thrive, and chronic diarrhoea lasting for more than 1 month are major criteria, while generalized lymphadenopathy, persistent oral candidiasis, repeated common infections, persistent cough, generalized dermatitis and confirmed maternal HIV infection are minor criteria. A case of AIDS is defined as two major and two minor criteria in the absence of any other causes of immunosuppression including cancer, severe malnutrition or other aetiologies (WHO 1986).

Table 17.3 Centers for Disease Control (1987b) classification of HIV-1 infection in children under 13 years of age

I.   Class P-0: Indeterminate infection (perinatally exposed seropositive infants under 15 months with unknown infection status)
II. Class P-1: Asymptomatic infection (patients meeting one of the definitions for HIV infection but without symptoms, subclassification based upon immunological testing of serum immunoglobulins, T-cell subsets, and CBC)
   Subclass A: Normal immune function
   Subclass B: Abnormal immune function
   Subclass C: Immune function not tested
III. Class P-2: Symptomatic infection
   Subclass A: Non-specific findings (includes children with two or more of the following for > 2 months: fever, failure to thrive, hepatosplenomegaly, lymphadenopathy, parotitis, and diarrhoea)
   Subclass B: Progressive neurological disease
   Subclass C: Lymphoid interstitial pneumonitis
   Subclass D: Secondary infectious diseases
     Category D-1: Specified secondary infectious diseases listed in the Centers for Disease Control (CDC) surveillance definition for AIDS (PCP, systemic CMV, disseminated toxoplasmosis, etc.)
     Category D-2: Recurrent serious bacterial infections (sepsis, meningitis, pneumonia, visceral abscess, and bone/joint infections)
     Category D-3: Other specified secondary infectious diseases (persistent thrush > 2 months, disseminated zoster, or two or more episodes of herpetic stomatitis)
   Subclass E: Secondary cancers
     Category E-1: Specified secondary cancers listed in the CDC definition for AIDS (Kaposi's sarcoma, B-cell non-Hodgkin's lymphoma or primary lymphoma of the brain)
     Category E-2: Other cancers secondary to HIV-1
   Subclass F: Other diseases possibly due to HIV-1 infection (hepatitis, cardiomyopathy, nephropathy, haematological and dermatological diseases)

CBC, complete blood count; PCP, *Pneumocystis carinii* pneumonia; CMV, cytomegalovirus

CLINICAL MANIFESTATIONS

The majority of children infected with HIV perinatally develop HIV-associated symptoms within the 1st year of life (Krasinski et al 1989, Scott et al 1989). In most cases, early symptoms are non-specific, but some children will present with more severe AIDS-defining illnesses (see Table 17.4). Clinicians caring for children should be familiar with the common manifestations of paediatric HIV infection. HIV should be suspected in the child who is born to a mother with risk behaviours associated with acquisition of HIV infection. In addition, the presence of two or more non-specific signs (see Table 17.4), recurrent or severe infec-

Table 17.4 Clinical manifestations associated with HIV-1 infection in children

Non-specific findings
  failure to thrive
  generalized lymphadenopathy
  hepatomegaly
  splenomegaly
  chronic/recurrent diarrhoea
  parotitis
HIV-associated conditions
  progressive encephalopathy
  lymphoid interstitial pneumonitis
  cardiomyopathy
  thrombocytopenia
  nephropathy
  malignancy
  hepatitis

Infectious complications
Bacterial
  pyogenic
  Mycobacterium tuberculosis
  atypical mycobacterium
Viral
  herpes simplex
  herpes zoster
  measles
  cytomegalovirus
  Epstein-Barr virus
Protozoal
  Pneumocystis carinii
  Toxoplasma gondii
  cryptosporidiosis
  Isospora belli
Fungal
  Candida, mucocutaneous and invasive
  Cryptococcus

tions, or the presence of opportunistic infection or other AIDS-defining illnesses should alert the clinician to the possibility of HIV infection. Other causes of immunodeficiencies in infants and children including primary immunodeficiencies and congenital infections should be ruled out.

Non-specific findings

Early and common findings seen in most HIV-infected children include oral candidiasis, splenomegaly, hepatomegaly, lymphadenopathy, chronic and recurrent diarrhoea, parotitis and failure to thrive. Most infants with HIV infection frequently have two or more of the above findings. Generalized lymphadenopathy (lymph nodes > 1 cm in two or more non-contiguous sites) and hepatomegaly with or without splenomegaly are common findings early in infants with HIV infection.

INFECTIOUS COMPLICATIONS

Bacterial infections

Paediatric patients with HIV infection have an increased susceptibility to bacterial infections, particularly to those pathogens with polysaccharide capsules. This increased susceptibility is likely due to the child's lack of prior experience with these organisms and the immune dysfunction that accompanies HIV infection. Decreased antibody responses to specific antigens have been documented in certain children with HIV infection (Bernstein et al 1985, Pahwa et al 1986, Borkowsky et al 1987) Multiple and recurrent serious bacterial infections is an AIDS-defining condition in children but not in adults. In our population of over 500 infected children at the University of Miami/Jackson Memorial Hospital Medical Center in Miami, Florida, *Streptococcus pneumoniae* is the most common pathogen, but *Haemophilus influenza* type b, *Staphylococcus aureus* and *Salmonella* species are also reported. Pneumonia, urinary tract infection, otitis media, sinusitis, meningitis and bacteraemia are common manifestations.

Upper respiratory tract infections are common with otitis media occurring in a large number of young children with HIV infection. In our experience, some of these children may develop chronic infection with perforation of the tympanic membrane and drainage. Acute otitis media occurs commonly in children with progressively declining CD4+ lymphocyte counts. In one study of 28 HIV-infected children, 80% had experienced more than five episodes of otitis media by 3 years of age (Barnett et al 1992). Commonly isolated organisms from the middle ear in recurrent cases of otitis media are *S. epidermidis*, *S. pneumoniae*, Enterococcus, *E. coli*, *Pseudomonas aeruginosa*, and *Candida albicans* (Williams 1987, Krasinski et al 1988).

Mycobacterium tuberculosis

Since 1985 there has been an increase in HIV-related tuberculosis cases (Chaisson & Slutkin 1989, Reider et al 1989). Organisms with multiple drug resistance patterns have been reported in some urban areas (CDC 1991a). With the rise in numbers of cases of *Mycobacterium tuberculosis* and the number of resistant strains in the HIV-infected population there is need for careful monitoring of HIV-infected patients for this disease (Braun & Cauthen 1992, Jones et al 1992, Khouri et al 1992). Persons with HIV infection frequently live in the inner city where conditions are poor with overcrowding, homelessness, intravenous drug abuse and poverty, conditions which are also ideal for the spread of tuberculosis. Progressive primary pulmonary disease is the most common clinical manifestation in children with HIV infection, but extrapulmonary disease is also prevalent. In a series of nine children diagnosed with *Mycobacterium tuberculosis* at our institution, the median age at presentation of tuberculosis was 42 months with a median survival time of 20 months after diagnosis. The common presenting symptoms include prolonged fever, anorexia and cough. Only one of nine children under investigation had a positive tuberculin skin test (PPD) (Khouri et al 1992). Tuberculosis in HIV-infected children may be difficult to diagnose since other illnesses may mimic the signs and symptoms of tuberculosis. A good epidemiologic history is important to find if other family members have tuberculosis. Lack of response to broad spectrum antibiotics, persistence of respiratory symptoms, fever, and a radiographic picture of hilar or paratracheal lymphadenopathy with a consolidation suggest pulmonary infection with *Mycobacterium tuberculosis*. The diagnosis of tuberculosis is confirmed by a positive culture from the gastric washings (GW) or bronchoalveolar lavage (BAL). Bronchoalveolar lavage is a more sensitive diagnostic technique and also facilitates the detection of other respiratory pathogens. Isoniazid (INH), rifampin and pyrazinamide are used for initial treatment pending culture results, unless there is the possibility of a drug-resistant organism. In such a case, at least four drugs should be used. Therapy should continue for a minimum of 9 months or more depending on the site and type of infection. All children who present with a diagnosis of tuberculosis should be offered testing for HIV infection (CDC 1989).

Tuberculin-positive HIV-infected children who have no signs of active disease should receive prophylactic INH for at least 9 months. All household contacts and children should be screened for active disease and, if documented, this should be appropriately treated. Those without active disease should be put on prophylactic treatment with INH and re-evaluated in 3 months.

Mycobacterium avium intracellulare complex

Mycobacterium avium intracellulare complex (MAC) is a slow-growing mycobacterium that usually presents as a systemic illness and/or gastrointestinal disease in adults and children with advanced HIV infection. MAC infection has been reported in approximately 8% of paediatric AIDS patients (Horsburgh & Selik 1989). This infection usually occurs in severely immunocompromised children with absolute CD4 + lymphocyte counts of less than 100/mm^3. Clinical symptomatology includes weight loss, fever, abdominal pain and anaemia. This condition is associated with a high morbidity and mortality rate. Drug regimens using various combinations of ethambutol, rifampin, rifabutin, clofazimine, ciprofloxacin and amikacin help reduce symptoms. Clarithromycin is an antibiotic which has shown promise for treatment. Use of Rifabutin has been approved for the prevention of disseminated MAC in adult patients with advanced HIV infection. There is limited experience with this drug in children.

Parasitic infections

Parasitic infestations are a common cause of opportunistic infection seen in HIV infection in both children and adults. In the developed world, *Pneumocystis carinii* pneumonia is the most important infection in HIV-infected patients.

Pneumocystis carinii pneumonia

Pneumocystis carinii pneumonia (PCP) is the most frequent opportunistic infection in HIV-infected children and is associated with a high mortality rate. In contrast to adults with *Pneumocystis carinii* pneumonia, infants and children with perinatal HIV infection commonly present with PCP during the first few months of life, and PCP may be the initial presenting illness. The median age at diagnosis is 5–7 months (Scott et al 1989, Connor et al 1991). Clinically PCP presents as a progressive respiratory disease with tachypnea, low-grade fever, cough and dyspnea. PCP is characterized by a foamy alveolar exudate containing organisms on histopathological section. The diagnosis of the disease includes the demonstration of the organism in the lung parenchyma or bronchial secretions. Specimens can be obtained by bronchoalveolar lavage, deep endotracheal suction and by open lung biopsy, the most sensitive method available. The chest radiograph picture shows bilateral perihilar infiltrates which progress to involve the periphery. Lactate dehydrogenase levels are elevated. Blood gas analysis is useful in monitoring the progression and extent of disease.

The differential diagnosis of diffuse interstitial pneumonia includes miliary tuberculosis, lymphoid interstitial pneumonitis, cytomegalovirus infection and other viral infections. Aggressive treatment coupled with prophylaxis against PCP has reduced the morbidity and mortality associated with this opportunistic infection. The drug of choice for treatment is trimethoprim–sulphamethoxazole. Therapy should continue for 2–3 weeks. Pentamidine isethionate is an alternative drug for those patients who are unable to tolerate trimethoprim–sulphamethoxazole or who fail treatment. Another drug, Ataquivone (566C80), has recently been licensed in the USA for use in the treatment of acute PCP in adults. Supportive therapy includes oxygen and in some cases assisted ventilation may be required. Use of corticosteroids in adults with moderate to severe PCP has shown marked benefits in clinical outcomes (Gagnon et al 1990, Bozzette et al 1990). In a report of two children managed with antimicrobials and corticosteroids there was marked improvement in their clinical condition (Plebani et al 1989). PCP carries a poor prognosis, with a median survival after diagnosis of 2 months or less (Scott et al 1989, CDC, 1991b, Kovacs et al 1991, Connor et al 1991). The mortality rate of PCP if left untreated is almost 100%. Patients completing therapy for acute PCP should receive prophylaxis to prevent further episodes (see section on prophylaxis).

Toxoplasma gondii

Maternal screening for *Toxoplasma* antibodies will identify infants at risk for congenital infection with this organism. Congenital toxoplasmosis occurs mostly in infants born to mothers who have active parasitaemia during gestation (Remington et al 1990). Most of these infants are born with subclinical infection, and presenting features include chorioretinitis and central nervous system involvement. Mitchell and colleagues (1990) reported four young infants dually infected with HIV and *Toxoplasma gondii* transplacentally. Diffuse central nervous system toxoplasmosis was found at autopsy in three of the four infants. The authors suggest that in populations of women seropositive for *Toxoplasma*, chronic parasitaemia may be more common in women co-infected with HIV than in women seronegative for HIV. *Toxoplasma* infection is treated with pyrimethamine, sulfadiazine and folinic acid supplement. Detection of toxoplasmosis in the neonatal period mandates early initiation of therapy.

Viral infections

Viral infections are usually recurrent or chronic. The herpes family of viruses are the most commonly reported in paediatric AIDS. Infection with herpes simplex is seen as gingivostomatitis and perineal lesions. The course may be prolonged with more aggressive lesions. Management of herpes lesions includes intravenous, oral or topical acyclovir. Recurrence of lesions with scarring is common. Varicella Zoster presenting in a dermatomal distribution is seen in some children and may be chronic with hyperkeratotic changes.

Respiratory syncytial viruses and adenoviruses cause severe disease in immunocompromised children. Measles is a common childhood infection and may have an atypical presentation in HIV-infected children. It may present with the classical picture or may be more fulminant with severe pneumonia and absence of rash (CDC 1988a). The presence of multinucleated giant cells with nuclear inclusions in bronchoalveolar fluids suggests measles infection. Intramuscular or intravenous immunoglobulin given shortly after exposure to measles may modify the clinical course of disease (American Academy of Pediatrics 1988).

Cytomegalovirus (CMV) infection in children with HIV infection usually is disseminated and involves multiple organ systems. CMV retinitis, hepatitis, pneumonitis, oesophagitis and colitis have been reported. CMV encephalitis runs a progressive course. The isolation of CMV from body fluids and the presence of inclusion bodies is suggestive of CMV disease. Ganciclovir is the drug of choice in the management of CMV infection, but there is little experience with treatment in children. Foscarnet, a newer antiviral, has shown promising results in the treatment of CMV retinitis in adults.

Fungal infections

Fungal infections are seen at most stages of HIV infection. Oral thrush and monilial diaper rash are commonly encountered in the course of paediatric HIV infection. Oral thrush presents as creamy plaques or erythema of the mouth. It may become chronic and difficult to eradicate. Management of oral thrush includes the use of topical antifungal agents such as mycostatin or clotrimazole troches. In more severe cases, ketoconazole is administered. *Candida* oesophagitis is the second most common opportunistic infection in children, and typically presents with fever, difficulty in swallowing, vomiting and weight loss. Differential diagnosis should include cytomegalovirus and herpes simplex as other aetiologies of esophagitis. A presumptive diagnosis can be made by barium swallow. If there is no response to therapy, oesophagoscopy with biopsy and culture should be performed. *Candida* oesophagitis is treated with ketoconazole orally for 14 days. Fluconazole has been used successfully in a few patients. Predisposing factors for fungal infections include low CD4 + lymphocyte counts and repeated antibiotic treatment. Disseminated candidiasis is rare but can occur in advanced HIV infection and is often associated with nosocomial acquisition. Studies show an association between persistent granulocytopenia (< 100 cells/mm^3), low absolute numbers and percentages of T helper lymphocytes and incidence of disseminated candidiasis (Pizzo et al 1982 Leibovitz et al 1991). Intravenous amphotericin B is the drug of choice in disseminated candidiasis.

HIV-ASSOCIATED CONDITIONS

Central nervous system

There is a broad spectrum of central nervous system abnormalities associated with HIV infection ranging from mild developmental delay to a progressive encephalopathy. Several studies have estimated that 50–90% of all HIV-infected children present with some CNS abnormality (Epstein et al 1986, Belman et al 1988). HIV encephalopathy results from direct infection of the central nervous system with the virus (Resnick et al 1985). HIV-associated encephalopathy presents with mental and motor delay, development of pyramidal tract signs and loss of developmental milestones. Early signs include weakness of the lower limbs, progressing to the upper limbs and trunk. Clinical signs including microcephaly, ataxia and seizures may be observed. The course of disease may be static or progressive. The diagnosis of CNS involvement entails a complete history and physical examination including a neurological examination. A thorough evaluation of developmental milestones using age-appropriate neuro-developmental tests should be done. Computerized tomography of the brain may show cerebral atrophy or basal ganglia calcifications. It may be helpful to do a baseline CT scan of the brain shortly after the diagnosis of HIV is made for comparison if central nervous system abnormalities occur later. Comparison of serial head circumferences may show an acquired microcephaly. Cerebrospinal fluid findings include mild pleocytosis and elevated protein. Based on the frequency of central nervous system abnormalities and developmental delay, all at risk and infected children should have developmental testing as part of routine care. Early intervention may alter the course of disease. Zidovudine therapy has stabilized and improved neurological symptoms.

Lung

Lymphoid interstitial pneumonia is the most common HIV-associated pulmonary condition seen in children. The etiology of this disease is uncertain but both HIV and Epstein-Barr virus have been serologically and virologically linked to lymphoid interstitial pneumonitis as possible causative agents (Katz et al 1992). Usually insidious in onset, cough is the earliest symptom. Other associated symptoms include clubbing, generalized lymphadenopathy with hepatosplenomegaly and hypergammaglobulinaemia. The chest radiograph shows bilateral interstitial reticulonodular infiltrates, with or without hilar adenopathy, which are persistent for at least a 2-month period. The histological picture shows mononuclear interstitial infiltrates composed of immunoblasts, plasma cells and CD8+ lymphocytes. The diagnosis is usually made on the basis of radiographic findings. Confirmatory diagnosis is made by lung biopsy. Other pathogens which can cause bilateral interstitial infiltrates should be ruled out. The course may be stable or progressive leading to chronic lung disease. Bronchodilators chest physiotherapy and oxygen therapy are part of the treatment of more severe disease. Management includes oxygen and steroid therapy in patients with oxygen tension less than or equal to 65 mmHg. Prednisone is given in a dose of 2 mg/kg per day for 2 weeks and then tapered incrementally to 0.5 mg/kg per day as oxygenation improves. Steroids can be discontinued after improvement in oxygenation occurs. This condition has a better prognosis than most other AIDS-defining illnesses in children, with a median survival after diagnosis of 72 months (Scott et al 1989, Tovo et al 1992)

Cardiac findings

Structural and functional abnormalities of the heart have been described in HIV infection. A progressive left ventricular dilatation with compensating hypertrophy is a common cardiac finding in HIV-infected children (Lipshultz et al 1992). Focal myocarditis and pericarditis are commonly seen at autopsy. The cardiac manifestations in HIV-infected children have been attributed to the direct effect of the virus based on a case report that identified HIV DNA and RNA in the cardiac tissue (Lipshultz et al 1990). Others have implicated other infections and possible cardiotoxic effects of such drugs as pentamidine, ganciclovir and interferon-α-2a (Deyton et al 1989, Cohen et al 1990, Stein et al 1991). A recent study by Lipshultz and associates (1992) suggests that there

is no correlation between zidovudine therapy and cardiac dysfunction.

Nephropathy

HIV-associated nephropathy, with proteinuria and moderate decrease in renal function has been described in more than 30% of children with perinatally acquired HIV infection (Connor et al 1988, Strauss et al 1991). HIV nephropathy may sometimes be the first manifestation of HIV infection. The histopathological presentation in most HIV-infected children includes mesangial hypercellularity, focal segmental glomerulosclerosis (FSS), and minimal change glomerulonephritis (Ingulli et al 1991, Strauss et al 1989). Most HIV-infected children present with proteinuria, pyuria, haematuria and urinary tract infections. Some cases progress to nephrosis with oedema and renal failure. Therapy with prednisone has not usually been helpful in reversing the course of FSS. In a recent study remission of proteinuria was achieved in three patients treated with cyclosporin (Ingulli et al 1991). In the same study the authors found a higher predisposition (8/47) to developing HIV-associated nephropathy in patients who had received intravenous immunoglobulin therapy than those who did not (7/117). The pathophysiology of HIV-associated nephropathy is not well understood. Considering the numerous drugs used in the management of HIV infection, drug-induced nephropathy must be considered. However, some children have presented with nephrosis as their initial HIV-associated illness and have not had prior exposure to multiple drugs.

NEOPLASMS

Malignancy is reported in less than 2% of all cases of paediatric AIDS. With prolonged survival of infected children neoplastic transformation may be more frequently seen in the future. In contrast to adults, Kaposi's sarcoma is infrequently reported in paediatric AIDS cases. A disseminated lymphadenopathic form of Kaposi's sarcoma involving mostly lymph nodes, the liver, thymus, mesentery and gastrointestinal tract and rarely with skin manifestations is seen in children with HIV infection (Buck et al 1983). Other neoplasms reported include Hodgkin's disease, non-Hodgkin's lymphoma, pulmonary leiomyosarcoma and Burkitt's lymphoma/B-cell leukaemia. Primary CNS lymphoma has been reported as a cause of intracranial mass lesions in HIV-infected children (Horowitz & Pizzo 1990).

TREATMENT

Treatment considerations for the child with HIV infection need to be individualized and the choice of specific therapies is determined by the clinical status and the degree of immunocompromise. In the early years of the epidemic, treatment was largely supportive. Close medical follow-up, nutritional support and aggressive diagnosis and treatment of infection were the major modalities of treatment and continue to be important adjuncts in the care of these children. As more has been learned about the spectrum of disease and the natural history of HIV infection in children, there has been a greater focus on prophylaxis against specific infections and treatment with antiretroviral drugs and immunomodulators. The licensing of zidovudine and didanosine and the availability of other drugs through multicentre clinical drug trials has significantly changed the treatment of the child with HIV infection.

Prophylaxis

Pneumocystis carinii pneumonia (PCP) is the most common serious opportunistic infection reported in children with AIDS. In children with perinatally acquired infection, it may be the presenting illness with or without other signs or symptoms of HIV infection. In perinatal HIV infection, PCP is commonly diagnosed between 3 and 7 months of age and is the most common AIDS-defining illness in those children who progress to AIDS during the 1st year of life (Scott et al 1989, CDC 1991b, Connor et al 1991). The mortality from PCP is high and the median survival in reported studies is 2 months or less (Scott et al 1989, Connor et al 1991, CDC 1991b, Kovacs et al 1991). Because of the high prevalence and mortality associated with PCP in HIV-infected infants and children, it is important to identify all infants who are at risk for PCP early, so prophylaxis can be initiated.

Table 17.5 Age-adjusted levels of CD4 + lymphocyte counts for initiation of *Pneumocystis carinii* prophylaxis (PCP) in children at risk[*] and infected, and initiation of antiretroviral therapy for HIV-infected children

| Age | CD4 + lymphocyte count (cells/mm^3) | |
	Pneumocystis carinii prophylaxis	Antiretroviral
6–11 months	1500	1750
12–23 months	750	1000
24 months–5 years	500	750
6 years–older	200	500

[*] Any child with a history of PCP, and children with a CD4 + percentage less than 20% should be started on PCP prophylaxis

Guidelines for initiation of PCP prophylaxis in children at risk for or known to be infected with HIV were published by the US Public Health Service based on the recommendations of a panel of experts in paediatric HIV care. The recommendations were based on the available data correlating CD4 + lymphocyte counts and the development of PCP in HIV-infected children and the recently published information on normal lymphocyte age-adjusted values in uninfected infants and children. Prophylaxis is recommended for the 'at-risk' or infected infant greater than 1 month

Table 17.6 Recommended drug regimens for *Pneumocystic carinii* pneumonia prophylaxis (from CDC 1991b)

Recommended regimen (children > 1 month of age):
Trimethoprim–sulphamethoxazole (TMP–SMX)150 mg TPM/m^2 per day with 750 mg SMX/m^2 per day given orally in divided doses twice a day (b.i.d) three times per week on consecutive days (e.g. Monday–Tuesday–Wednesday)

Acceptable alternative TMP–SMX dosage schedules:
1. a 150 mg TMP/m^2 per day with 750 mg SMX/m^2 per day given orally as a single daily dose three times per week on consecutive days (e.g. M–T–W)
2. b 150 mg TMP/m^2 per day with 750 mg SMX/m^2 per day orally divided b.i.d and given 7 days per week
3. c 150 mg TMP/m^2 per day with 750 mg SMX/m^2 per day given orally divided b.i.d and given three times per week on alternate days (e.g. M–W–F)

Total daily dose should not exceed 320 mg TMP and 1600 mg SMX

Alternative regimens, if TMP–SMX is not tolerated
1. Aerolized pentamidine > 5 years of age, 300 mg given via Respirgard II jet nebulizer monthly

2. Intravenous pentamidine, 4 mg/kg given every 2 or 4 weeks

3. Dapsone (> 1 month of age), 1 mg/kg given orally once daily (do not exceed 100 mg)

of age utilizing the age-adjusted absolute CD4+ lymphocyte counts outlined in Table 17.5. In addition, any child with a CD4+ percentage of 20% or less and children with a history of prior PCP should receive PCP prophylaxis. The recommended antibiotic regimens and alternative regimens for PCP prophylaxis are outlined in Table 17.6. Trimethaprim–sulphamethoxazole is the drug of choice. There are no studies evaluating PCP prophylaxis in HIV-infected children, but it is known that prophylaxis effectively prevents PCP in other immunocompromised populations, i.e. children with cancer. As in any patient where multiple drug therapy is instituted, drug interactions must be considered. Pentamidine and didanosine should not be administered concomitantly since they both predispose to pancreatitis.

Antiretroviral agents

Over the past few years, several antiviral agents with activity against HIV-1 have been developed and tested in clinical trials in both adults and children. At present, two agents, zidovudine and didanosine, are licensed for use in children under 13 years of age in the United States. Another drug, zalcitabine (dideoxycytidine, ddC) is licensed for use as combination therapy with zidovudine in adolescents and adults.

There is a general consensus that early antiretroviral treatment will be beneficial and prevent progression of HIV disease. All children treated with antiretroviral therapy should have a definitive diagnosis of HIV infection. Clinical trials of treatment in asymptomatic children are just beginning and because of the development of resistance to antiretroviral drugs and the limited drugs available, widespread treatment of the asymptomatic child with a normal age-adjusted CD4 lymphocyte count is not generally recommended. The treatment of the HIV-infected child may be complex, particularly if the child has advanced disease, and it is recommended that the child's physician consult with a specialist in HIV paediatric care in decisions regarding initiation of treatment, prophylaxis and changing therapies. Recently a panel of experts was convened by the National Pediatric HIV Resource Center to make recommendations regarding guidelines for use of antiretroviral therapy and the

medical management of the HIV-infected child. Recommendations were made regarding the use of CD4+ lymphocyte counts in therapeutic decisions for use of antiretroviral agents. In general, the age-adjusted CD4+ lymphocyte counts recommended for commencing antiretroviral therapy in the otherwise asymptomatic or mildly symptomatic child are generally 250 cells greater than the threshold for PCP prophylaxis (see Table 17.5). The percentage of CD4+ cells is an additional indicator for initiation of antiretroviral therapy in an otherwise asymptomatic or mildly symptomatic child. Antiretroviral therapy should be instituted at a CD4 percentage of 30% in the first 12 months of life, 25% between ages 12 and 24 months of age and 20% in children older than 2 years of age.

Zidovudine (ZDV) was the first antiviral licensed by the Food and Drug Administration for use in children. Phase I and II studies of ZDV have demonstrated clinical benefit and good tolerance of the drug. Clinically, children have shown weight gain and subjective improvement in activity, with decrease in the size of the liver and spleen. In addition, improvement in developmental milestones and intellectual capacity has been demonstrated (Pizzo et al 1988, McKinney et al 1990, Pizzo & Wilfert 1990). Laboratory parameters have shown normalization of immunoglobulin levels, an increase in CD4+ lymphocyte counts and a decrease in p24 antigen levels.

The dosage for ZDV is 180 mg/m^2 per dose given every 6 h for infants and children over 1 month of age. This dose is higher than that usually administered to adults. There are ongoing clinical trials comparing the standard dose of ZDV to a lower dose, 90 mg/m^2 per dose. At the present time the higher dose is maintained because of its proven beneficial effect on central nervous system infection with HIV. The drug is indicated for use in children with symptomatic HIV infection. Table 17.5 gives age-specific CD4+ lymphocyte counts at which therapy should be begun in asymptomatic or mildly symptomatic children infected with HIV. Bone marrow toxicity with resultant anaemia and neutropenia is reported in both adults and children. The anaemia usually responds to dose reduction, or transfusions may be administered to maintain the haemoglobin level. The bone marrow toxicities are more frequent with higher doses of drug. Complete blood counts should be done monthly and liver function tests should be done every 3 months while a child is on therapy.

Dideoxyinosine (ddI), another nucleoside analogue with activity against the reverse transcriptase of HIV-1 was recently approved for use in HIV-infected children aged 6 months and older who have developed resistance to or are intolerant to ZDV. Clinical trials in symptomatic children show that ddI is well tolerated and its beneficial effects include weight gain; a decrease in size of lymph nodes, liver and spleen; a decline in p24 serum antigen levels and an increase in CD4+ lymphocyte counts (Butler et al 1991). The dose of didanosine is 200 mg/m^2 per day given orally in divided doses every 12 h. For children over 1 year of age, it is important to give a two-tablet dosage to provide adequate buffering for optimal absorption of the medication. The adverse effects include pancreatitis in approximately 5% of the children treated at doses of >270 mg/m^2 per day, and depigmentation at the periphery of the retina which is not associated with visual impairment has been reported in a few children. Peripheral neuropathy has not been reported in children at the recommended dosing levels. A complete blood count, amylase level and lipase should be monitored monthly. Didanosine should not be administered with pentamidine since both drugs predispose to pancreatitis.

Zalcitabine (Dideoxycytidine (ddC)) is also a nucleoside analogue that is active against HIV-1. It is presently approved for use as combination therapy with ZDV in adolescents and adults with HIV infection. There is currently insufficient information to recommend this drug for use in children. Trials of ddC in younger children are limited, but one study showed that it was safe in low doses on an alternating regimen with ZDV (Pizzo et al 1990). A clinical trial using zalcitabine monotherapy in children who have progressive disease while on ZDV or who become intolerant to ZDV has been recently closed to accrual and results are not yet available. Clinical trials using combination therapy with zalcitabine and ZDV in children are presently underway.

Combination therapy has been shown to be effective in adults and is also likely to be effective in children. Several clinical trials of combination therapy are presently underway. These include monotherapy with ZDV or didanosine, compared with combinations of ZDV plus Didanosine and ZDV plus zalcitabine. It is hoped that combination therapy will limit the emergence of drug resistant strains of virus.

In the United States there are several centres for AIDS Clinical Drug Trials in paediatric patients. These trials are critical to evaluation of new therapies and children and pregnant women should have access to such programmes as feasible.

INTRAVENOUS GAMMAGLOBULIN THERAPY (IVIG)

Early uncontrolled studies using IVIG in HIV-infected children showed a decrease in the occurrence of serious bacterial infections (Calvelli & Rubenstein 1986, Siegel & Oleske 1986). More recently a multicentre, double blind placebo, controlled clinical trial of intravenous immunoglobulin compared to intravenous albumen (placebo) was conducted. In children receiving IVIG the time to development of serious infections was prolonged in those with a base line CD4+ cell count of >200/mm^3 (NICHD 1991). Survival rates however were not affected by use of IVIG. The greatest effect of IVIG was seen in prevention of *S. pneumonia* infection and clinically diagnosed pneumonia. There are no published guidelines for use of IVIG but at our institution the following conditions warrant IVIG therapy: hypogammaglobulinaemia; two or more episodes of serious bacterial infection; two episodes of presumptive or proven bacterial pneumonia; significant impairment of B cell function with decreased or absent antibody formation following immunization. The usual dose of IVIG is 400 mg/kg per dose given every 4 weeks.

PROGNOSIS AND OUTCOME

Improvements in management and therapy have improved survival of HIV-infected infants and children. In our population of 275 children living with HIV infection followed at the University of Miami/Jackson Memorial Hospital Medical Center, 50% are 4 years of age or older and the perinatally acquired cases range from 1 month to 13 years of age. Natural history studies have provided important information on the clinical and laboratory parameters correlated with survival. Clinical predictors of survival in children include age at onset of disease and the type of clinical manifestation. With the exception of lymphoid interstitial pneumonia, most other AIDS-defining illnesses are associated with poor survival. Such conditions include the development of an opportunistic infection, particularly *Pneumocystis carinii* pneumonia, and progressive encephalopathy (Krasinski et al 1989, Scott et al 1989, Blanche et al 1990, Tovo et al 1992).

An early age at clinical diagnosis of HIV is related to poor prognosis in infants and young children with HIV infection. In a cohort of 172 HIV-infected children, more than 80% developed clinical disease within the first 2 years of life with the majority presenting within the 1st year and median survival from time of diagnosis was 38 months (Scott et al 1989). The recent Italian study by Tovo and colleagues (1992) found a higher median survival (96.2 months). The higher figure was attributed to the fact that the earlier studies had considered only children with overt clinical signs of HIV infection.

Two patterns of clinical presentation have been described in HIV-infected children (Blanche et al 1990). The first pattern is an early presentation, with development of severe disease within the 1st year of life and associated with a poor prognosis. PCP, progressive encephalopathy and failure to thrive are common findings. The second pattern presents with a slower progression of disease usually associated with a lymphoproliferative process, with lymphoid interstitial pneumonia, lymphadenopathy, hepatosplenomegaly and parotitis. It is not clear why some infected children are relatively free of symptoms for long time-periods (5–10 years) even though the infection was acquired in utero or at birth.

Several laboratory parameters have been correlated with a poor survival. These include a low CD4 + lymphocyte count compared to age-related standards, the absence of lymphocyte proliferative responses to antigens and mitogens, increases in the level of p24 antigen and the loss of antibody to HIV-specific proteins (Blanche et al 1986, Epstein et al 1986, Borkowsky et al 1989, de Martino et al 1991, Geffin et al 1992).

PSYCHOSOCIAL ASPECTS/SUPPORTIVE CARE

The psychosocial impact of HIV infection on both the patient and the family is devastating and frequently disruptive to the normal family life. Despite the length of time that the disease has been recognized, most families find the diagnosis difficult to cope with and they fear discrimination and rejection by society. The mother may experience guilt and anger associated with the knowledge that she may transmit HIV to her newborn. Counselling about the disease process is essential for the entire family. Frequently, there is more than one infected member of the family. Other family members, especially the mother's sexual partner and her other children should be tested for HIV infection. Thus, the whole family needs medical and psychosocial intervention.

Supportive care is an important component of the management of the HIV-infected child and this can be co-ordinated by the child's physician. Since HIV infection is a chronic illness with multisystem involvement, a multidisciplinary care team is frequently necessary. The medical team should be made up of both paramedical and social–health care workers – i.e. nurses, counsellors, social workers, case managers, nutritionists, physical therapists, play therapists, respiratory therapists and speech therapists.

A designated case manager who is well versed in the language and cultural norms of the family should act as an advocate for the HIV-infected family. They should make periodic visits to the home and evaluate the family's immediate needs and assure compliance with medical visits. Monthly visits in addition to weekly phone communications should be encouraged. Confidentiality is essential based on the existing laws in a particular jurisdiction.

The issue of foster care or respite care frequently arises because of illness in the mother or loss of the parent(s) related to AIDS. Planning for care of children should be encouraged and frequently other family members will be willing to assume the care of a child in the event of a parent's death. Legal guardianship should be obtained for the child if possible. Potential foster parents should be counselled as to the medical needs and prognosis of the child, as well as the legal aspects of caring for an HIV-infected child.

Children with HIV infection should be encouraged to participate in day-to-day childhood activities as much as they are able. It is important that the child be treated as normally as possible. HIV infection should not be a deterrent to attending school unless the child is too ill to participate in normal school activities. There is no obligation for the school to be informed of the child's diagnosis, although there may be some benefits to selected people within the school knowing the diagnosis.

THE FUTURE

Significant advances have been made in the diagnosis and treatment of HIV infection in infants and children. The natural history of children continues to evolve, particularly with the increased use of PCP prophylaxis and the availability of antiretroviral therapy. Our challenge for the future is to prevent perinatal transmission, to develop new and better therapies for opportunistic infections and HIV-associated complications, and to improve outcome and prognosis.

REFERENCES

American Academy of Pediatrics 1988 Measles. In: Peters G (ed) The report of the committee on infectious diseases (Red Book), 21st edn. Elk Grove Village, IL, p 277–289

American Academy of Pediatrics 1991 AIDS and infections. In: Peter G, Lepow M L, McCracken G H, Phillips C F (eds) Report of the committee on infectious diseases. Elk Grove Village, Illinois, p 115–130

Barnett E D, Klein J O, Pelton S I, Luginbuhl L M 1992 Otitis media in children born to human immunodeficiency virus-infected mothers. Pediatr Infect Dis J 11: 360–364

Belman A L, Diamond G, Dickson D et al 1988 Pediatric acquired immunodeficiency syndrome. Neurologic syndromes. Am J Dis Child 142: 29–35

Bernstein L J, Ochs H D, Wedgewood R J et al 1985 Defective humoral immunity in pediatric acquired immunodeficiency syndrome. J Pediatr 107: 352

Blanche S, LeDeist F, Fisher A et al 1986 Longitudinal study of 18 children with perinatal LA V/HTL V III infection: attempt at prognostic evaluation. J Pediatr 109: 965–970

Blanche S, Tardieu M, Duliege A et al 1990 Longitudinal study of 94 symptomatic infants with perinatally acquired immunodeficiency virus infection. Evidence for a bimodal

expression of clinical and biological symptoms. Am J Dis Child 144: 1210–1215

Borkowsky W, Steele C J, Grubman S et al 1987 Antibody responses to bacterial toxoids in children infected with human immunodeficiency virus. J Pediatr 110: 563

Borkowsky W, Krasinski K, Paul D et al 1989 Human immunodeficiency virus type-1 antigenemia in children. J Pediatr 114: 940–945

Bozzette S A, Sattler F R, Chin J et al 1990 A controlled trial of early adjunctive treatment with corticosteroids for Pneumocystis carinii pneumonia in the acquired immunodeficiency syndrome. N Eng J Med 323: 1444–1450

Braun M M, Cauthen G 1992 Relationship of the human immunodeficiency virus epidemic to pediatric tuberculosis and Bacillus Calmette-Guerin immunization. Pediatr Infect Dis J 11: 220–227

Buck B E, Scott G B, Valdez-Dapena M et al 1983 Kaposi's sarcoma in two infants with acquired immunodeficiency syndrome. J Pediatr 103: 911–913

Butler K M, Husson R N, Balis F M et al 1991 Dideoxyinosine in children with symptomatic human immunodeficiency virus infection. N Eng J Med 324: 137–144

Calvelli T, Rubenstein A 1986 Intravenous gamma-globulin in infant acquired immunodeficiency syndrome. Pediatr Infect Dis J 5: S207–210

Centers for Disease Control 1982 Unexplained immunodeficiency and opportunistic infection in infants – New York, New Jersey, California. MMWR 31: 665–667

Centers for Disease Control 1987a Revision of the CDC surveillance definition for acquired immunodeficiency syndrome. MMWR 36 (suppl 1): 1–15S

Centers for Disease Control 1987b Classification system for human immunodeficiency virus (HIV) infection in children under 13 years of age. MMWR 36: 225–236

Centers for Disease Control 1988a Measles in HIV-infected children, United States. MMWR 37: 183–188

Centers for Disease Control 1988b Use of BCG vaccine in the control of tuberculosis: a joint statement by the ACIP and the advisory committee for the elimination of tuberculosis. MMWR 37: 663–675

Centers for Disease Control 1989 Tuberculosis and human immunodeficiency virus infection: recommendation of the advisory committee for the elimination of tuberculosis (ACET). MMWR 38: 236–238, 243–250

Centers for Disease Control 1991a Nosocomial transmission of multidrug-resistant tuberculosis among HIV-infected persons – Florida and New York, 1988–1991. MMWR 40: 585–591

Centers for Disease Control 1991b Guidelines for prophylaxis against Pneumocystis carinii pneumonia for children infected with human immunodeficiency virus. MMWR 40: 1–13

Centers for Disease Control 1992a HIV infection and AIDS – Georgia, 1991. MMWR 41: 876–878

Centers for Disease Control 1992b HIV infection, syphilis, and tuberculosis screening among migrant farm workers – Florida, 1992. MMWR 41: 723–725

Chaisson R E, Slutkin G 1989 Tuberculosis and human immunodeficiency virus infection. J Infect Dis 159: 96–100

Chin J 1990 Epidemiology. Current and future dimensions of the HIV/AIDS pandemic in women and children. Lancet 336: 221–224

Cohen A J, Weiser B, Afzal Q, Fuhrer J 1990 Ventricular tachycardia in two patients with AIDS receiving ganciclovir (DHPG). Aids 4: 807–809

Connor E, Gupta S, Joshi V et al 1988 Acquired immunodeficiency syndrome-associated renal disease in children. J Pediatr 39: 39–44

Connor E, Bagarazzi M, McSherry G et al 1991 Clinical and laboratory, correlates of Pneumocystis carinii pneumonia in children infected with HIV. JAMA 265: 1693–1708

De Martino M, Tovo P, Galli L, Gabiano C et al 1991 Prognostic significance of immunologic changes in 675 infants perinatally exposed to human immunodeficiency virus. J Pediatr 119: 702–709

De Martino M, Tovo P, Tozzi A E et al 1992 HIV-1 transmission through breast-milk: appraisal of risk according to duration of feeding. AIDS 6: 991–997

Deyton L R, Walker R E, Kovacs J A et al 1989 Reversible cardiac dysfunction associated with interferon alpha therapy in AIDS patients with Kaposi's sarcoma. N Eng J Med 321: 1246–1249

Epstein L G, Sharer L R, Oleske J M et al 1986 Neurologic manifestations of human immune deficiency virus infection in children. Pediatrics 78: 678–687

European Collaborative Study 1991 Children born to women with HIV-1 infection: natural history and risk of transmission. Lancet 337: 253–260

Gagnon S, Boota A M, Fischl M A, Baaier H, Kirksey O W, La Voie L 1990 Corticosteroids as adjunctive therapy for severe Pneumocystis carinii pneumonia in the acquired immunodeficiency syndrome: a double-blind, placebo-controlled trial. N Engl J Med 323: 1444–1450

Geffin R, Hutto C, Lai S et al 1992 Correlation of HIV-1 antibody reactivity and survival in perinatally infected children (abstract). Presented at The New York Academy of Sciences Conference. Pediatric AIDS: Clinical, Pathologic and Basic Science Perspectives, Nov 18–21, Abstr PI-5

Gwinn M, Pappaioanou M, George J R et al 1991 Prevalence of HIV infection in childbearing women in the United States: surveillance using newborn blood samples. JAMA 265: 1704–1708

Horowitz M E, Pizzo P A 1990 Cancer in the child infected with the human immunodeficiency syndrome (editorial). J Pediatr 116: 730–731

Horsburgh C R, Selik R M 1989 The epidemiology of disseminated non tuberculous mycobacterium infection in the acquired immunodeficiency syndrome (AIDS). Am Rev Resp Dis 139: 4–7

Hutto C, Parks W P, Shenghan L et al 1991 A hospital based survey of perinatal infection with human immunodeficiency virus type 1. J Pediatr 118: 347–353

Ingulli E, Tejani A, Fikrig S et al 1991 Nephrotic syndrome associated with acquired immunodeficiency syndrome in children. J Pediatr 119: 710–716

Jones D S, Malecki J M, Bigler W J, Witte J J, Oxtoby M J, 1992 Pediatric tuberculosis and human immunodeficiency virus infection in Palm Beach County, Florida. AmJ Dis Child 146: 1166–1170

Katz B Z, Beckman A M, Shapiro E D 1992 Serologic evidence of active Epstein Barr virus infection in Epstein Barr virus associated lymphoproliferative disorders of children with acquired immunodeficiency syndrome. J Pediatr 120: 228–232

Khouri Y F, Mastrucci M T, Hutto C, Mitchell C D, Scott G B 1992 Mycobacterium tuberculosis in children with human immunodeficiency virus type 1 infection. Pediatr Infect Dis J 11: 950–955

Kovacs A, Frederick T, Church J et al 1991 CD4 T-lymphocyte counts and Pneumocystis carinii pneumonia in pediatric HIV infection. JAMA 265: 1698–1702

Krasinski K, Borkowsky W, Bonk S et al 1988 Bacterial infection in human immunodeficiency virus-infected children. Pediatr Infect Dis J 7: 323–328

Krasinski K, Borkowsky W, Holzman R S 1989 Prognosis of human immunodeficiency virus infection in children and adolescents. Pediatr Infect Dis J 8: 216–220

Landesman S, Weiblen B, Mendez H et al 1991 Clinical utility of HIV-UgA immunoblot assay in the early diagnosis of perinatal HIV infection. JAMA 226: 3443–3446

Leibovitz E, Rigaud M, Chandwani S et al 1991 Disseminated fungal infection in children infected with human immunodeficiency virus. Pediatr Infect Dis J 10: 88–94

Lipshultz S E, Fox C H, Perez-Atayde A R et al 1990 Identification of human immunodeficiency virus-1 RNA and DNA in the heart of a child with cardiovascular abnormalities and congenital acquired immunodeficiency syndrome. Am J Cardiol 66: 246–250

Lipshultz S E, Orav J E, Sanders S P et al 1992 Cardiac structure and function in children with human immunodeficiency virus infection treated with zidovudine. N Eng J Med 327: 1260–1265

McKinney R E, Pizzo P A, Scott G B et al 1990 Safety and tolerance of intermittent intravenous and oral zidovudine therapy in human immunodeficiency virus-infected pediatric patients. J Pediatr 116: 640–647

Mitchell C D, Erlich S S, Mastrucci M T et al 1990 Congenital toxoplasmosis occurring in infants perinatally infected with human immunodeficiency virus 1. Pediatr Infect Dis J 9: 512–518

National Institute of Child Health and Human Development Intravenous Immunoglobulin Study Group 1991 Intravenous immune globulin for the prevention of bacterial infections in children with symptomatic human immunodeficiency virus infection. N Engl J Med 325: 73–80

Novello A C, Wise P H, Willioughby A, Pizzo P A 1989 Final report of the United States Department of Health and Human Service secretary's work group on pediatric human immunodeficiency virus infection and disease: content and implications. Pediatrics 84: 547–555

Oleske J, Minnefor A, Cooper R, et al 1983 Immune deficiency in children. JAMA 249: 2345–2349

Oxtoby M J 1990 Perinatally acquired immunodeficiency virus infection. Pediatr Infect Dis J 9: 609–619

Pahwa S, Firkring S, Menez R et al 1986 Pediatric acquired immunodeficiency syndrome: demonstration of B lymphocyte defects in vitro. Diagn Immunol 4: 24

Pizzo P A, Robichaud K J, Gill F A, Witebsky F G 1982 Empiric antibiotic and antifungal therapy for cancer patients with prolonged fever and granulocytopenia. Am J Med 72: 101–111

Pizzo P A, Eddy J, Fallon J et al 1988 Effects of continuous intravenous administration of zidovudine (AZT) in children with symptomatic HIV infection. N Eng J Med 319: 889–896

Pizzo P A, Bulter K, Balis F et al 1990 Dideoxycytidine alone and in alternating schedule with zidovudine in children with symptomatic human immunodeficiency virus infection. J Pediatr 117: 799–808

Pizzo P A, Wilfert C M 1990 Treatment considerations for children with human immunodeficiency virus infection. Pediatr Infect Dis J 9: 690–699

Plebani A, Clerici Schoeller M, Pietrogrande M C, Bardare

M, Careddu P 1989 Steroids in Pneumocystis carinii pneumonia in HIV seropositive infants. Eur J Pediatr 148: 579–584

Quinn T C, Kline R L, Halsey N et al 1991 Early diagnosis of perinatal HIV infection by detection of (viral-specific IgA antibodies. JAMA 266: 3439–3442

Reider H L, Cauthen G M, Bloch A B et al 1989 Tuberculosis and acquired immunodeficiency syndrome – Florida. Arch Intern Med 149: 1268–1273

Remington J, Desmonts G 1990 Toxoplasmosis. In: Remington J, Klein J(eds) Infectious disease of the fetus and newborn infant Saunders, Philadelphia, p 89–195

Report of a consensus workshop, Siena, Italy, January 17–18 1992 Early diagnosis of HIV infection in infants. J Acq Immune Def Synd 5: 1169–1178

Resnick L, Di Marzo-Veronese, F, Schupbach J et al 1985 Intra-blood–brain barrier synthesis with AIDS or AIDS-related complex. N Eng J Med 313: 1498–1504

Rubinstein A, Sicklick M, Gupta A et al 1983 Acquired immunodeficiency with reversed T4/T8 ratios in infants born to promiscuous and drug-addicted mothers. JAMA 249: 2350–2356

Scott G B, Buck B E, Leterman J G, Bloom F L, Parks W P 1984 Acquired immunodeficiency syndrome in infants. N Engl J Med 310: 76–81

Scott G B, Hutto C, Makuch R W et al 1989 Survival in children with perinatally acquired human immunodeficiency virus type I Infection. N Eng J Med 321: 1791–1796

Siegel F P, Oleske J M 1986 Management of the acquired immunodeficiency syndrome: is there a role for immune globulin? In: Movell A, Nydeggar AE (eds) Clinical use of intravenous immunoglobulins. Academic Press, Harcourt Brace Jovanovich, London, p 373–384

Stein K M Fenton C, Lehany A M, Okin P M Kligfield P 1991 Incidence of QT interval prolongation during pentamdine therapy of Pneumocystis carinii pneumonia. Am J Cardiol 68: 1091–1094

Strauss J, Abitbol C, Zilleruelo G et al 1989 Renal disease in children with acquired immunodeficiency syndrome. N Eng J Med 321: 625–630

Strauss J, Montane B, Zilleruelo G et al 1991 Persistent abnormal proteinuria in children of HIV positive mothers (abstr 2097). Pediatr Res 29: 352A

Tovo P A, De Martino M, Gabiano C et al 1992 Prognostic factors and survival in children with perinatal HIV-1 infection. Lancet 339: 1249–1253

Van de Perre P, Simonon A, Msellati P et al 1991 Postnatal transmission of immunodeficiency virus type 1 from mother to infant: a prospective cohort study in Kigali, Rwanda. N Engl J Med 325: 593–598

Williams M A 1987 Head and neck findings in pediatric acquired immune deficiency syndrome. Laryngoscope 97: 713–716

World Health Organization 1986 Acquired immunodeficiency syndrome (AIDS). Wkly Epidemiol Rec 61: 69–73

World Health Organization 1987 Special Programme on AIDS and Expanded Programme on Immunization. Joint statement consultation on human immunodeficiency virus (HIV) and routine childhood immunization. Wkly Epidemiol Rec 62: 297–304

18. Contraception and safer sex

M. Potts, S. F. Crane and J. B. Smith

INTRODUCTION

In *De Morbo Gallico* (1564) Gabriel Fallopio gave the first description of the condom in the Western world. It was a linen sheath fitted over the glans penis. He was writing at a time when syphilis was spreading rapidly, casting a shadow over the known world in a way similar to today's AIDS epidemic. In 1993, over 400 years later, attention is again focused on safer sex. The threat of AIDS is changing sexual and contraceptive behaviour and, to a lesser extent, family planning experience is feeding back into the control of HIV.

In the decade that AIDS has been the focus of intensive scientific study, the natural history of the disease has been unravelled in considerable detail and the molecular structure of the virus is known virtually atom by atom. A good deal of work is being conducted with the goal of developing a vaccine: however, HIV has the potential to double several times in the global population before a vaccine reaches large-scale use (Potts et al 1991). There is even a slight but grim possibility that a vaccine might be delayed for a very long time, or might prove impossible to develop.

It also seems likely that although palliative treatments will continue to improve, extending the life expectancy of those with HIV infection, a genuine pharmacological cure is unlikely. Therefore, during the critical exponential growth of the global HIV epidemic we are currently witnessing, our only defence lies in:

- Educating people about the nature of the disease and its routes of spread
- The treatment of other bacterial and viral sexually transmitted diseases (STDs) that are known to be risk factors in HIV transmission and acquisition, particularly genital ulcer diseases
- The promotion and distribution of condoms and other barrier methods to prevent transmission of HIV and other STDs.

One of the few pieces of good news in relation to AIDS is that the discipline of family planning has extensive information about the technical, clinical and acceptability aspects of barrier methods of contraception, and proven efficient distribution systems have been developed. Those who work in family planning are also experienced in the politics of making contraceptive choices available. The bad news is that the spread of HIV inevitably will affect the use of certain methods of contraception for family planning purposes. While barrier methods protect against HIV, concern has risen that some other methods might facilitate HIV transmission.

CONDOMS

AIDS is unique in that its spread could be greatly slowed tomorrow if there was a widespread volition to change sexual behaviour and a universal commitment to mutual monogamy. In reality, most human beings have more than one sexual partner in a lifetime and in many societies sexual partner change is moderately rapid (Johnson et al 1992). From a public health point of view it would seem rational to educate people to be selective in their sexual partners and to use condoms: 'if you can't be chaste be careful', is sound advice. Observational data also suggest that it is advice a community will heed (ASCF Investigators 1992).

A minority of people, some in decision-making

positions, believe with considerable conviction and deep sincerity that the distribution of condoms, rather than controlling the spread of disease, actually encourages people to have multiple sexual partners and therefore has the potential to accelerate the spread of AIDS. The two sides promoting these conflicting interpretations of condom distribution approach the topic from such different directions and with such strong feelings that there is little exchange of ideas but a great deal of conflict. Lack of unanimity slows distribution, inhibits promotion and undermines use.

The limited empirical data that do exist suggest it is reasonable both to counsel people to have fewer sexual partners and to distribute condoms. For example, a 1990 study of prostitutes and their clients in Lampang, a northern province of Thailand, showed a reasonably high use of condoms (77–79%). At the same time 60% of men claimed they were having sex with prostitutes less frequently than they had 1 year earlier. Certainly, HIV has spread rapidly in Africa where condom use is very low, but relatively slowly in countries such as the United Kingdom and China where condoms are available without restriction (Potts & Short). In the 1960s, those who worked in family planning tried to give the condom a 'clean' image, separate from venereal disease. Today, large-scale contraceptive distribution programmes are asking how they can more effectively prevent HIV. Condom promotion is often limited by state law, internal regulation or custom. In Ireland, the sale of condoms except through a limited number of requested outlets is a crime and in 1992 the Irish FPA was fined £500 for selling a condom in the Dublin Virgin Megastore. Other constraints on use are not always as obvious but they can still exert a deterrent to adopting the method. For example, the 1954 Commercial Television Act in Britain permitted anything and anyone to be advertised except for 'undertakers, astrologers and contraceptive manufacturers', while even today The New York Times encourages AIDS prevention in its editorials, but makes condom advertising on other pages almost impossible. The WHO/ Global Programme on AIDS claims to be a world leader in AIDS but has little time for the mechanics of condom distribution and has spent under 1% of its AIDS budget on buying condoms. Indeed, shortage of condoms – or

plain non-availability – is common in many countries with a high prevalence of HIV, such as Zambia, Tanzania or Uganda. If the spread of HIV is to be slowed then there must be:

- An adequate supply of high quality condoms
- At a price which is accessible to most people
- Without any restrictions on promotion, other than those common to the sale and distribution of any high-volume, lower-cost item.

Condoms can be purchased in bulk in the USA for about 4 cents apiece and on the global market for between 2 and 3 cents, freighted and delivered to a recipient country. Local production becomes economical at a volume of 20 million pieces or more a year, but local production does not, of itself, solve the main problem for many people in the developing world: a condom is just too expensive to buy. A Bombay prostitute may earn a dollar for each act of sex and wind up keeping 20 cents: a 3-cent condom (plus the cost of promotion and distribution), whether made locally or overseas, is not going to solve her problems. If latex condoms are to be used in developing countries on a scale with any real chance of having an epidemiological impact on the spread of HIV then local governments and the international donor community will have to subsidize their use for the foreseeable future. Success in AIDS prevention is going to be expensive – although it will be a lot cheaper than the alternative of inaction. Everything that can be said about condoms also applies to female barrier methods.

The modern latex condom is a simple, low technology device produced by dipping ceramic mandrels in high quality latex and then heat-curing and vulcanizing it on a continuous production line. Condoms can be plain or coloured. They can be unlubricated or lubricated; lubricants include silicon and aqueous solutions containing the spermicide nonoxynol-9. The commonest causes of holes in condoms are dust and foreign bodies on the mandrels, so that holes are literally cast into the condom. Many manufacturers test condoms individually by passing an electric current through metallic mandrels dipped in saline, although the test can be set at any level of quality. National and international testing standards are based on inflating a sample of condoms with air until they burst. Both the final pressure prior to bursting and the rate of flow during inflation measure the physical integrity of the condom. Condoms are also filled with 300 ml of water and rolled on blotting paper in order to check for holes. There are genuine differences in adult penis size and currently manufacturers make an Asian condom smaller than that for the rest of the world. Studies are being conducted into the need for a third large condom for Africa.

Condoms break in approximately one in a hundred acts of intercourse (Albert et al 1991). Some sexual practices, such as the belief in 'dry sex' found in parts of Africa, or anal intercourse, subject condoms to higher than usual strains and are associated with more breakages. To date, no correlation has been established between the manufacturers' quality control tests and actual failure during sexual intercourse; the tensile strength of condoms does not predict rupture (Geofi et al 1991). Oil-based lubricants, such as vaseline, can severely weaken latex condoms within 1 min of application. Condoms also have a poor shelf-life, especially when stored and distributed in tropical countries: one-fifth of couples in Bangladesh reported breakage and this could be the result of poor storage and transport (Ahmed et al 1990).

Animal 'skins' are a premium product, mostly sold in the USA. One of the many reprehensible chapters in the history of HIV control has been the almost total failure to develop simple, obvious, achievable and much-needed new barrier methods for men and women. The caecum of a sheep's gut is removed in Australian slaughter-houses, exported to Puerto Rico to have a rubber ring sewn in and sold as a premium product in the USA. This medieval product probably persists because the loose, baggy feeling is more acceptable than the conventional tight-fitting latex condom. The natural membrane is tough but has holes in it larger than HIV.

The contemporary latex condom is the product of a long history of technical refinement and has probably reached a stable end-point with few or no improvements or alterations in sight. Several companies are experimenting with a plastic condom. The potential advantages of a plastic device are that it would overcome problems of shelf-life, might be stronger than a latex condom

and would be compatible with a wide range of lubricants. In addition, a plastic condom would be open to a number of variations in design and the capital investment needed for a low-volume commercially viable product would be less than for latex devices.

Although condoms are universally recommended as prophylaxis against disease, the number of clinical and epidemiological situations where effectiveness against HIV or STD transmission has been demonstrated is remarkably limited. Such trials have been very difficult to conduct, even with bacteriological STDs. In the case of HIV, there are particularly serious ethical questions surrounding the design of any studies. It is hardly acceptable to randomly allot a prophylaxis for a lethal disease.

Even data on pregnancy rates for condoms are limited. In the Oxford Family Planning Association study of contraceptive methods (1968–74), non-smoking, low parity women aged 25–39 years who had used condoms for more than 4 years had a pregnancy rate of 0.6 per 100 women-years of use, while high parity women aged 25–34 years who smoked and had used the method for less than 2 years had a risk of 14.7 (Vessey et al 1988). Extrapolations to HIV protection are difficult because a woman is at risk of pregnancy for perhaps 60 days in the year, while so far as we know HIV can be acquired or transmitted on each and every act of intercourse involving a discordant couple. Direct observation on STDs, HIV and condom use point to an unambiguous protective effect (Feldblum et al 1980, American Public Health Association 1988). For example, none of 127 HIV-negative wives of HIV-positive haemophiliac men studied in Germany seroconverted (Evler et al 1989), but even approximate measurements of the percentage reduction in risk are likely to remain uncertain for the foreseeable future.

Organized family planning programmes have a quarter of a century's experience of promoting and distributing contraceptives. The most cost-effective way of distributing condoms in developing countries has been through social marketing programmes. These use existing retail outlets and sell the product at a price which is adjusted to the needs of society and which provides an incentive for the distributor.

FEMALE BARRIER METHODS

As all female mammals make a greater investment in pregnancy than do males (Stein 1991), there are biological reasons why women are sometimes more sensible than men when it comes to taking sexual risks. Certainly, a need to study current methods and develop new ones exists. It is thought that the risk of HIV transmission is greater from a man to a woman than vice versa, and one of the most important gaps in information about HIV transmission is the anatomical route taken for infection in the woman. Is it through the cervical canal, the cervical epithelium or the vaginal wall? Monkeys that have been hysterectomized still acquire the simian immunodeficiency virus (Alexander 1992, personal communication), so perhaps the virus can traverse intact epithelium, possibly being taken up by dendritic cells. But it is also biologically possible that erosions would make HIV transmission easier.

The question is of more than academic interest, because if the cervix is the primary route, then the diaphragm or cervical cap could protect against HIV transmission. A recent analysis of 5681 women attending a STD clinic in Denver found female barrier methods provided greater protection than condoms against *Neisseria gonorrhoea*, *Trichomonas vaginalis* and *Chlamydia* (Rosenberg et al 1992). It is impossible, at present, to apportion the results between the possible effect of the barrier covering the cervix, a spermicide killing the pathogen or better compliance with female than male methods (Table 18.1). Perhaps the explanation of the relatively poor performance of condoms in the Denver study is that women are more consistent in inserting a female method prior to intercourse than couples are in using condoms once the man has an erection.

As bacterial and other viral STDs are a powerful risk factor in HIV transmission, then the use of female barrier methods has an obvious indirect value in HIV control (in one study a diaphragm and spermicide reduced gonorrhoea rates by half, Austin et al 1984), but there is no way, given current knowledge, of assessing whether they will be as good, better, or worse than a condom in directly affecting HIV transmission.

The newest female barrier method of contraception is the female condom. It is a lubricated polyurethane bag with a soft ring that remains external to the vulva and a stiffer, loose internal ring that enables the woman to manoeuvre the device into the posterior fornix (Bounds et al 1992). It is on sale in parts of Europe and was approved by the US Food and Drug Administration (FDA) in 1992. On common sense grounds, it should, if inserted and correctly used, provide a high degree of protection against HIV, although it is likely to be many years before clinical data are available to validate reasoned speculation. It is a welcome additional choice for HIV and STD prevention as well as a useful method of contraception, although it has the disadvantage that, in addition to any problem of widespread acceptability, and for developing countries a relatively high price, it is also visible to the male partner.

In approving the female condom, the US FDA used pregnancy failure rates as a surrogate for HIV infection to assess new barrier methods. In addition to the gross difference in the size of HIV and sperm, there is another more important, but less visible problem. Fertilization is a risk for only a few days during each ovulatory cycle, but infection, as far as is known, can take place at any unprotected intercourse. However, the risk of conception at the time of ovulation is high (perhaps 20–50% for one at-risk intercourse), while the possibility of HIV transmission during a single coital act is low (perhaps 0.2% in an otherwise healthy couple). Therefore a method with a modest to high pregnancy rate could still have a substantial impact on HIV and other STD transmission.

Table 18.1 Female methods of contraception and sexually transmitted diseases (STDs): relative risk of STD infection when using barrier methods*

| | Relative risk | | | |
	Sponge	Diaphragm	Condom	Referent†
Gonorrhoea	0.31	0.32	0.7	1.0
Trichomoniasis	0.29	0.24	0.86	1.0
Chlamydia	0.64	0.25	0.93	1.0
Candidiasis	1.2	1.88	1.02	1.0

* A relative risk < 1 denotes protection; a relative risk > 1 (as in *Candida* infection) means the condition becomes more common; † the referent group involved 4332 women who used no method or had a tubal ligation, which is assumed not to protect against STD infection. (Modified from Rosenberg et al 1992)

GAPS AND OPPORTUNITIES

One of the many reprehensible chapters in HIV control has been the almost total failure to develop simple, achievable and much-needed new barrier methods for men and women. There is a clear and present need for a method women can use to protect themselves against HIV infection, particularly when they have reason to suspect their partner may not be sexually monogamous but they cannot convince him to use a condom. Tens of millions of women fall into this category, from prostitutes to battered women and wives of men in loving partnerships, but who may – with justice – worry about what their husbands are doing when away on long business trips or labouring on a distant building site. If barrier methods are to be used in sufficient scale to slow the spread of HIV, then an essential step in reaching the necessary prevalence will be to widen the range of methods available. A consistent and important lesson in family planning has been that high prevalences can only be achieved by making a variety of contraceptives available; the same policy is likely to be true for HIV and STD prevention.

It is probable that a simple, cheaper, more acceptable device than natural skins could be fabricated from one of a range of modern plastics. By the end of 1990 Family Health International had spent over $1 million of United States Agency for International Development money in the pursuit of this goal, and had produced prototype devices that more than half of couples preferred to latex condoms. Unfortunately, the momemtum gained in this critical project seems to have been lost.

The advantages of a plastic condom, in addition to broadening choice and therefore increasing prevalence, include:

- A better shelf life than latex condoms
- The potential of greater strength
- Compatibility with any lubricant (latex condoms are rapidly damaged (10–60 s) by oil-based lubricants)
- Defect-free production
- Potential of equal or greater acceptability
- Greater acceptability for anal intercourse
- The possibility of re-use and therefore low price.

SPERMICIDES

A good many chemical agents, including many that are already approved for use as spermicides or as skin disinfectants, kill HIV rapidly. The Denver study suggests consistency of use may be important for female methods, but it is also possible to argue that such a method might be less effective than a condom. What if, as is also possible, it proved easier to use, and some proportion of current condom users switched to, the less effective, more user-friendly method? The answer seems to be that, unless the difference in effectiveness was great and the rejection of condoms extreme, the new method would make a considerable contribution to HIV control (Figure 18.1).

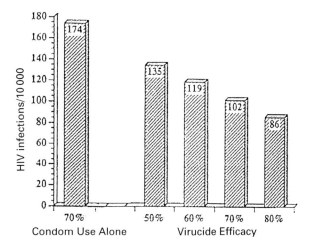

Figure 18.1 HIV infections in clients: 60% condom use with 35% virucide use. From Sokal D C, King T D N 1991 Modelling the efficacy of vaginal viricides: a simple projection. Family Health International, North Carolina, USA. October 1991 (unpublished)

Nonoxynol-9 (N-9), chlorhexidine, iodine and a variety of other antibacterial agents will kill HIV, and most other bacterial and viral diseases in the laboratory. The formulation of a product may be almost as important as the chemical entity chosen. Free virus and lymphocytes are inactivated in minutes by low pH (3.6–6) found in healthy vaginal secretions, while semen is alkaline (pH 7–8) and provides the optimum environment for HIV. This may explain why transmission from women to men is lower than from men to women (Voeller & Anderson 1992). In developing an effective vaginal virucide for HIV prevention, account must be taken of the fact that semen is the best buffer known in nature and vaginal pH jumps from 4.5 to 7 within seconds of ejaculation. Vaginal douching, while condemned by some commentators (Berer 1992), could be beneficial by removing the man's ejaculate and lowering the pH.

Two major clinical trials of nonoxynol-9-containing spermicides on STDs have been conducted in Bangkok, in a well designed placebo cross-over trial using the Today sponge, containing 1 g N-9 (Rosenberg et al 1987). A significant reduction in gonorrhoea and *Chlamydia* occurred but there was a rise in *Candida* infections. A similar study in the USA confirmed the results (Louv et al 1988).

The sponge, however, does not appear to protect against HIV spread. A study of Nairobi prostitutes, also using the sponge with 1 g of N-9, found no protective effect and a possible increased risk (Kreus et al 1992) of HIV transmission from men to women. This could have been an artifact in a limited study, or the result of vaginal damage due to the spermicide (or the mechanism of using the sponge) that accelerated transmission, counterbalancing any direct virucidal effect of N-9. These findings have been sufficiently disturbing to curtail possible recommendations for the use of the sponge as a prophylactic against HIV infection.

A study by Roddy and others on monogamous women not exposed to HIV infection who used the Today sponge every 4 h showed that although there was no subjective evidence of vaginal irritation, repeated high doses of N-9 were associated with small areas of epithelial sloughing which, in turn, might provide a route for HIV transmission from a man to a woman (Niruthisard et al 1991). It may well be that 1 g of N-9 in the sponge used on more than one occasion within 24 h represents an overdose (the Nairobi prostitutes averaged 34 partners a week). Less frequent use might be effective; in a group of African prostitutes offered condoms and N-9 suppositories, the risk of seroconversion was reduced by 80% in users of N-9 (Zekeng et al 1991).

The present state of affairs is highly unsatisfactory and research is urgently needed to determine doses and formulations of spermicides which might be appropriate for 'normal' marital intercourse or for use by commercial sex workers. In one Bombay brothel, for example, the house rule is that a woman should not spend more than 7 minutes with her client. In the Lampang study, 20% of the prostitutes had one client a night, 10% had five clients and one in 20 had eight or more clients. The average was 3.3. The UK Medical Research Council is developing a research strategy in this field.

Lea's Shield is a new barrier method, currently undergoing clinical trial in the USA. It is a silicone device that fills the posterior fornix and has an anterior loop moulded into the device which both stops rotation and facilitates removal. One size fits all and it is planned for over-the-counter sale. It should be easier to make available than a diaphragm and it is used with a spermicide. Like the diaphragm, it should reduce STD infection and common sense suggests it would have a similar impact on HIV as other female barrier methods – whatever that is finally proved to be.

OTHER METHODS OF CONTRACEPTION

The AIDS epidemic has begun to change the face of family planning and will do so even more in the future. Currently HIV-positive women are using oral contraceptives, intrauterine devices and sterilization as well as condoms (Johnstone et al 1990). Many want children. Could oral contraceptives, for example, retard the spread of HIV by thickening cervical mucus, or could they accelerate it, for example, by increased prevalence of cervical erosions, which might make infection with the virus more likely?

Until we know more about transmission, it is difficult to predict whether an intrauterine device (IUD) might increase a woman's risk of acquiring or even transmitting HIV. IUDs produce an increase in leukocytes in the endometrium and make menstrual bleeding longer and heavier. It is difficult, however, to envisage a data set that might demonstrate a difference in HIV incidence in IUD users. IUDs are uncommon where HIV prevalence is highest and random allotment of IUDs to women at risk of HIV would be unethical.

The problems which arise in this area are hard to answer and even when information is available, policy-setting, at the individual and community level, is going to be demanding. Research in these areas is pitifully inadequate and currently a good many people in family planning merely hope the issue will go away; it will not.

Tubal ligation, vasectomy and especially vacuum aspiration of abortion could transmit HIV if instruments were inadequately sterilized. Fortunately, HIV is easily killed and current aseptic and sterile regimens appear adequate.

If an adverse relationship between any specific method and HIV transmission were to be unequivocally confirmed, then, where HIV prevalence is low, screening methods might be devised to identify groups with high-risk behaviour, to whom condoms or alternative methods should be recommended; where prevalence is high, screening might define those at least risk (e.g. married couples of a specified age without a history of STDs), for whom use of the method might remain reasonable.

CONCLUSION

When dealing with a disease that doubles its prevalence in certain groups in less than 1 year and in the rest of the population in 2–3 years, then opportunities missed and time wasted translate into human death on a frightening scale.

Prior to 1980 condoms received remarkably little scientific investigation and, while they were regarded as a useful prophylactic against STDs and as a licit contraceptive method, use in the Western world was probably declining. Following the explosion of AIDS, more has been written about condoms in a decade than in the previous 400 years. Use in the developed world has gone up by 30–50% but not at the same level that these devices have hit the news headlines, become the focus of media attention, or the subject of locker-room jokes. Other barrier methods, including the use of spermicidal and virucidal agents used vaginally, have considerable potential to help slow HIV spread, but inadequate work has been conducted to enable clinical guidelines to be established.

REFERENCES

Ahmed G, Liner E C, Williamson M E, Schellstede W P 1990 Characteristics of condom use and associated problems: experience in Bangladesh. Contraception 42: 523–532
Albert A, Fletcher R A, Graves W 1991 Condom use and breakage among women in a municipal hospital family planning clinic. Contraception 43: 167–176
Alexander N 1992 Personal communication
American Public Health Association, Family Health International and Centres of Disease Control 1988 Condoms for prevention of sexually transmitted disease. MMWR 37: 133–137
ASCF Investigators 1992 AIDS and sexual behaviour in France. Nature 360: 407–409
Austin H, Luv K, Alexander J 1984 A case control study of spermicides and gonorrhoea. J Am Med Soc 251: 2822
Berer M 1992 Adverse effects of nonoxynol-9. Lancet 340: 616
Bounds W, Guillebaud J, Newman G B 1992 Female condom (Femidom): a clinical study of its use, effectiveness and patient acceptability. Br J Fam Planning 18: 36–41
Evler P, van Loo B, Kamradt T 1989 No more seroconversions among spouses of patients in the Bonn haemophiliac chart study. V International Conference in AIDS, Montreal, June. Abstr TAP 107
Feldblum, P J, Fortney J A 1980 Condoms, spermicides and the transmission of human immunodeficiency virus: a review of the literature. Am J Public Health 78: 52–54
Geofi J E, Shelley G, Donovan B 1991 A study of the relationship between tensile testing of condoms and breakage in one. Contraception 43: 177-185
Johnson A M, Wadsworth J, Wellings K, Bradshaw S, Field J 1992 Sexual lifestyles and HIV risk. Nature 360: 410–412
Johnstone F. Macallum L, Riddell R 1990 Contraceptive use in HIV infected women. Br J Fam Planning 16: 106–108
Kreus J, Ngugi E, Holmes K et al 1992 Efficacy of nonoxynol-9 contraceptive sponge use in preventing heterosexual acquisition of HIV in Nairobi prostitutes. JAMA 268: 477–482
Louv W C, Austin H, Alexander W J, Stagno S, Checks J 1988 A clinical trial of nonoxynol-9 for preventing gonococcal and chlamydia infections. J Infect Dis 158: 518–523
Niruthisard S, Roddy R C, Chutivongse S 1991 The effects of frequent nonoxynol-9 use on the vaginal and cervical mucosa. Sex Trans Dis 18(3): 176–179
Potts M, Anderson R M, Boily M C 1991 Slowing the spread of human immunodeficiency virus in developing countries. Lancet 338: 1–5
Potts M, Short R V 1989 Condoms for the prevention of HIV transmission: cultural dimensions. AIDS 3: 5259–5263
Rosenberg M T, Rojananapithayakorn W, Feldblum P F, Higgins J F 1987 Effect of the contraceptive sponge on chlamydial infection, gonorrhoea and candidiasis. JAMA 257: 2308–2313
Rosenberg M T, Davidson A J, Chan J M, Judson F H, Douglas J M 1992 Barrier contraceptives and sexually transmitted diseases in women: a comparison of female-dependent methods and condoms. Am J Public Health 82: 669–674
Stein Z A 1991 HIV prevention: the need for methods women can use. Am J Public Health 80: 460–462
Vessey M, Villard-Mackintosh L, McPherson K, Tates D 1988

Factors determining use-effectiveness of the condom. Br J Fam Plan 14: 40–43

Voeller B, Anderson D J 1992 Heterosexual transmission of HIV. JAMA 267: 1917–1918

Zekeng L et al 1991 HIV infection and barrier contraceptive use among high-risk women in Cameroon. Presented at International Society for Sexual Disease Research

19. Other sexually transmitted disease: cervical intraepithelial neoplasia

Katherine D. LaGuardia

INTRODUCTION

For the practitioner who cares for women with HIV infection, cervical intraepithelial neoplasia (CIN) has become a central management issue in maintaining the health of the reproductive tract. The appearance of an abnormal smear early on in the care of the infected woman is now an expected occurrence. The smear triggers a chain of events for the provider and patient and both become engaged in the persistent, worrisome battle to keep cervical disease from progressing. We know enough about CIN and its behaviour in the presence of HIV to be worried. Since Bradbeer in 1987 first published evidence supporting an association, clinicians and scientists have been reaffirming and refining the significance of the link.

But over the past 5 years in which it has become increasingly clear that women with HIV are more than 10 times as likely to develop CIN as those who are not infected (some studies indicate a risk 100-fold higher than that of the general population), we still understand very little about pathogenesis beyond immunosuppression theory. We have not significantly improved diagnostic or treatment modalities, and we have learned very little about oncogenesis in the process.

The clinician interested in tackling the problem of cervical disease and HIV is starting with very little to work with. We do not know much about the cervico-vaginal environment and why or how it might be susceptible to HIV in the first place. We do not know much about the lymphocytic characteristics of vaginal secretions, how antigens are usually processed, and whether this has any relationship to HIV susceptibility. We do not even know where HIV enters in the lower reproductive tract. There is much theoretical knowledge that on first glance appears attractive, but each theory has its refutation. Women have become infected post-hysterectomy and after a monogamous (on their part) relationship. While breaks in vulvo-vaginal mucosal barriers and access to the endometrial wall via the cervix offer logical explanations for how the how the virus could enter, the point is, we really do not know.

The confusion about the female genital tract and HIV and CIN is compounded by the role of human papillomavirus (HPV). HPV has been studied extensively in the gynaecological, oncological and virological literature. Its association with CIN and immunosuppression has been well established (Sillman 1984, Carson 1986). It is also acknowledged that HPV has a complex and yet to be fully understood role in the development of CIN in the presence of HIV. Is it a cofactor for enhanced susceptibility to the virus? Or is it a form of opportunistic infection in the face of immunosuppression? Does HPV accelerate CIN in the HIV-infected woman? There are theories in response to these queries, but there is no clear answer.

In summary, we face many more questions than answers about the relationship of HIV with CIN and HPV. It is hoped that this chapter will provide some understanding of what we know and stimulate some research on what we do not know.

WHAT WE KNOW

Epidemiology of CIN and cervical cancer

Cervical intraepithelial neoplasia or squamous intraepithelial lesion (SIL) of the cervix is a relatively rare phenomenon but has been shown to vary by population. For the purposes of this chapter, CIN will be used in reference to intraepithelial disease of the cervix; CIN I is considered a low-grade lesion and CIN II and III are considered high-grade lesions. Carcinoma in situ is encompassed within CIN III. Table 19.1 explains the corresponding terminology using the old system of reporting and the new (Bethesda) system.

Table 19.1 Terminologies of epithelial cell abnormalities of the cervix

Squamous intraepithelial lesions (SIL)	Cervical intraepithelial lesions (CIN)
Low-grade SIL	
cellular changes associated with HPV	CIN I
mild dysplasia	
High-grade SIL	
moderate dysplasia	CIN II
severe dysplasia	CIN III
carcinoma in situ	CIN III

HPV, human papillomavirus

While very few large-scale studies have been done in the general population, a large study in Canada (Meisels & Morin 1981) of over 230 000 women screened showed a prevalence rate of 0.4% for CIN and 0.04% for invasive cancer. However, another study by Bickell and colleagues (1991) of prevalence of CIN in a jailed population in the USA, revealed that 8% of the women screened had abnormal Pap smears. And, Briggs and co-workers (1980) demonstrated the high association of cervical dysplasia with sexually transmitted disease (STD). In a population of women attending STD clinics in Seattle, Washington, USA, the prevalence of abnormal Pap smears was 11.4%. Cervical cancer has actually declined steadily over the past 30 years (see Figures 19.1 and 19.2), and this is largely attributed to the efficacy of the Pap smear in early detection of disease. Yet in some populations the incidence of CIN has been shown to be alarmingly high. As a result of the shifts in prevalence of CIN among different populations, cervical cancer is once again a cause for concern. High risk populations are considered to be those with multiple sexual partners, a history of STDs, and those infected with HIV. This is in addition to

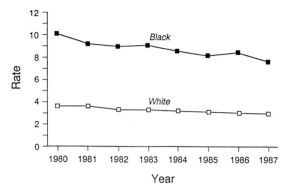

Figure 19.1 Age-adjusted cervical cancer rates per 100 000 women, by race and year; USA 1980–1987 (adapted from MMWR 1990 39:15)

the other well recognized risks – early onset of sexual activity, cigarette smoking and certain dietary deficiencies. Sexual activity and its attendant risks are independently associated with cervical cancer, leading many to claim cervical cancer as a sexually transmitted disease.

The association of cervical cancer with sexual activity is derived largely from the epidemiologic data on HPV and CIN and invasive disease. In addition, the behavioural characteristics of women who develop cervical cancer reinforce the sexual transmission hypothesis. In a study by Peters and colleagues (1986), age at first coitus (coitarche), number of partners, and interval between menarche and coitarche were the most significant risk

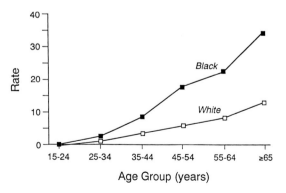

Figure 19.2 Cervical cancer mortality rates per 100 000 women, by race and age-group; USA 1980–1987 (adapted from MMWR 1990 39:15)

Table 19.2 Invasive cervical cancer (Los Angeles County): risk by selected characteristics of sexual history (adapted from Peters et al 1986)

Characteristic		Matched relative risk	
Age at first intercourse (years)	< 16	16.1	$p < 0.001$
	16–19	2.9	
	20–22	1.0	
	≥ 23 / never	1.0	
Years between menarche and first coitus (coitarche)	< 1	26.4	$p < 0.001$
	1–5	6.9	
	6–10	3.1	
	≥ 11 / never	1.0	
Total number of sexual partners	0–1	1.0	$p < 0.001$
	2–3	2.1	
	4–9	3.5	
	≥ 10	2.6	

factors for development of cervical cancer. (See Table 19.2).

While the association between CIN and invasive disease is not disputed, there is remarkably little known about the natural history of the disease. Most women in Western societies develop cervical cancer in their 50s and 60s. It is the third most common gynaecological malignancy in the USA, but the most common world-wide. Women in the Third World, particularly Africa, develop cervical cancer at young ages (30s and 40s) and because of lack of medical resources to diagnose and treat, they die younger and in greater numbers. In the USA, the mean age for development of carcinoma in situ (CIN 3) is 35 years. In 1990, there were 13 500 cases of cervical cancer and 50 000 cases of CIN 3. How long is the latent period of premalignant disease? What triggers the chain of reactions? What enhances these reactions? Why is it that some women have been reported with the disease in their 20s and others not until their 50s? Clearly, the development of cervical cancer is a multifactorial event, involving demographic characteristics (racial and socio-economic), sexual behaviour and biological response. The seed and soil concept is the most compelling argument for the mechanism by which the disease begins. Behaviour and demographics alone cannot explain pathogenesis. It appears that an agent (seed) is introduced into the female genital tract (soil) that has potentially biologically transforming charac-

teristics. This agent is now widely believed to be HPV. The biological response to this agent is determined by a number of cofactors which can theoretically enhance its carcinogenic potential. These cofactors include cigarette smoke (nicotine concentrates in the lower genital tract and is thought to reduce immune response), other STDs such as herps simplex virus (HSV) and infections which produce a local cervicitis (*Chlamydia*, gonorrhoea), other forms of immunosuppression, and the relative balance of sex steroids in the female.

The association of cervical cancer with a short interval between menarche and coitarche lend support to the theory that the presence of cervical ectopy (or eversion) enhances entry of a variety of pathogenic agents (eg. HPV, HIV, HSV, *Trichomonas*, *Chlamydia*). In the early postmenarchal years adolescents have a relatively oestrogen-dominant system and anovulation is not uncommon. The columnar epithelium that characterizes cervical ectopy may not recede into the endocervical–cervical canal as it typically does. The exposure of columnar epithelium to the vaginal canal predisposes the cervix to chronic low-grade inflammation and hence to other organisms.

The typical morphological changes in the cervical canal throughout the female's life promote the transformation of exposed columnar epithelium to squamous epithelium. From the late fetal period through reproductive life the columnar mucosa tends to be displaced distally while retracting after menopause (oestrogen withdrawal). The 'ideal' squamocolumnar junction (where the two cell types meet to form the transformation zone) is situated at the external os. In cases of cervical ectopy the junction is situated outside the os, on the ecto cervix. This may be congenital, hormonally induced (most strikingly in diethylstilboestrol exposure), or a result of cervical trauma, usually childbirth. Whatever the cause, the presence of cervical ectopy enhances the entry of infectious agents. Cervical ectopy may well be the 'soil' that supports the entry of the 'oncogenic seed' that is now widely acknowledged to be HPV.

It is important to note that not all women with cervical ectopy develop HPV or CIN. Furthermore, not all women with HPV will develop CIN. And, while we don't have the studies to demonstrate it, it is likely that not all women with CIN will go on to develop invasive disease if left untreated. But we can now predict who is statistically at risk and have a better sense of the significance of the risk factors.

CIN and its association with HIV

Because of the multifactorial aetiology of cervical dysplasia and cervical cancer, the behaviour that puts women at risk for HIV may also increase their risk for cervical cancer. Because of the confounding variables frequently present in women with HIV and CIN, any epidemiological studies of this relationship need to adjust for such factors as sexual behaviour, STDs and cigarette smoking. In 1992, there is little doubt that CIN is more common among women with HIV and the virus is felt to be an independent risk factor. Investigators have found varying prevalence rates of CIN among

lation groups (i.e. African sex workers and inner city drug users). However, reports emerging over the past 2 years reveal a striking consistency in prevalence of CIN among HIV-infected women. Feingold and associates (1990) showed a 40% prevalence of CIN in infected women vs a 9% prevalence in a comparable uninfected group. Maiman and his colleagues (1991) demonstrated a 41% prevalence of CIN among HIV-positive women. In addition they have shown relationships in the reverse direction (1990, 1991). They inquired, within a subpopulation or disease group, how many have been infected by HIV? In a group of women attending a colposcopy clinic, 10% were HIV-seropositive and of 32 women with invasive cervical cancer 19% were HIV-infected. Even though these studies were conducted in a high seroprevalence region of the USA, the findings reinforce the epidemiological association of HIV with CIN and cervical cancer. They also serve

Table 19.3 HIV infection and cervical disease: literature review

Author	Year/Country	Prevalence of cervical dysplasia among HIV-infected women
Bradbeer C	1987/UK	64% ($n=9$)
Tarricone NJ	1990/US	40.6% ($n=32$) (biopsy specimens)
Schafer A et al	1991/Germany	41% vs 9%* ($n=187$)
Hiller KF et al	1989/?	15% ($n=58$)
Kreiss J et al	1989/Kenya	2% ($n=125$)
LaGuardia KD et al	1991/USA	48% ($n=44$)
Schrager LK et al	1989/USA	31% vs 4% HIV− ($n=35$)
Marte C et al	1992/USA	48% vs 10% HIV− ($n=35$, Kings County Hospital)
		32% vs 5% HIV− ($n=35$, Community Health Project)
		23% vs 10% HIV− ($n=65$ Cook County Hospital)

* HIV-positive vs HIV-negative intravenous drug users; −, negative; +, positive

infected women (Table 19.3). These rates may be largely determined by the health of the population studied, the methods by which cervical samples were collected and analysed, and the size of the population studied. The prevalence rates of CIN have ranged from 2% in Nairobi (Kreiss et al 1989) to 64% in London (Bradbeer 1987). The studies examining risk among HIV-infected women have by and large been designed to compare HIV-seropositive women with seronegative women of comparable risk. While this design allows for comparison within a population group, the differences within that population group need to be carefully controlled for confounding variables and the conclusions may not be comparable to other popu-

to remind us of the importance of stressing HIV counselling in these populations.

Research on this subject over the past 3 years has focused primarily on disease prevalence. There have been very few studies on the natural history of CIN in the presence of HIV. Natural history studies give us a sense of how clinically significant statistical associations are, and how disease progresses over time. Does the disease progress rapidly in the infected woman? What is the typical course of the disease? While there have been sporadic reports of very young women with HIV who develop cervical cancer, we really have very little understanding of the nature of the association – is it insidious or relatively fulminant? One interesting

Table 19.4 Pap smear in relation to seroconversion in 47 patients; adapted from Provencher et al 1988

Pap smear findings ($n = 47$)	Relation to seroconversion	
	Before (%)	After (%)
Normal	88.1	40.6
Hyperkeratosis	1.7	15.2
Parakeratosis	0.4	6.2
Trichomonas	23.3	40.6
Herpes	0.8	4.6
Atypia	8.3	29.6
Human papillomavirus (suggestive of)	0.8	20.3
Dysplasia	0.8	17.1
Carcinoma in situ	—	3.1
Rule out invasion	—	4.6

attempt to gain insight into this question is the study by Provencher and colleagues (1988). This is the first published study on the natural progression of cervical disease in HIV-infected women. A subgroup of women ($n = 47$) on whom Pap smear data were available before and after seroconversion was evaluated (see Table 19.4). While the study does not control for date of seroconversion or frequency of Pap smear, one does get a sense of the severity of disease progression post-seroconversion. Clearly more studies are needed that examine the latent period of preclinical disease in the infected woman and the difference in rate of progression of disease post-seroconversion.

CIN and CD4 counts in HIV

The vast majority of studies which have examined HIV and CIN have demonstrated a relationship between immune depletion and severity of disease. Marte and colleagues (1992) compared infected women with CD4 counts greater than $600/mm^3$ to women with counts less than $400/mm^3$ and found a prevalence of abnormal smears of 21% and 45%, respectively. Maiman and co-workers (1991) demonstrated that infected patients with CIN had an average CD4 count of $221/mm^3$ compared to an average count of $408/mm^3$ among those without CIN ($p < 0.06$). In a study done at the New York Hospital–Cornell University Medical Center, of 44 infected women, those with CD4 counts less than $200/mm^3$ had a prevalence of CIN of 61% compared to 38.4% among those with counts greater than $200/mm^3$ (LaGuardia 1991) (see

Figure 19.3). Schafer and colleagues (1991) also confirmed that frequency and severity of dysplasia appear to increase with diminishing CD4 cell counts.

While the study design and sample size have varied among investigators, it appears quite clear that CIN becomes clinically apparent as CD4 counts drop.

Mode of CIN and acquisition of HIV

There does not appear to be any clinically or statistically significant difference in mode of acquisition of HIV and the development of CIN. This has been confirmed by a series of abstracts from the VIII International Conference in Amsterdam as well as previously published work. The mode of acquisition of HIV among those with CIN tends to mirror that of the general demographics of HIV in women. Nor is immune status (or progression of disease) particularly related to mode of acquisition. There is probably greater need for work in this area, however.

Correlation of cervical cytology and colposcopically directed biopsies in the HIV-infected woman

The report by Tarricone and colleagues in 1990 at the VI International Conference on AIDS indicated that there was poor correlation between cytologic cervical screening and colposcopically directed biopsies. The study examined 32 HIV-infected women. While only 9.4% ($n = 3$) had abnormal cytology on Pap smear, 84% ($n = 27$) had abnormal histology by biopsy; 13 of these patients revealed CIN (40%) and 14 had cervicitis (44%). Excluding cervicitis from this analysis, there was a discrepancy between cytology and histology of 9.4% vs 40%. Maiman and colleagues who reported on this (1991) also noticed a poor correlation between cytology and histology. While few other investigators have chosen to examine this finding in closer detail, the study's findings have not been replicated and there is much evidence to support the Pap smear as a positive predictor of disease. In our study of 44 patients at the New York Hospital–Cornell University Medical Center, we found a close correlation between cytology and

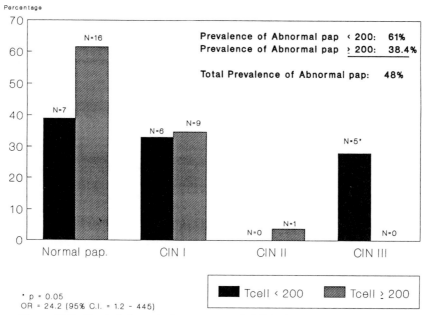

Figure 19.3   Cervical disease by immune status in HIV-infected women; the New York Hospital–Cornell Medical Center, June 1991

histology by cone biopsy, five of 44 patients underwent cone biopsy during the study period and there was close to 100% correlation with the Pap smear (see Table 19.5).

While the finding of Tarricone and associates (1990) and Maiman's group (1992) has not been widely confirmed, there has been broad concern in the health care delivery sector about how to manage HIV-infected women gynaecologically. We receive several phone inquiries from medical providers requesting that their referred patients undergo colposcopy and biopsy at first visit. The informed consumer will also bring this up at consultation in our clinic.

We feel at this point there is little evidence to

support the cost and discomfort associated with routine colposcopy. A review of the sensitivity and specificity of the Pap smear is in order and may help explain the confusion in this area.

The Pap smear has an acceptable false-positive rate. It is rare for a Pap smear to be reported as positive and no neoplasm found on colposcopic examination. One of the most important causes for false-positive smears is mislabelling the specimen. Laboratories could overread the specimen due to failure to recognize changes associated with HPV or artifact associated with air-dried specimens. Proper handling and labelling of specimens has the largest impact on reducing false-positives.

A distinct disadvantage of the Pap smear, however, is its false-negative rate, ranging from 15 to 40% (Stafl et al 1973, Richart 1980). A false-negative report indicates a cervical neoplasia has been missed. The most common cause for this is the failure of the person taking the sample to place abnormal cells on the slide. This can result from inexperience or more likely, missing a lesion near the cervical os or in the endocervical canal. A rare cause of false-negatives is laboratory error – labs are much more likely to 'over-read' a Pap smear.

There is no reasonable biological explanation

Table 19.5   Relationship of cervical cytology to cone biopsy histology among HIV-infected women (sample = 5/44); the New York Hospital–Cornell Medical Center, June 1991

Cervical cytology	T cells	Cone histology
CIN III*	86	carcinoma in situ
CIN III*	199	carcinoma in situ
CIN I†	107	no residual disease
CIN III*	104	severe dysplasia
CIN III*	52	severe dysplasia

* Rule out high-grade dysplasia; † rule out low-grade dysplasia

why HIV-infected women would have unique features that would lead to a higher rate of false-negative readings on cytology. And in fact, the data overwhelmingly support the fact that HIV-infected women have higher than expected rates of abnormal findings on Pap smear.

The community level of concern and a certain confusion in the literature, however, suggest a large-scale study should be done to resolve the matter.

HIV infection, CIN and the role of HPV

The interaction of human papillomavirus in the presence of HIV infection with the development of CIN has generated much work in the area of the oncogenic potential of HPV. With regard to HIV, there appear to be two schools of thought:

1. In the face of immunosuppression associated with HIV, HPV entry into cervical cells is enhanced and this presents the key stimulus for the development of CIN.
2. In the face of a fairly ubiquitous virus – reports of its prevalence in the general population range from 30 to 90% – the development of a subclinical infection is not unlikely. However, certain factors including viral type and degree of immunosuppression may promote the subsequent development of CIN.

Background

The question that remains unclear is whether it is the virus or host that promotes the development of progressive cervical disease. Certainly as HPV infection has resurfaced as an agent of concern in the development of cervical cancer, a multitude of studies have examined both host characteristics and the relationship of HPV to CIN. Ludwig and colleagues (1981) demonstrated that as many as 70% of lesions classified as CIN I were in fact condylomas. Reid and co-workers (1984) drew attention to the morphological continuity linking condylomas with CIN and they and others emphasized the gradual morphologic transition from benign condylomas to high-grade CINs.

Today we know much more about HPV and its relationship to the development of cervical cancer.

The papillomaviruses are small, non-enveloped viruses with icosahedral capsids consisting of 72 capsomeres. Their DNA is double-stranded and they reproduce in the nucleus of the host cell. They tend to exist as episomes rather than integrating into host DNA. More than 70 subtypes of HPV have been identified over the past 10 years and are associated with infection at various anatomical sites (feet, hands, anus, vulva, cervix and vagina). Twenty-two viral subtypes associated with anogenital tract disease have been identified.

At the present time there is no tissue culture system which has been developed to support the growth of HPV. Laboratory identification depends on methods other than viral isolation. Common methods used include:

- Electronmicroscopy (for assembled virions)
- Immunocytochemistry (for viral antigens)
- Molecular hybridization (for viral genome) – Southern Blot technique
- In situ hybridization (viral genome)
- Polymerase chain reaction (for viral antigens)

The most commonly used and highly sensitive technique for identifying viral type is the Southern blot method. Commercially available probes can detect the sequences present in the known subtypes. It is important to note that there are probably more than the 70 identified subtypes and the commercial probes may not identify infection if an unusual subtype is present. The advantages of in situ hybridization technique over that of the molecular hybridization is that paraffin block sections can be used. This allows one to look retrospectively at biopsy material.

HPV and CIN

It is now widely recognized that three basic groups of HPV subtypes are associated with genital tract condylomas. The first group is associated with benign disease and is considered as low oncogenic risk. This group includes HPVs 6/11/42/43/44. Types 6 and 11 are commonly found in vulvar condyloma acuminata in women, and rarely in flat aceto white lesions of the cervix.

The second group of HPVs are considered of high oncogenic potential and are frequently detected in high-grade CIN lesions and anogenital tract cancers. These include types 16, 18, 45 and 56. Of these, HPV 16 is the most common and has been associated with 50–80% of all high-grade CIN lesions (Koutsky et al 1992, Cuzick et al 1992, Lorincz 1992).

Interestingly, HPV 16 has also been detected in studies of women with normal cervical cytology. Schneider and colleagues (1992) followed 21 women with a history of negative Pap smears for 5 years before entry into the study. They were sampled monthly for 1 year and analyses of cervical cytology and polymerase chain reaction for HPV 16 was performed. The point prevalence of HPV 16 ranged from 14 to 33% in the group of patients. Only one patient with evidence of HPV 16 went on to develop CIN within the 5-year follow-up. Interestingly, HPV 16 was detected much more commonly in the luteal phase of these subjects. Other investigators have also documented similar findings of HPV infection in the absence of cytologic abnormality (Toon et al 1986, Meanwell et al 1987). These findings in a presumably healthy population suggest that the oncogenic potential of certain HPV subtypes (particularly 16) is enhanced by other cofactors.

The three other viruses in this group (HPV 18, 45, 56) are quite similar to one another at the molecular level. HPV 18 has been detected in approximately 20% of squamous cell carcinomas of the cervix and is the predominant cell type in endocervical adenocarcinomas. HPV 18 is rarely found in asymptomatic women or in high-grade CIN. The fact that HPV 18 is rarely found in precursor lesions to invasive disease has led to speculation that it is a particularly virulent form associated with rapidly developing cancers (Lorincz et al 1992).

The third group of viruses includes types 31, 33, 35, 39, 51 and 52. They are molecularly similar to HPV 16 and are found in high-grade CINs but are rare in invasive disease.

It is not within the scope of this chapter to discuss the theories on oncogenic transformation caused by the HPVs. It appears quite clear that HPV is necessary but not sufficient for the production of neoplasia. A series of events are required to induce transformation from a normal cell to a neoplastic cell. The E6/E7 proteins encoded in the HPV genome are thought to play a critical role in this transformation and function in a similar manner to the oncoproteins produced by other DNA tumour viruses, including SV40 and adenovirus. Briefly, the theory is that E6 and E7 proteins antagonize the host tumour suppressor proteins p53 and pRB, thereby deregulating cell growth (Werness et al 1990).

As we learn more about this virus, it becomes increasingly important to begin to document the natural history of its infection. From the time of exposure, how long does it take for clinically significant disease (i.e. CIN) to appear? A very important study by Koutsky and colleagues (1992) addresses the temporal relation between HPV infection and appearance of CIN I or II. In a prospective cohort study of 241 women attending a STD clinic, Pap smear, colposcopic, HPV typing, cervical culture and serological data were obtained every 4 months for an average of 25 months. At 2 years the cumulative incidence of CIN was 28% among women with a positive test for HPV and 3% among those without detectable HPV DNA. The risk was highest among those with type 16 or 18 (relative risk = 11). Other findings which correlated with the development of CIN were young age at first intercourse, and the presence of antibodies to *Chlamydia trachomatis* and cytomegalovirus, and cervical infection with *Neisseria gonorrhoea*. The authors point out that the time from detection of HPV to the development of CIN is remarkably short in this population. The development of CIN with a history of past or present cervical infections by STDs was independent of infection with HPV. The authors suggest that detection of HPV may have been obscured by these infections and that other cervical infections interact with HPV to enhance the development of CIN.

Clearly this was an unusual population to study. They were a STD population and also at high risk for HIV but no HIV data are reported in the study. The study shows a more fulminant course of HPV-induced intraepithelial disease. One cannot help but think other factors were also at work.

So, in summary, HPV has been extensively studied in reference to the development of CIN. It appears to be highly prevalent in the general population; certain subtypes appear more oncogenic than others; and yet the documentation of these subtypes in asymptomatic women indicates that infection alone is insufficient to cause CIN. The natural history of HPV-associated CIN remains to be fully defined and understood, particularly in reference to the HIV-infected woman.

HIV, and HPV and the Development of CIN

One of the few indisputable facts about HPV and HIV is that there is a very high correlation between HIV infection and HPV infection. This correlation strengthens as HIV disease progresses and as CIN appears. Feingold and colleagues (1990) demonstrated that of 22 women with symptomatic HIV infection, 11 (50%) had CIN on cervical cytology and 10 of these 11 were also HPV-positive. Among 13 asymptomatic HIV-infected women only three (23%) had such cytologic lesions. These findings reinforce the concept that cervical neoplasia is more likely as HIV disease progresses (or as CD4 counts fall) and supports the theory that HIV-induced immunosuppression exacerbates HPV-mediated cervical cytologic abnormalities.

Schrager and associates (1989) first reported on the prevalence of HPV infection in HIV-infected women with documented CIN. In a case-control study of infected women and uninfected women at risk (partners of HIV-seropositive men), CIN was documented in 31% ($n = 11/35$) and 4% ($n = 1/23$) of women respectively. They were not stratified by severity of disease. The presence of HPV was reported in nine of the 35 infected women (26%) and in one of the 23 uninfected women (4%). The authors neglected to mention whether the HPV cases were associated with the CIN cases nor did they document HPV by typing or histologically. None the less, the relationship appeared.

Johnson and colleagues (1992) contributed an important study which documented a very high correlation between low CD4 counts ($< 200/mm^3$), presence of HPV (particularly HPV 18) and the presence of CIN. It should be noted however, that none of the severely immunosuppressed patients had evidence of CIN II or III despite the high prevalence of HPV types 16 and 18 (60%). In the relatively immunocompetent group (CD4$> 209/mm^3$) there was one case of CIN II among 22 patients and yet only 9% had evidence

of HPV 16/18 by dot blot. These findings do prompt one to ask some questions. Why is the most virulent form of HPV found among the most immunocompromised? And why is there not a stronger relationship to presence of high-grade cervical neoplasia? Clearly, there is a need for a prospective cohort study similar to Koutsky's in this kind of population.

In our cross-sectional study of 44 infected women in 1991, there was strong correlation between the presence of HPV, high-grade cervical dysplasias and immunodepletion (see Figure 19.4).

It is important to ask, given the evidence of a relationship between HPV and HIV, whether patients with documented HPV are more likely to have been exposed to HIV. Matorras and colleagues (1991) found an HIV seroprevalence of 16.3% among a group of women with either genital or cervical condyloma. It is notable that 53.3% of the HIV-positive group had a past history of STDs compared to 28.4% in the control group (HIV-negative/HPV-positive). Again, further work in this area is necessary to understand the interplay of risk factors for development of CIN. It is quite possible that the molecular changes effected by the HPV genome enhance susceptibility to entrance of HIV. It would be valuable to conduct HIV seroprevalence studies among patients with high-grade CIN, HPV or both. Such a study would prompt further work in mechanisms of viral entry and viral interaction in the genital tract.

Management of the patient with CIN

There is now a broad consensus on how frequently HIV-infected women should be followed gynaecologically (Minkoff & DeHovitz 1991, Maiman et al 1991). What remains under dispute is whether routine colposcopy should be performed at each visit. Maiman and colleagues (1991) are proponents of this management approach. However, as discussed earlier, there are too few studies on which to structure a management approach based on their recommendations.

In the New York Hospital–Cornell University Medical Center, we feel the Pap smear provides an adequate initial screening of any existing cervical abnormalities and we use this as the primary screen-

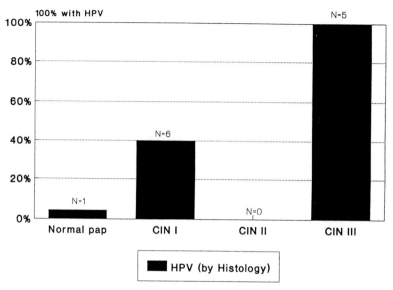

Figure 19.4 Prevalence of human papillomavirus (HPV) according to cervical cytology; the New York Hospital–Cornell Medical Center, June 1991

ing tool to guide further intervention. Patients should be seen every 6 months for cervical cytology, cultures or DNA probe testing for *Chlamydia* or gonorrhoea (if they are sexually active), and for general visual inspection of the lower genital tract.

If the Pap smears show any abnormality (beyond inflammation), the patients are brought back in for colposcopy. We strongly advocate that the same providers performing the gynaecologic care also perform the colposcopy, biopsy and any subsequent treatment.

Patients with evidence of low or high-grade dysplasia of the cervix undergo a thorough colposcopic examination of the cervix with directed biopsies and an endocervical curettage. If biopsy material does not correlate with the Pap smear, either a repeat colposcopic examination should be performed of a broader area of the cervico-vagina vault, or a cone biopsy may be necessary. Biopsy material should confirm Pap smear findings. If the biopsy is normal or of lower grade than the Pap, one should presume the lesion has been missed. It then rests with the practitioner to find the lesion.

Because HIV-related CIN and HPV tend to present as multifocal and multisite disease, the standard approach to examining the cervix may no longer hold. It has been traditionally taught that 95% of intraepithelial disease of the cervix orig-

inates from the transformation zone. While studies have not been performed in our HIV population on frequency of disease within the T-zone, our clinical experience and that of others (Maiman et al 1991) indicate that CIN can be found in multifocal sites across the cervix.

There are some who advocate a thorough examination of the cervix, vagina and vulva with acetic acid (5%) application. Any and all aceto white areas should be biopsied. We do not yet subscribe to this approach. Again, the Pap smear is our primary guide and visual inspection of the lower genital tract is a sufficient beginning.

As disease progresses, and anyone working in this field has witnessed its progression, more aggressive steps in evaluation and treatment may be instituted. In terms of diagnostics, we rely on the colposcopic examination and ability to visualize the squamocolumnar junction to determine whether cone biopsy is required.

HPV typing has not yet become standardized clinical practice. Part of the reason for this is the high prevalence of HPV found in women with normal cytology. It is not yet known how predictive the presence of HPV is for the subsequent development of disease. We know it is highly associated with CIN, but it currently has limited predictive value.

Table 19.6 An algorithm for managing the abnormal Pap in the HIV-infected woman

Cytology	Colposcopic findings	Histology		Therapy	Follow-up
CIN I	adequate SCJ	ECC neg	→ biopsy > Pap	cryotherapy	q3 months
			→ biopsy = Pap	cryotherapy	
			→ biopsy < Pap	repeat colposcopy and include vagina	5FU vs q3 months Pap
CIN II/III	adequate SCJ	ECC neg	→ biopsy > Pap	cone	q3 months Pap until negative
			→ biopsy = Pap	cryotherapy	q3–6 months Pap
			→ biopsy < Pap	repeat colposcopy and include vagina	colposcopy q3 months, cone acceptable
CIN I	inadequate SCJ	ECC neg		cryotherapy	q3 months Pap
CIN II/III	inadequate SCJ	ECC neg		cone	q3–6 months Pap
CIN I	adequate SCJ	ECC pos	→ biopsy > Pap	cone	q3 months Pap
			→ biopsy = Pap	cryotherapy	HPV typing, Pap q3 months
			→ biopsy < Pap	repeat colposcopy	consider cone
CIN II/III	adequate SCJ	ECC pos	all biopsies = >	cone	Pap 3 months

SCJ = squamocolumnar junction; ECC = endocervical curettage; neg = negative; pos = positive; 5FU = 5-fluorouracil; HPV = human papillomavirus; CIN = cervical intraepithelial neoplasia

Cervicography may well become an extremely valuable adjunctive diagnostic tool in both evaluating the risk of disease development and monitoring its progression. Cervicography provides a photographic record of the cervix under colposcopic examination. While the examiner may note certain pertinent findings (T-zone, aceto white areas) the degree of ectopy is often difficult to describe, the shape of the T-zone may alter over time, and the cervix may change in morphology over time. While currently expensive, it is a modality that provides invaluable information to providers following women for a period of time. For example, the woman with frank ectopy, chronic cervicitis, and a Pap smear suggestive of low-grade dysplasia may warrant more aggressive follow-up than a woman with a normal squamocolumnar junction and low-grade dysplasia. Cervicography aids in recording these distinctions.

So, in summary, women with HIV should be seen at least twice a year for Pap smear and cultures and examination. The management of patients who manifest signs of HPV infection or whose Pap smear begins to progress varies by clinician and appears related to clinical experience. In the uninfected woman, there are those who do not treat subclinical HPV, or do not perform cone biopsies for CIN I. The question we face in HIV/AIDS is whether a more aggressive approach should be taken. An algorithm for care is suggested in Table 19.6.

Management of HPV and the abnormal Pap smear

There is no universally accepted approach to the abnormal Pap smear. Every provider has their own nuance in treatment and much is based on clinical experience and sense of confidence in diagnosis as well as maintaining patient follow-up. Patient follow-up is a key component of Pap smear management. If one feels confident a patient will be returning for frequent and regular Pap smears, the practitioner is much more likely to act conservatively. On the contrary, the patient who finds it exceedingly difficult to keep her appointments is more likely to prompt an aggressive approach to put an end to any potential problem. This generally means that the non-compliant patient is likely to go to cone biopsy sooner than her compliant counterpart.

The technologies that are now available for surgical treatment of neoplasias provide an ever-increasing array of choices for the gynaecologist. They also allow one to tailor one's management in a more refined way. The current technologies in use for ablation of intraepthelial diseases are:

- Cryotherapy (nitrous oxide, $-90°C$ or carbon dioxide, $-60°C$)
- LASER therapy
- LEEP cautery (loop electrosurgical excisional procedure)
- Cold knife cone

These therapeutic interventions are listed in order of increasing invasiveness. Cryotherapy, LASER, and LEEP can be done in an ambulatory setting, although patient toleration of both LASER and LEEP is variable. LASER in an outpatient setting should be limited to cervical ablations and superficial ones at that. A LASER cone is reserved for the operating room. Patients' toleration of LEEP in an outpatient setting is limited. Reports of cone biopsies by LEEP in the office merit further study.

The best tolerated procedure in the office is cryotherapy. Patients feel minimal discomfort. Recurrence of disease, when properly used, is low (15%) – although may be higher among HIV-infected women. There has also been an association of cryotherapy and pelvic inflammatory disease post-procedure. For these reasons we instruct patients to avoid intercourse for 4 weeks following cryotherapy. In over 100 cases of cryotherapy we have not seen any post-procedure complications.

The cold knife cone remains the gold standard in both diagnosis and therapy of CIN. It is a minor surgical procedure that is not without risk. The incidence of post-cone haemorrhage and infection is approximately *10–15%*. The incidence of postoperative morbidity in an HIV population is unknown, but is undoubtedly higher – particularly in the face of severe immunosuppression. In 1992, the tendency at our institution is to avoid the cold knife cone in HIV-seropositive women. With the advent of LEEP, the practitioner in this field can obtain an adequate diagnostic specimen and effect therapy as well. Cone biopsy is now reserved for the perplexing diagnostic cases or for the non-compliant patient.

There is a great need to study the comparative benefits of LASER, cold knife cone and LEEP among HIV-infected women. The anecdotal reports of HIV particles recovered and cultured from the plume of LASER smoke has prompted many to move away from LASER toward cryotherapy and LEEP. In the absence of hard data for either case, the practitioner using LASER should *always* wear a heavy fibre face mask. Despite the advent of these technologies the specimen produced for examination by the pathologist is best preserved in the cold knife specimen. There is obviously no heat damage and cellular destruction in the cold cone. While ability to identify histologic lesion apparently does not differ among the different approaches, the histologist has the most thorough view of the epithelial layers in a fresh specimen. The advantages of heat damage conferred by LASER and LEEP are that therapeutic goals may be achieved better than with the knife. The heat radiation goes beyond the immediate target area. Long-term studies of these modalities are needed. They are probably not all equal in efficacy and may well serve different functions in management of disease.

CONCLUSION – WHAT WE DO NOT KNOW

The field of HIV infection in the reproductive tract presents some fascinating and important opportunities to study the immunology of the vagina, the mechanisms of viral entry in mucosal tissue, and the morphologic changes associated with viral infection. A number of research questions are prompted by the growing interest in the field. As more data emerge on the relationship of HIV to CIN, more questions arise. And increasingly, these questions focus on the fundamental mechanism of disease at the molecular level and the interactions that occur at the cellular level. Additionally, now that we understand that there is a relationship between HIV, HPV, CIN and immunocompetence, there is a desire to refine that understanding. Pertinent areas of future study in the HIV-infected woman include:

- Natural history of CIN
- HPV type prevalence and its relationship to CIN
- Influence of hormonal control on immunoglobulin concentrations in cervico-vaginal secretions and susceptibility to cervical infections
- Interaction of exposure to other STDs with the subsequent development of CIN

• Relationship of HIV load in cervico-vaginal secretions or tissue and the subsequent development of cervical disease. Does HIV act synergistically with other agents to promote cellular change at the local level?
• The impact of virucidal agents and other vaginal barrier methods on reducing cervical disease and HIV susceptibility.

The list of needed research could go on rather extensively. There is a fundamental need to improve our understanding of mucosal immunity and the molecular changes that occur in the presence of HIV and HPV.

The vagina and cervix have the advantage of being accessible organs. They are subject to disease processes to which many other organ systems are also vulnerable. We have an opportunity to improve the understanding of mechanisms of infection, disease progression, oncogenesis and neoplastic transformation by studying the lower genital tract in the female. As a result, we also are offered a tremendous opportunity to study preventative strategies and begin thinking about effective interventions to reduce HIV transmission, HPV infection, and the subsequent development of CIN.

Let us hope by the end of this decade we can report on a vast improvement in knowledge about the female genital tract and successful interventions to reduce susceptibility to disease.

REFERENCES

Bickell N A, Vermund S H, Holmes M 1991 Human papillomavirus, gonorrhea, syphilis, and cervical dysplasia in jailed women. Am J Public Health 81(10): 1318–1322

Bradbeer C 1987 Is infection with HIV a risk factor for cervical intraepithelial neoplasia? (letter) Lancet 2: 1277–1278

Briggs R M, Holmes K K, Kiviat N, Barker E, Eschenbach D A, DeJong R 1980 High prevalence of cervical dysplasia in STD clinic patients warrants routine cytologic screening. Am J Public Health 70: 1212–1214

Carson L F, Twigg L B, Fukushima M et al 1986 Human genital papilloma infections: an evaluation of immunologic competence in the genital neoplasia–papilloma syndrome. Am J Obstet Gynecol 155: 784–789

Cuzick J, Terry G, Ho L et al 1992 Human papillomavirus type 16 DNA in cervical smears as predictor of high-grade cervical cancer. Lancet 339: 959–960

Feingold A, Vermund S H, Burk R D et al 1990 Cervical cytologic abnormalities and papillomavirus in women infected with human immunodeficiency virus. J Acq Immune Defic Synd 3: 896–903

Hiller K F, Lutz R, Baur S, Stauber M 1989 High rates of cervical dysplasias, cervical intraepithelial neoplasias (CIN) and human papilloma virus infection in HIV infected female patients. V International Conference on AIDS, Montreal, June 4–5;5: 231, Abstr MBP60

Johnson J C, Burnett A F, Willet G D et al 1992 High frequency of latent and clinical human papillomavirus cervical infections in immunocompromised human immunodeficiency virus-infected women. Obstet Gynecol 79(3): 321–327

Koutsky L A, Homes K K, Critchlow M S et al 1992 A cohort study of the risk of cervical intraepithelial neoplasia grade 2 or 3 in relation to papillomavirus infection. N Engl J Med 327(18): 1272–1278

Kreiss J, Kiviat N, Plummer F, Ngugi E, Waiyaki P, Holmes K 1989 HIV, human papillomavirus, and cervical dysplasia in Nairobi prostitutes. V International Conference on AIDS, Montreal, June 4–9;5: 230, Abs MBP53

LaGuardia K D, McGuinness K, Hunter D 1991 Cervical disease among HIV-infected women by immune status. VII International Conference on AIDS, Florence, Italy, Abstract MC 97

Lorincz A, Reid R, Jenson A B et al 1992 Human papillomavirus infection of the cervix: relative risk associations of 15 common anogenital types. Obstet Gynecol 79(3): 328–337

Ludwig M E, Lowell D M, LiVolsi V A 1981 Cervical condylomatous atypia and its relationship to cervical neoplasia. Am J Clin Pathol 76: 255

Maiman M, Fruchter R G, Serur E 1988 Prevalence of human immunodeficiency virus in a colposcopy clinic (letter). JAMA 260(15): 2214

Maiman M, Fruchter R G, Serur E et al 1990 Human immunodeficiency virus infection and cervical neoplasia. Gynecol Oncol 38: 377–382

Maiman M, Tarricone N, Viera J et al 1991 Colposcopic evaluation of human immunodeficiency virus-seropositive women. Obstet Gynecol 78(1): 84–88

Marte C, Kelly P, Cohen M et al 1992 Papanicolaou smear abnormalities in ambulatory care sites for women infected with human immunodeficiency virus. Am J Obstet Gynecol 166(4): 1232–1237

Matorras R, Ariceta J M, Rementeria A et al 1991 Human immunodeficiency virus-induced immunosuppression: a risk factor for human papillomavirus infection. Am J Obstet Gynecol 164(1): 42–44

Meanwell C A, Cox M F, Blackledge G, Maitland N J 1987 DNA in normal and malignant cervical epithelium: implications for the aetiology and behavior of cervical neoplasia. Lancet 1: 703

Meisels A, Morin C 1981 Human papilloma virus and cancer of the uterine cervix. Gynecol Oncol 12: 5111–5123

Minkoff H L, DeHovitz J A 1991 Care of women infected with the human immunodeficiency virus JAMA 266(16): 2253–2258

Morbidity and Mortality Weekly Report 1990 Black–white differences in cervical cancer mortality – United States, 1980–1987. Vol. 39: 245–248

Peters R K, Thomas D, Hagan D G, Mack T M, Henderson B E 1986 Risk factors for invasive cervical cancer among Latinas and non-Latinas in Los Angeles County. J Natl Cancer Int 77(5): 1063–1077

Provencher D, Valme B, Averette H E et al 1988 HIV status and positive papanicolaou screening: identification of a high risk population. Gynecol Oncol 31: 184–188

Reid R, Crum C P, Herschman B R, Fu Y S, Braun L, Shah K V, Agronow S J, Stanhope C R 1984 Genital warts and cervical cancer III Subclinical papillomaviral infection and cervical neoplasia are linked by a spectrum of continuous morphologic and biologic change. Cancer 53: 943

Richart R M 1980 The patient with an abnormal pap smear – screening techniques and management. N Engl J Med 302: 332

Schafer A, Friedmann W, Mielke M, Schwartlander B, Koch M A 1991 The increased frequency of cervical dysplasia–neoplasia in women infected with the human immunodeficiency virus is related to the degree of immunosuppression. Am J Obstet Gynecol 164(2): 593–599

Schneider A, Kirchhoff T, Meinhardt G et al 1992 Repeated evaluation of human papillomavirus 16 status in cervical swabs of young women with a history of normal papanicolaou smears. Obstet Gynecol 79(5): 683–688

Schrager L K, Friedland G H, Maude D et al 1989 Cervical and vaginal squamous cell abnormalities in women infected with human immunodeficiency virus. J Ac Immune Defic Synd 2: 570–575

Sillman F, Stanek A, Sedlis A et al 1984 The relationship between human papilloma virus and lower genital intraepithelial neoplasia in immunosuppressed women. Am J Obstet Gynecol 150: 300–308

Stafl A, Friedich E G Jr, Mattingly R F 1973 Detection of cervical neoplasia – reducing the risk of error. Clin Obstet Gynecol 16: 238

Tarricone N J et al 1990 Colposcopic evaluation of HIV seropositive women (Abstr). VI International Conference on AIDS San Francisco, June 20–24, 2: 378

Toon P G, Arrand J R, Wilson L P, Sharp D S 1986 Human papillomavirus infection of the uterine cervix of women without cytological signs of neoplasia. Br Med J 293: 1261

Werness B A, Levine A J, Howley P M 1990 Association of human papillomavirus types 16 and 18 E6 proteins with p53. Science 248: 76–79

BIBLIOGRAPHY

Agosti J M 1991 HIV infection in women J Gen Intern Med 6: 380–381

Anderson J E, Kann L, Holtzman D et al 1990 HIV/AIDS knowledge and sexual behavior among high school students. Fam Plann Perspect 22(6): 252–255

Baggish M S, Campion M J, Ferenczy A S et al 1992 Ways of using LEEP for external lesions. Contemp Obstet, Gynecol 37(5): 138–182

Baker D A, Douglas J M, Buntin D M et al 1990 Topical podofilox for the treatment of condylomata acuminata in women. Obstet Gynecol 76(4): 656–659

Benedet J L, Anderson M B, Matisic J P 1992a A comprehensive program for cervical cancer detection and management. Am J Obstet Gynecol 166(4): 1254–1259

Benedet J L, Miller D M, Nickerson K G 1992b Results of conservative management of cervical intraepithelial neoplasia. Obstet Gynecol 79(1): 105–110

Berry S M, Fine N, Bichalski J A 1992 Circulating lymphocyte subsets in second- and third-trimester fetuses: comparison with newborns and adults. Am J Obstet Gynecol 167(4): 895–900

Beutner K R, Conant M, Freidman-Kien A E et al 1989

Patient-applied podofilox for treatment of genital warts. Lancet 1: 831–834

Bottles K, Reiter R C, Steiner A L et al 1991 Problems encountered with the Bethesda system: the University of Iowa experience. Obstet Gynecol 78(3): 410–413

Bradbeer C S, Heyderman E 1989 The risk of progression of cervical dysplasia in women with HIV. V International Conference on AIDS, Montreal, June 4–9;5: 231, Abstr MBP58

Cates W, Stone K M 1992 Family planning, sexually transmitted diseases and contraceptive choice: a literature update – part I Family Planning Perspectives. 24(2): 75–84

Centers for Disease Control 1991 Risk for cervical disease in HIV-infected women – New York City. JAMA 265(1): 23–24

Centers for Disease Control 1992 HIV/AIDS surveillance: US AIDS cases reported through December 1991, Atlanta, GA. US Department of Health and Human Services, Public Health Service

Covico J M, McCormack W M 1990 Vulvar ulcer of unknown etiology in a human immunodeficiency virus-infected woman: response to treatment with zidovudine. Am J Obstet Gynecol 163(1): 116–118

Delvenne P, Engellenner W J, Ma S F, Mann W J, Chalas E, Nuovo G J 1992 Detection of human papillomavirus DNA in biopsy-proven cervical squamous intraepithelial lesions in pregnant women. J Reprod Med 37(10): 829–833

Editorial 1992 Cervical cancer screening: quest for automation. Lancet 339: 963–964

Forrest B D 1991 Women, HIV, and mucosal immunity. Lancet 337: 835–836

Friedmann W, Schafer A, Schwartlander B 1989 Cervical neoplasia in HIV-infected women V International Conference on AIDS, Montreal, June 4–9;5: 600, Abstr WCP53

Gayle J A, Selik R M, Chu S Y et al 1990 Surveillance for AIDS and HIV infection among black and hispanic children of childbearing age, 1981–1989. MMWR 39(SS-3): 23–30

Goff B A, Atanasoff P, Brown E et al 1992 Endocervical glandular atypia in papanicolaou smears. Obstet Gynecol 79(1): 101–104

Henry M J, Stanley M W, Cruikshank S 1989 Association of human immunodeficiency virus immunosuppression with human papillomavirus infection and cervical intraepithelial neoplasia. Am J Obstet Gynecol 160: 352–353

Hoegsberg B, Abulafia O, Sedlis A 1990 Sexually transmitted diseases and human immunodeficiency virus infection among women with, pelvic inflammatory disease. Am J Obstet Gynecol 163(4): 1135–1139

Jones M H, Jenkins D, Cuzick J et al 1992 Mild cervical dyskaryosis: safety of cytological surveillance. Lancet 339: 1440–1443

Keijser K G, Kenemans P, Petronella H et al 1992 Diathermy loop excision in the management of cervical intraepithelial neoplasia: diagnosis and treatment in one procedure. Am J Obstet Gynecol 166(4): 1281–1287

Kirby A J, Spiegelhalter D J, Day N E 1992 Conservative treatment of mild/moderate cervical dyskaryosis: long-term outcome. Lancet 339: 828–831

Koss L 1992 Human papillomaviruses and genital cancer. Female Patient 17: 25–30

Lifson A R, Hessol N A, Buchbinder S P et al 1992 Serum β_2-microglobulin and prediction of progression to AIDS in HIV infection. Lancet 339: 1436–1443

Mandelblatt J, Schechter C, Fahs M et al 1991 Clinical implications of screening for cervical cancer under medicare. Am J Obstet Gynecol 164(2): 644–651

Marcus A C. Crane L A, Kaplan C P et al 1990 Clinical commentary: screening for cervical cancer in emergency centers and sexually transmitted disease clinics. Obstet Gynecol 75(3): 453–455

Marks G, Richardson J L, Maldonado N 1991 Self-disclosure of HIV infection to sexual partners, Am J Public Health 81(10): 1321–1322

Massachusetts Medical Society 1992 Current trends: hysterectomy prevalence and death rates for cervical cancer – United States, 1965–1988. MMWR 41(2): 17–31

Morbidity and Mortality Weekly Report 1991 Risk for cervical disease in HIV-infected women – New York City. Vol. 39: 846–849

Munoz N, Bosch F X 1989 Epidemiology of cervical cancer. In: Munoz N, Bosch F X, Jensen O M (eds) Human papillomavirus and cervical cancer International Agency for Research on Cancer (WHO), Lyon, France, p 9–39

New York State Department of Health, Albany, NY 1992 Methods of personal protection for women to reduce transmission of HIV through vaginal intercourse. Policy statement: AIDS Institute

Niruthisard S, Roddy R, Chutivongse 1992 Use of nonoxynol-9 and reduction in rate of gonococcal and chlamydial cervical infections. Lancet 339: 1371–1375

Pomerantz R J, de la Monte S, Donegan P et al 1988 Human immunodeficiency virus (HIV) infection of the uterine cervix. Ann Intern Med 108(3): 321–327

Report of the 1991 Bethesda workshop 1992 The revised Bethesda system for reporting cervical/vaginal cytologic diagnoses. J Reprod Med 37(5): 383–386

Richart R M 1991 The significance of the human papillomavirus infections in the 1990's. Obstetri Gynecol Forum 5(5): 2–15

Sehgal A, Singh V, Bhambhani S et al 1991 Screening for cervical cancer by direct inspection. Lancet 338: 282

Seidman S N, Mosher W D, Aral S O 1992 Women with multiple sexual partners: United States, 1988. Am J Public Health 82(10): 1388–1394

Spitzer M, Brandsma J L, Steinberg B 1990 Detection of conditions related to human papillomavirus. J Reprod Med 35(7): 697–703

Sweeny P, Onorato I M, Allen D 1992 Sentinel surveillance of human immunodeficiency virus infection in women seeking reproductive health services in the United States, 1988–1989 Obstet Gynecol 79(4): 503–510

US Department of Health and Human Services, Preventative Services Task Force 1989 Screening for cervical cancer. In: Guide to clinical preventative services: an assessment of the effectiveness of 169 interventions. Williams and Williams, Baltimore, MD, p 59–62

Vermund S H, Kelley K F, Klein R S, Feingold A R, Schreiber K, Munk G, Burk R D 1991 High risk of human papillomavirus infection and cervical squamous intraepithelial lesions among women with symptomatic human immunodeficiency virus infection. Am J Obstet Gynecol 165(2):392–400

Wright T C, Gagnon S, Ferenzy A 1991 Excising CIN lesions by loop electrosurgical procedure. Contemp Obstet Gynecol 36(3): 56–74

20. Gynaecological problems in women infected with the human immunodeficiency virus

K. H. McCarthy and S. G. Norman

This chapter considers the range of gynaecological conditions that may be of special importance to the HIV-infected woman and the woman with AIDS. The significance of these conditions, which to most HIV-seronegative women are miserable and dispiriting but hardly life-threatening, are twofold. If, for instance, chronic vaginal and pelvic infection is more common in HIV-seropositive women, and if this association is causal rather than casual, then there is an argument for including such pathology in the catalogue of AIDS-defining diseases. Recently recurrent vulvovaginal *Candida* has been classified as a condition 'attributable to HIV infection and/or indicative of a defect in cell mediated immunity' (CDC 1991). It will not be an AIDS-defining condition. Such a classification has implications for women seeking health care, especially in the USA. Second, just as immune suppression seen in HIV infection may contribute to the prevalence of (perhaps) abnormally aggressive or recurrent premalignant (and malignant) disease of the cervix, so it may lead to other abnormally severe, or rapidly progressive disease in the pelvis, particularly infection. As evidence mounts that HIV-seropositive women should undergo regular screening for cervical disease, probably by colposcopy rather than by simple Papanicolaou smear (Maiman et al 1991) there is an argument for regular screening for other pelvic disease.

Other issues facing the gynaecologist involve the significance of HIV infection and menstrual disorders, especially amenorrhoea and infertility. The latter has a moral as well as a physical dimension when considering reproduction in women with what at present, at least, appears to be a relentlessly progressive and ultimately fatal condition.

We feel that there are enormous difficulties in confidently establishing a causal association between HIV infection and common gynaecological complaints. Unlike the otherwise rare opportunistic infections and unusual tumours that are a marker of HIV infection, the conditions reviewed here are common. Establishing a direct link to HIV infection would require a controlled trial with many patients who, in general, place themselves at risk of many gynaecological conditions independent of their serostatus. Such a longitudinal study would need to run over probably several years bearing in mind the mean interval of about a decade (or possibly longer) between infection and progression to AIDS (Rutherford et al 1990). The problems of ensuring adequate follow-up in a group of mobile and often underprivileged women is daunting.

This article considers the evidence linking HIV infection with genital infection, pelvic pain and menstrual disorders, and discusses the problems of the infertile HIV-seropositive woman who wishes to have children. Pelvic infections generally classed as sexually transmitted diseases are considered elsewhere.

VAGINAL INFECTIONS

Candida

Generalized fungal infections are an important cause of morbidity and mortality in both male and female HIV-seropositive individuals. However, in addition to oropharyngeal and oesophageal infection, HIV-seropositive women appear to be at increased risk of vaginal candidiasis which is recurrent, difficult to treat, and the severity of which is related to the CD4 lymphocyte count (Iman et al

1990). Rhoads and colleagues (1987) described a group of 29 HIV-seropositive women, 25% of whom gave a history of chronic refractory vaginal candidiasis requiring almost constant intravaginal antifungal treatment. All these patients also had oral candidiasis and CD4 depletion. However, this need not always be the case. Iman and co-workers (1990) studied 66 predominantly White intravenous drug-using (IVDU) HIV-seropositive women followed for a mean of 14 months. Half of these patients had new or more frequently recurrent vaginal candidiasis which was of increased duration and severity, and many recalled that such changes predated their formal HIV diagnosis. Of the 25 women who also suffered oral candidiasis, only two had not previously experienced vaginal involvement. The location and severity of moniliasis was related to CD4 lymphocyte count. The most severely compromised patients (CD4 count $< 0.03 \times 10^6/l$) suffered oesophageal candidiasis, but those patients who had vaginal *Candida* had CD4 lymphocyte counts that did not differ significantly from unaffected seropositive women. Although the data are uncontrolled, the strong link between CD4 lymphocyte count and location and severity of candidiasis lends credence to them. Other data, though cross-sectional in nature, also support the increased prevalence of vaginal *Candida* amongst HIV-seropositive women (Friese et al 1989, Stein et al 1991, Anastos et al 1992). In HIV-positive women where candidal infection is limited to the vagina, conventional local treatment with clotrimazole or nystatin is applicable. In resistant cases ketoconazole 400 mg daily with monthly prophylactic courses has been indicated (Sobel 1986). There is recent evidence of resistance to fluconazole in the treatment of oral *Candida* (Cameron et al 1992) and thus we might expect that giving prophylactic antifungals would result in vulvovaginal *Candida* infection that is more resistant to standard treatments. The efficacy of fluconazole and ketoconazole has been compared in oropharyngeal candidiasis in AIDS patients (DeWit et al 1989). There is no reason to suspect that fluconazole will be less effective in treating vaginal infection in HIV-seropositive women when it has been shown to be of use against more serious infections (Lang et al 1990).

Other vaginal and cervical infections

Cross-sectional studies suggest a consistently high incidence of other vaginosis in HIV-seropositive women. Again controlled data are sparse. Infections with *Gardnerella* and *Trichomonas* are commonplace. Our own data drawn from a group of 61 HIV-seropositive women followed prospectively indicate a substantial carriage rate for *Candida*, *Gardnerella* and anaerobes. Our group differs from others studied in that the women do not derive from a population screened in a genitourinary clinic and a minority have been infected by IVDU. This contrasts with other studies that have mainly involved drug-using populations. Our preliminary data suggest that about $\frac{1}{3}$ of HIV-seropositive women screened will have a vaginal infection, $\frac{2}{3}$ of which will be *Candida* and the remainder *Gardnerella* or anaerobic infection. So far a small control group of HIV-seronegative women ($n = 17$) drawn from women presenting for counselling and testing, as they believed themselves to be at risk of HIV infection, showed 5/17 were infected, all of whom carried *Candida*. Clearly these numbers are too small to draw conclusions.

Stratification by CD4 lymphocyte count reveals no difference in degree of immunosuppression between HIV-seropositive women with and without vaginal infection. Classification by risk factors reveals that 50% of African women have a vaginal infection, but this falls to 33% amongst Caucasian women infected through IVDU and only 10% amongst Caucasian women infected heterosexually.

Examination of CD4 lymphocyte counts by risk group shows that African women and IVDU have significantly lower median CD4 counts (247 vs 505) and it is tempting to attribute the high infection rate amongst African women to this apparently more marked immunosuppression. However, reanalysis of CD4 lymphocyte counts between African women with and without vaginosis shows no significant difference in these parameters.

No conclusions can be drawn from these data relating CD4 count or risk category with risk of vaginosis. However, repeated episodes of vaginosis may, as is the case for cervical abnormalities (especially in women with other acknowledged risk factors) be a marker for possible HIV infection and testing should be considered.

PELVIC INFLAMMATORY DISEASE

Rigorous study of the aetiology of pelvic inflammatory disease (PID) in HIV-seropositive women is lacking because of the difficulty in controlling for sexual behaviour. There is, however, ample evidence to associate the presence of one sexually transmitted disease (HIV) with more mundane organisms (Piot et al 1987, Greenblatt et al 1988, Cameron et al 1989). Safrin and colleagues (1990) have shown a rise in HIV seropositivity amongst women admitted with a clinical diagnosis of PID from 0 to 6.7% over 4 years from 1985. A history of IVDU remained the most powerful marker for high risk of HIV infection (Safrin et al 1990). Hoegsberg and associates (1990) have reported rates of HIV infection of nearly 14% in Brooklyn, where the background rate of HIV infection amongst the young and sexually active is high (2%) but much less than that seen amongst patients admitted as an emergency with PID. In this group of women with PID an unexpectedly low total white cell count was associated with HIV infection and the authors postulated that in such patients there is an HIV-mediated blunting of the normal response to infection. Surgical intervention was required more often in the HIV-seropositive group, suggesting more severe infection. However, there is no conclusive evidence that the course or severity of PID is significantly different in HIV-seropositive and -seronegative women. Again, long-term follow-up of cohorts of HIV-infected and uninfected women with similar life-styles is required to show whether HIV infection at any stage of immunocompromise will lead to reactivation of dormant, chronic pelvic infection. The treatment of such infections follows the guidelines for PID in seronegative women. Therapy in severe cases with a cephalosporin, metronidazole and tetracycline is instituted in precisely the same manner, depending on the nature of the organisms isolated.

An increasingly prevalent mode of presentation of HIV is pulmonary tuberculosis, though extrapulmonary TB is disproportionately common. Although most studies show that organisms infecting the female genital tract are not unusual, the association of both pulmonary and extrapulmonary TB with HIV infection points to the fact that pelvic tuberculosis may become a significant finding. At present treatment of PID seems to follow, in general, that currently recommended.

MENSTRUAL DISORDERS

There is a suggestion that women infected with HIV may have an increased frequency of disorders of menstruation. Chronic disease, weight loss and stress-related illness are recognized causes of oligo- and amenorrhoea, so one might postulate that HIV-infected women may be subject to such variations in their menstrual cycle. It is unknown whether the HIV virus has any direct effect on ovarian or uterine function, or indirect action by influencing the endocrine system.

The great majority of HIV-infected women are of reproductive age and will have a range of menstrual disorders common to this age group. Very few data have been published on menstruation in HIV-positive women, and that which has is often uncontrolled, making it impossible to draw firm conclusions. Of 145 women referred for a gynaecological assessment, of whom 63% were not referred with a specific problem, only 34% had a completely normal examination. The most common presenting problems were menstrual abnormalities and vaginal irritation (Matnur-Wagh et al 1992). One study amongst IVDU reports an increased prevalence of amenorrhoea (24% vs 13%) and intermenstrual bleeding (18% vs 6%) in HIV-seropositive compared with -seronegative women (Warne et al 1991). Although the women studied were IVDUs, a group in which menstrual irregularities are common, they were matched to HIV-seronegative IVDUs. The difference observed does, therefore, suggest an alteration due to HIV infection. A recent report suggests that HIV-infected women recognized an increase in menstrual loss after HIV diagnosis compared to their menstrual loss prior to HIV diagnosis (Patrik et al 1992). The numbers in this study were small and there was no comparative control group; also, to accurately assess menstrual loss, objective measurement rather than self-reported changes is desired, particularly when the diagnosis of HIV infection will have an important psychological influence. Clearly, further prospective controlled trials are needed to determine what effect, if any, HIV infection has on menstrual function.

INFERTILITY

Many people may be surprised to find a discussion of infertility in a book concerning HIV infection in women. HIV-infected couples do, however, choose to become pregnant and have children (Johnstone et al 1990). There does not appear to be an increased rate of termination of pregnancy amongst HIV-infected pregnant women compared to seronegative women of similar backgrounds (Selwyn et al 1989). Those who discover their diagnosis whilst pregnant often do not opt for termination of pregnancy despite counselling on the risk of vertical transmission and prognosis of HIV infection. Safe sex is advised to prevent or reduce transmission of HIV from an infected individual to his or her uninfected partner. Safer sex in couples where both are infected may also be important, as the transmission of more aggressive strains of HIV, other viral infections or sexually transmitted diseases may act as cofactors in HIV progression.

Where pregnancy is desired, couples are advised to limit unprotected intercourse to around the time of ovulation which can be estimated by the use of ovulation kits and recording daily temperature. In the case of the uninfected male, artificial insemination by partner can be performed with the advantages of protecting the man from risk of infection, and can be performed without involving medical staff.

It is possible that with the rise in the number of women who are becoming infected and with the increase in frequency of PID associated with HIV infection, more women will present with tubo-ovarian disease for infertility treatment or will be found to be HIV-positive at the initial infertility assessment. A recent anonymous HIV seroprevalence study of 182 couples undergoing infertility treatments found that 2.6% of men and 0.6% of women were HIV-seropositive (Bray et al 1991). All individuals found to be HIV-positive had a history of STDs, and a history of multiple sexual partners was common.

Infertility treatment of HIV-positive couples raises many ethical considerations. Vertical transmission does occur and the WHO estimates that by the year 2000 this mode of transmission will account for 5–10 million HIV-infected children world-wide. The rate of vertical transmission has been estimated as 13% in the Western world, by the recent European Collaborative Study (1991). Higher rates have been reported (Italian multicentre Study 1988, Hira et al 1989), which may in part be explained by the different populations studied and rates of breast-feeding. Detection of HIV in utero is not practical and although there are some predictors of subsequent neonatal infection, such as advanced HIV infection in the mother and breast-feeding (European Collaborative Study 1991), a substantial risk of neonatal infection exists which cannot be reliably determined until the infant is 15–18 months old.

If a couple, in which one or both partners are HIV-infected, are seeking infertility treatment and are completely aware of the implications of their actions, do the medical staff have a right to deny investigation and treatment? If treatment is considered, is there a distinction between prescribing Clomiphene or performing tubal surgery and performing in vitro fertilization? Gynaecologists may find the first ethically more comfortable, although the aim of all procedures is conception.

If treatment is performed and is successful, is the doctor liable to the child and does the child have a case against the doctor or medical team, or indeed its parents? These issues were presented and discussed in a recent article (Smith et al 1991) prompted by a real case of a couple undergoing infertility investigations, at which time they were discovered to be HIV antibody-positive. Legally the specialist is liable to the child (a parallel being negligent obstetrical care leading to brain damage), but in this situation is not liable for the action of 'wrongful life' which may be brought by the child (Mckay 1982). Due to the natural history of HIV infection the action of a child against its parents is not a practical consideration.

The issue of risks to health care workers in treating HIV-infected couples for infertility has been raised as a reason for not providing this service (Smith et al 1991). Whilst the concern regarding occupational exposure is warranted, it should not be the determining factor in excluding patients from such investigation and treatment.

The investigation and treatment of HIV-infected couples with infertility will remain contentious and will depend not only on each individual case but also on the view taken by the attending gynaecologist and the availability of resources.

CONCLUSIONS

This chapter has highlighted the lack of information available regarding common gynaecological problems which, although not life-threatening, may cause substantial morbidity amongst HIV-infected patients, particularly if they have in addition other HIV-related problems. It appears that HIV-infected women are at increased risk of common vaginoses which are aggressive, resistant to treatment, or may require increased intervention. Clearly it is vital that all HIV-positive women have regular screening for genital infections, and that prompt and adequate treatment is instigated. Data on menstrual function are very sparse. Amenorrhoea may be more common and if long-term raises questions as to the use of hormone replacement therapy. Further prospective studies with large numbers and comparative controls are required to observe whether HIV infection is causal in disorders of menstrual function.

The dilemma surrounding the management of infertile patients known or discovered to be HIV-seropositive will not disappear but will receive further attention as the number of heterosexually infected individuals continues to rise and the natural history of HIV infection is altered by medical intervention. Clearly there is a need for gynaecologists to be both increasingly aware of conditions that present to them that may be markers for underlying HIV infection, and to be more involved in the management of known HIV-positive women to ensure that adequate gynaecological care is given.

REFERENCES

Anastos K, Deuenberg R, Solomon L, Rein S 1992 Relationship of CD4 cell counts to cervical cytologic and gynaecologic infections in 150 HIV infected women.

Proceedings of VIII International AIDS Conference, Amsterdam. Abstr no TuBO532

Bray M A, Minkoff H, Soltes B et al 1991 Human immunodeficiency virus-I infection in an infertile population. Fertil Steril 56: 16–19

Cameron D W, Simonsen J N, D'Costa J D et al 1989 Female to male transmission of human immunodeficiency virus type 1: risk factors for seroconversion in men. Lancet 2: 403–407

Cameron M L, Schell W A, Waskin H A et al 1992 Azole resistant candida albicans oesophagitis and oral candidiasis in patients with AIDS. Proceedings of VIII International AIDS Conference, Amsterdam, Abstr PUB7085

Centres for Disease Control 1991 Revised classification system for HIV infection and disease in adolescents and adults (draft) 1991: 4. In Mitchell J L, Tucker J, Loftman P O, Williams S B 1992 HIV and women: current controversies and clinical relevance. J Women's Health 1: 35–39

De Wit S, Weerts D, Goossens H, Chumeck N 1989 Comparison of fluconazole and ketoconazole for oropharyngeal candidiasis in AIDS. Lancet 1: 746–747

European Collaborative Study 1991 Children born to women with HIV-1 infection: natural history and risk of transmission. Lancet 337: 253–260

Friese K, Rossol S, Voth R, Hess G et al 1989 Epidemiological, infectiological and immunological results from the HIV-ambulance of the Dept of Obstetrics and Gynaecology. Proceedings of the Vth International Conference on AIDS, Montreal. Abstr no WDP54

Greenblatt-R M, Lukehart S A, Plummer F A et al 1988 Genital ulceration as a risk factor for human immunodeficiency virus infection. AIDS 2: 47–50

Hira S K, Kamanga J, Bhat G J et al 1989 Perinatal transmission of HIV-1 in Zambia. Br Med J 299: 1250–1252

Hoegsberg B, Abulafia O, Sedlis A et al 1990 Sexually transmitted diseases and human immunodeficiency virus infection among women with pelvic inflammatory disease. Am J Obstet Gynecol 163: 1135–1139

Iman N, Carpenter C C, Mayer K et al 1990 Hierarchical pattern of mucosal candida infection in HIV seropositive women. Am J Med 89: 142–146

Italian Multicentre Study 1988 Epidemiology, clinical features and prognostic factors of paediatric HIV infection. Lancet 2: 1043–1045

Johnstone F D, Brettle R P, MacCallum L R et al 1990 Women's knowledge of their HIV antibody state: its effect on their decision whether to continue the pregnancy. Br Med J 300: 23–24

Lang O S, Greene S I, Stevens D A 1990 Thrush can be prevented in AIDS/ARC patients: randomised double-blind placebo controlled study of 100 mg fluconazole daily. Proceedings of 6th International AIDS Conference, San Francisco. Abstr no 2165

McKay vs Essex Area Health Authority 1982 AER 771

Maiman M, Tarricone N, Vieira J et al 1991 Colposcopic evaluation of human immunodeficiency virus seropositive women. J Obstet Gynecol 78: 84–88

Matnur-Wagh V, Roche N, Stein J et al 1992 Gynaecologic findings in an HIV positive out patient population. Proceedings of VIII International AIDS Conference, Amsterdam. Abstr no PoB 3057

Patrik S, Smith R, Kitchen V et al 1992 Menstrual abnormalities in HIV seropositive women. Proceedings of the VIII International Conference on AIDS, Amsterdam. Abstr no PoB3062

Piot P, Plummer F A, Rey M et al 1987 Retrospective seroepidemiology of AIDS virus infection in Nairobi populations. J Infect Dis 155(6): 1108–1112

Rhoads J L, Wright C, Redfield R R, Burke D S 1987 Chronic vaginal candidiasis in women with human immunodeficiency virus infection. JAMA 257: 3105–3107

Rutherford G W, Lifson A R, Hessol N A et al 1990 Course of HIV-1 infection in a cohort of homosexual and bisexual men: an 11 year follow up study. Br Med J 301: 1183–8

Safrin S, Dattel B J, Hauer L, Sweet R L 1990 Seroprevalence and epidemiologic correlates of human immunodeficiency virus infection in women with acute pelvic inflammatory disease. Obstet Gynecol 75: 666–670

Selwyn P A, Carter R J, Schoenbaum E E et al 1989 Knowledge of HIV antibody status and decision to continue or terminate pregnancy among intravenous drug users. JAMA 261: 3567–3571

Smith J R, Kitchen V S, Munday P E et al 1991 Infertility management in HIV positive couples: a dilemma. Br Med J 302: 1447–1450

Sobel J D 1986 Treatment of recurrent candida vaginitis. N Engl J Med 315: 1455–1488

Stein J, Roche N, Mathur-Wagh U et al 1991 Gynecologic findings in an HIV positive out patient population. Proceedings of the VII International Conference on AIDS, Florence. Abstr no MB2427

Warne P, Ehrhardt A, Schechter D et al 1991 Menstrual abnormalities in HIV+ and HIV− women with a history of intravenous drug use. Proceedings of VII International Conference on AIDS, Florence. Abstr no MC3113

21. Particular issues for African women

J. Anderson

INTRODUCTION

HIV infection and AIDS have imposed a massive burden on the populations of many countries in sub-Saharan Africa. Throughout Africa the major route of spread of infection is heterosexual intercourse. World Health Organization (WHO) statistics suggest that sub-Saharan Africa has the highest rates for HIV infection in the world, with an overall estimate of one woman in 40 being HIV-seropositive (Chin 1990). Both HIV-1 and HIV-2 are prevalent but existing data show that the main focus of HIV-1 infection remains in East and Central Africa. In some large urban areas between one-quarter and one-third of all adults aged 15–19 years are infected. The expansion of HIV from large urban areas into more rural parts of many countries in Africa is increasing and HIV-1 is now spreading into the populations of West Africa. Data available on HIV-2 suggest that it is still largely confined to West Africa. Studies of incidence of HIV are relatively few. Those that exist suggest that incidence is higher in groups of individuals with identified high risk behaviour patterns than in whole populations (Nkowane 1991).

Although modes of transmission of HIV are the same throughout Africa, it is increasingly clear that marked differences exist in the shape of the epidemic in different countries, reflecting the diversity of the continent and its inhabitants (Piot et al 1990). The same is true for individuals from the African continent, and the differences between countries, cultures and behaviour must be explored at an individual level.

The last 20 years have seen enormous political upheaval in many African countries. The economic situation has deteriorated and this has contributed to the phenomenon of migrant labour. Civil wars and political instability have been rife. In such situations sexually transmitted diseases traditionally flourish, and HIV has been no exception. Under such circumstances people may be forced to leave their homes and seek asylum and safety or attempt to earn their livelihood. Many African countries have links with areas of Europe reflecting historical colonial association which influence the patterns of migration. Britain has far-reaching traditional links with East Africa, Belgium with Zaire and France with several West African countries. Clinicians in Europe and the USA have developed skills in relation to their own HIV epidemics over the past decade. The problems facing women from sub-Saharan Africa may be unfamiliar to physicians working in the developed world. As travel increases and the epidemic develops, there will be more people from African countries seeking care with new needs which must be addressed.

This chapter aims to address some of the issues that may be relevant to women from Africa seeking medical services, and to their clinicians in the developed world.

NATURAL HISTORY AND CLINICAL MANIFESTATIONS

The clinical manifestations associated with HIV infection are the end result of a complex blend of many factors. These include the pathogens to which an individual has been exposed, the susceptibility of the host and the possible genetic variability of different strains of HIV. Little information is available on the natural history of HIV infection in Africa but it is clear that geographical variation exists in the way the disease manifests itself. Comparison of natural history studies of HIV in Africa with those carried out in either the USA or Europe shows a shorter survival time in people with AIDS in Africa (Anzala et al 1991, Mbaga et al 1990). Such discrepancies may reflect lack of diagnostic and clinical facilities in under-developed countries with limited health care, or may be related to a different natural history. There is clear evidence for variation in HIV-1 isolates from different parts of the world. Whether this has significance for the outcome of infection is not known (Cheingson-Popov et al 1992). Both HIV-1 and HIV-2 cause immunodeficiency syndromes in Africa. There is a suggestion that HIV-2 may be a less pathogenic virus than HIV-1. Comparisons of women infected with HIV-1 with those infected with HIV-2 in the Gambia showed that, although the immune system was abnormal in those women with HIV-2 infection, the abnormalities were less than in those women infected with HIV-1 (Pepin et al 1991). The recent interest in phenotypic difference in HIV may also be relevant to the natural history of the disease (Schellekens et al 1992).

The clinical picture of AIDS in Africa is domi-nated by dermatological and gastrointestinal symptoms, in various combinations with weight loss and fevers (Kreiss & Castro 1990). In African patients, skin pathology familiar in Caucasians may appear macroscopically different, and additional, unfamiliar pathology may be present. A distinctive pruritic rash is a very common com-plaint. It is associated with a generalized papular eruption which is usually symmetrical and prefers the extremities. Histological examination shows non-specific inflammation and the pathogenesis is not clear. The condition has been reported in up to 18% of HIV-seropositive patients in Kinshasa (Colebunders et al 1987). Herpes Zoster infection (HZV) is common amongst patients from Africa and elsewhere. The occurrence of HZV in people from regions of high HIV prevalence may be the first clue to underlying infection with the virus. Colebunders and colleagues (1988) quote a 91% positive predictive value of a history of HZV in identifying HIV-infected individuals in Africa. Nail and hair pathology is also commonly reported. Hair may become depigmented and straight (Ansary et al 1989). Blue–black nail pigmentation

associated with zidovudine therapy has been docu-mented more commonly in black patients taking the drug (Groark et al 1989). It may begin with the thumb nails and be followed by other finger nails and then toe nails. Patients may be upset by nail pigmentation which is recognized as being associated with zidovudine and thus implies their HIV status. It is cited by some black patients as a reason for not taking the drug.

Chronic diarrhoea is a major symptom in African patients with HIV infection. *Cryp-tosporidium* species and *Isospora* are amongst the commonest pathogens implicated (Colebunders & Latif 1991), but in many cases no specific cause is found. Intestinal biopsies rarely identify additional pathogens, but may show a non-specific inflam-matory reaction (Conlon et al 1990).

The infections which occur in people with HIV will reflect the microbial environment to which they have been exposed during their lifetime. For those who have spent much of their lives in Africa the microbial mix will differ from that in Europe or the USA and symptoms will require other diag-nostic algorithms. Fever in such patients may be due to pathogens unrelated to immunodeficiency, such as malaria. Non-opportunistic bacterial infec-tions are commonly described in HIV-positive individuals in Africa and are responsible for con-siderable morbidity and mortality (Gilks et al 1990, Pallangyo et al 1992). *Salmonella typhi-murium* septicaemia, frequently recurrent, is a common cause of enteric fever-like illness. It has also been implicated in haematogenous osteo-myelitis, a condition that has become much more common in adults with HIV disease in Africa (Jellis 1992).

Of conventional pathogens, *Mycobacterium tuberculosis* (TB) was recognized early in the epi-demic as a major HIV-related problem in Africa (Mann et al 1986). In parts of sub-Saharan Africa at least half the adult population has been infected with TB which may reactivate as immu-nodeficiency supervenes. A study from Zaire showed an incidence of TB in HIV-seropositive women of 3.6% per year which was 30 times higher than that in seronegative women (Badi et al 1990). This is consistent with the a 4.4% incidence of active TB per year reported in HIV-seropositive people in Zambia (Wadhawan et al 1990). Chemoprophylaxis of TB in HIV-positive tuberculin skin test (PPD)-positive people with a view to reducing the incidence of active TB is the American strategy (ACET 1989). Although this may be logistically difficult to manage in countries with limited resources, it is relevant for patients from Africa who are being treated in developed countries. Atypical mycobacteria such as *M. avium intracellulare* appear infrequently in African studies in comparison to the USA and Europe (Okello et al 1990). This may be due to the fact that patients in poorer countries succumb earlier to more virulent pathogens. Care must be exercised in extrapolating to African patients receiving advanced health care in Europe.

Pneumocystis carinii pneumonia (PCP) has been one of the major infections associated with HIV in the USA and Northern Europe. In Africa, PCP seems to occur less frequently in patients with AIDS (Lucas 1989). *Cryptococcus*, however, is particularly common in many African countries and may occur in up to 12% of AIDS patients (Desmet et al 1989). A comparison of opportunistic infections in patients from Africa and Belgium, all of whom were investigated in Belgium, showed significantly less PCP and cerebral toxoplasmosis in patients from Africa but higher frequency of cryptococcal meningitis and severe mucocutaneous herpes virus (Taelman et al 1988). Cytomegalovirus retinitis, another common clinical problem in the USA and Europe, is much less frequently seen in Africa. In Kinshasa the incidence in one series was 4% (Kawe et al 1990). However, the prevalence of antibodies to CMV has been shown to be similar in African and American patients with AIDS (Quinn et al 1987). The observed clinical difference may reflect the fact that patients in Africa succumb to the earlier manifestations of immunosuppression prior to the development of retinitis.

In many African countries the incidence of sexually transmitted diseases (STDs) is high. Infections associated with genital ulceration, particularly chancroid, are more common than in Europe (Nsanze et al 1981). Pelvic inflammatory disease is one of the commonest causes of admission to gynaecology wards in some African hospitals (Muir & Belsey 1980). The interrelationships between HIV and other STDs are

complex (Laga et al 1991), but in practical terms the sexually transmitted nature of HIV means that all women with HIV infection should be screened for coexisting STD and appropriate treatment initiated.

Kaposi's sarcoma has been strongly associated with HIV infection in the USA and Europe, especially in homosexual men. The incidence in women with HIV in developed countries has been very low. In Africa Kaposi's sarcoma has been well described long before the AIDS era (Taylor et al 1971). Before AIDS, African Kaposi's sarcoma occurred in a male to female ratio of 10 : 1. More aggressive disease, however, was noted to be more frequent in women than men (Kyalwazi 1981). Data from the Uganda Cancer Institute show a dramatic decrease in the male to female ratio from 14 : 1 in 1964–1968 to 4 : 1 in 1988–1990. Clinically diagnosed Kaposi's sarcoma in women with HIV infection in Malawi has increased dramatically from 1983 to 1986, and the male to female ratio has changed from 10 : 1 to 3 : 1 (Desmond-Hellmann & Katongole-Mbidde 1991). Kaposi's sarcoma must be considered in the differential diagnosis in women from Africa.

Despite the increased incidence of lymphoma in patients with HIV reported from Europe and the USA, no excess of lymphoma has been reported from African HIV-infected patients. Epstein-Barr virus (EBV), which is considered important in the aetiology of HIV-related adult lymphoma, is also implicated in African Burkitt's lymphoma. There is, however, no indication that Burkitt's lymphoma is any more prevalent in people with HIV infection in Africa (Lucas 1989).

LABORATORY MARKERS

In Britain increasing use is made of laboratory markers to inform prognosis and management, especially in people with asymptomatic infection. CD4 lymphocytes have been shown to have predictive value in assessing prognosis (Phillips et al 1992). As such investigations are costly and require sophisticated laboratory facilities, few data exist on CD4 counts from Africa in people with HIV infection. There is some evidence that expression of the T4 epitope shows some heterogeneity in black people (Tollerud et al 1990) which may influence the numbers of CD4 lymphocytes that are estimated during counting procedures. Further data are needed on the ranges of CD4 counts in women of African origin to help interpret the observed results.

P24 antigenaemia bears little relationship to the course of HIV disease in African patients. It is frequently absent, even in very advanced stages of infection (Brown et al 1991). Clinicians must be alert to the limitations of such tests in African women.

ISSUES FOR AFRICAN WOMEN IN DEVELOPED COUNTRIES

People who have lived in areas of Africa in which HIV is prevalent may have seen many, including some members of their own families, desperately sick and dying of AIDS. The possibilities for early diagnosis and intervention are few. As a consequence it is difficult for people to entertain the idea of asymptomatic HIV infection. The possibility of remaining physically well for long periods of time whilst being infected with HIV may be difficult to grasp. This will colour the way in which people react to the fact of being HIV-positive.

The perception of hospital care may also be very different from the European view. In countries with limited resources people may only seek hospital care in the final stages of disease. Admission to hospital may be presumed to inevitably herald death and may be partly responsible for some women's reluctance to be investigated. In a number of African hospitals friends and relatives are involved in the care of inpatients, providing food and performing many of the basic nursing duties. The Western hospital system may seem alien in comparison. The health services may not be easy to negotiate and women may feel uncomfortable about attending clinics for sexually transmitted disease.

Traditional medicines are frequently used for many conditions throughout Africa and HIV is no exception. Women may use a wide variety of preparations and it is important that doctors are aware of compounds that may be used.

HIV and AIDS in Africa, as in other parts of the world, are often associated with promiscuity and the use of prostitutes. Perceived immorality is attached firmly to these areas and the potential for stigmatization and discrimination is great. Many women from African countries who are HIV-seropositive feel this potential very keenly, both from within their own community and from the wider world. As a consequence, women may be very reluctant to reveal their diagnosis which makes support networks difficult to establish. Unlike some of the active patient groups that have traditionally provided strong advocacy for people with HIV and AIDS, the voice of these women is not often heard. Even the possibility of meeting other people from their own community may make women reluctant to attend clinics. Anxiety also concerns the possibility of information being relayed back to family or friends in Africa and the stigmatizing impact that could have. Thus for many reasons women may be unable to make use of such support and benefits that may be available.

Many East African women are in Britain as political refugees. Some have experienced highly traumatic events in their own country associated with war and violence, some of which may be very painful to discuss but which may have left deep scars. Family and friends have often been left behind in very difficult circumstances. There may be anxiety that various official bodies will be made aware of the woman's HIV status and thus bias her chances of staying in Britain. She may be waiting rulings on her immigration status and be faced with uncertainty about her future. Accommodation may be unsatisfactory if in temporary housing awaiting relocation. Financial worries can be considerable.

Language barriers may exist for African women, especially those from Francophone countries who are in the USA or Britain. Even for those from English-speaking countries, there may be difficulties. Finding suitable translators may not be easy, given the reluctance of many women to discuss either their HIV status or sexual matters with others.

Issues of pregnancy and child care are complex. Many women already have children. Some children may be with their mother, but others may still be in Africa with other family members and the woman may not know exactly where or how they are. The HIV status of the children may not be known and may be another source of anxiety for the mother. In some cases the first member of the family to fall ill may be the child, and knowledge of the woman's HIV status follows from the diagnosis of the child. Hospital services for HIV and AIDS in the USA and Europe have been largely utilized by young, single men and are not always easy for women and children to use. Finding regular carers for children when the mother has to spend time in hospital is vital. Women often prefer that their diagnosis is not made known to people involved in caring for their children. Helping to plan for children after the mother's death may need to encompass the wishes for children to return to the paternal extended family which has traditional responsibility.

For women who do not have children the issues of pregnancy need consideration. In many African cultures, fertility and child-bearing are crucial for the credibility of adult women in society. HIV infection poses fundamental questions for women about their present and future roles. Continued fertility may be perceived as essential for the continuation of a relationship. Data from Nairobi (Temmerman et al 1990) show that only a small proportion of HIV-infected women had informed their male partner of their serostatus and there was low use of barrier contraception.

It is important to remember that not all HIV-positive women from sub-Saharan Africa acquired their infection in Africa. Any woman who is having unprotected intercourse is at risk of acquiring HIV. African women may choose partners in Europe who have also come from high seroprevalence countries themselves and so may already be seropositive. Women need information on prevention of infection. A study of sexual behaviour in Ugandan university students showed that only a very small minority used condoms despite good knowledge of risks of HIV transmission and multiple sexual partners (Lule & Gruer 1991). Barriers to condom use have been identified in a number of African countries. These include their association with prostitution, sexually transmitted diseases and AIDS. Women are often powerless to insist on condom usage (Lamptey & Goodridge 1991)

Access to appropriate medical care and health education is crucial for all women who may have been exposed to HIV infection. For women from sub-Saharan Africa the need may be greater whilst the ability to access services may be less for reasons already discussed.

Information needs to be available in an accessible format and to be located in areas that women will visit in their day-to-day life. Confidentiality must be guaranteed. A balance must be struck between meeting the potentially considerable needs of women from Africa and allowing HIV to dominate the medical agenda.

REFERENCES

Advisory Committee for the Elimination of Tuberculosis 1989 Tuberculosis and human immunodeficiency virus infection: recommendations of the advisory committee for the elimination of tuberculosis. MMWR 38: 236–250

Ansary M A, Hira S K, Bayley A C et al 1989 A colour atlas of AIDS in the tropics. Wolfe Medical Publications, London, p28–54

Anzala A, Wambugu P, Plummer F A et al 1991 Incubation time to symptomatic disease and AIDS in women with known duration of infection. VII International Conference on AIDS, Florence. Abstr TuC 103

Badi N, Braun M, Ryder R et al 1990 A retrospective cohort study of the incidence of tuberculosis among child bearing women with HIV infection in Kinshasa Zaire. VI International Conference on AIDS, San Francisco. Abstr ThB 485

Brown C, Kline R, Atibu L et al 1991 Prevalence of HIV 1 p24 antigenaemia in African and North American populations and correlation with clinical status AIDS 5: 89–92

Cheingsong-Popov R, Callow D, Beddow S et al 1992 Geographic diversity of human immunodeficiency virus type 1: serologic reactivity to env epitopes and relationship to neutralisation. J Infect Dis 165: 256–261

Chin J 1990 Global estimates of AIDS cases and HIV infections. AIDS 4 (suppl 1): s277–283

Colebunders R, Mann J M, Francis H et al 1987 Generalised papular pruritic eruption in African patients with human immunodeficiency virus infection. AIDS 1: 117–121

Colebunders R, Mann J M, Francis H et al 1988 Herpes zoster and HIV infection in Africa. J Infect Dis 157: 314–318

Colebunders R L, Latif A S 1991 Natural history and clinical presentation of HIV infection in adults. AIDS 5 (suppl 1): s103–112

Conlon C P, Pinching A J, Perera C U et al 1990 HIV related enteropathy in Lusaka, Zambia: a clinical and histological study. Am J Trop Med Hyg 42: 83–88

Desmet P, Kayembe K D, De Vroey C 1989 The value of cryptococcal serum antigen screening among HIV positive/AIDS patients in Kinshasa Zaire. AIDS 3: 77–78

Desmond-Hellman S D, Katongole-Mbidde E 1991 Kaposi's sarcoma: recent developments. Aids 5(suppl 1): s135–142

Gilks C F, Brindle R J, Otieno L S 1990 Life threatening bacteraemia in HIV-1 seropositive adults admitted to hospital in Nairobi, Kenya. Lancet 336: 545–549

Groark S P, Hood A F, Nelson K 1989 Nail pigmentation associated with zidovudine therapy. J Am Acad Dermatol 21: 1032–1033

Jellis J E 1992 Haematogenous osteomyelitis. Surgery 10: 145–148

Kawe L W, Renard G, Le-Hoang P et al 1990 Manifestations ophtalmolgiques du SIDA en milieu Africain. A propos de 45 cas. J Fr Ophtalmol 13: 199–204

Kreiss J K, Castro K G 1990 Special considerations for managing suspected human immunodeficiency virus infection and AIDS in patients from developing countries. J. Infect. Dis. 162: 955–960

Kyalwazi S K 1981 Kaposi's sarcoma: clinical features experience in Uganda. Antibiot Chemother 29: 59–67

Laga M, Nzila N, Goeman J 1991 The interrelationship of sexually transmitted diseases and HIV infection: implications for the control of both epidemics in Africa. AIDS 5 (suppl 1): s55–63

Lamptey P, Goodridge G A W 1991 Condom issues in AIDS prevention in Africa. AIDS 5 (suppl 1): S183–191

Lucas S 1989 Missing infections in AIDS, Trans R Soc Trop Med Hyg 84 (S1): 34–53

Lule G S, Gruer L D 1991 Sexual behaviour and use of the condom among Ugandan students. Aids Care 3: 11–19

Mann J, Snider D E, Francis H et al 1986 Association between HTLV-iii/LAV infection and tuberculosis in Zaire. JAMA 256: 346

Mbaga J M, Pallangyo K J, Bakari M et al 1990 Survival time of patients with acquired immunodeficiency syndrome: experience in Dar es Salaam. E Afr Med J 67: 95–99

Muir D G, Belsey M A 1980 Pelvic inflammatory disease in the developing world. Am J Obstet Gynecol 138: 913–928

Nkowane B M 1991 Prevalence and incidence of HIV infection in Africa: a review of data published in 1990. AIDS 5 (suppl 1): s7–15

Nsanze H, Fast M V, D'Costa L J et al 1981 Genital ulcers in Kenya. Clinical and laboratory study. Br J Vener Dis 57: 378–381

Okello D O, Serwankambo N, Goodgame R et al 1990 Absence of bacteremia with Mycobacterium avium-intracellulare in Ugandan patients with AIDS. J Infect Dis 162: 208–210

Pallangyo K, Hakanson A, Lema L et al 1992 High HIV seroprevalence and increased HIV associated mortality among hospitalized patients with deep bacterial infections in Dar es Salaam, Tanzania. AIDS 6: 971–976

Pepin J, Morgan G, Dunn D et al 1991 HIV-2 induced immunosuppression among asymptomatic West African prostitutes: evidence that HIV 2 is pathogenic but less so than HIV 1. AIDS 5: 1165–1172

Phillips A N, Lee C A, Elford J et al 1992 The cumulative risk of AIDS as the CD4 lymphocyte count declines. J Acq Immune Defic Synd 5: 148–152

Piot P, Laga M, Ryder R et al 1990 The global epidemiology of HIV infection: continuity, heterogeneity and change. J Acq Immune Defic Synd 3: 401–412

Quinn T C, Piot P, McCormick J B et al 1987 Serologic and immunologic studies in patients with AIDS in North America and Africa. JAMA 257: 2617–2621

Schellekens P T, Tersmette M, Roos M L et al 1992 Biphasic rate of CD4 cell count decline during progression to AIDS correlates with HIV-1 phenotype. AIDS 6: 665–669

Taelman H, Clumeck N, Sonnet J et al 1988 Frequency of occurrence of opportunistic diseases among African and European AIDS patients diagnosed in Belgium. IV International Conference on AIDS, Stockholm. Abstr 5550

Taylor J F, Templeton A C, Vogel C L et al 1971 Kaposi's sarcoma in Uganda: a clinico pathological study. Int J Cancer 8: 122–135

Temmerman M, Moses S, Kiragu D et al 1990 Impact of a single session post partum counselling of HIV infected women on their subsequent reproductive behavior. AIDS Care 2: 247–251

Tollerud D J, Clark J W, Morris Brown L et al 1989 The influence of age, race and gender on peripheral blood mononuclear cell subsets in healthy non smokers. J Clin Immunol 9: 214–222

Wadhawan D, Hira S, Mwansa N et al 1990 Isoniazid prophylaxis among patients with HIV infection. VI International Conference on AIDS, San Francisco. Abstr ThB510

22. Nosocomial infection and infection control procedures

Anne Cockcroft

INTRODUCTION

Women with HIV infection will come into contact with health services in a number of ways: for diagnosis and monitoring; during pregnancy and labour in some cases; for treatment of HIV-related illness; and for treatment of unrelated conditions. Whenever HIV-infected people have clinical contact with health care workers, issues about the risk of transmission of infection will arise and must be addressed to ensure that they do not compromise the quality of care given. The author's experience is that it is not possible to talk to health care workers about the care of people with HIV infection without considering their own concerns about contracting the infection and discussing methods by which risks of occupational transmission can be minimized.

Women without HIV infection who come into contact with the health services may also have concerns about their risks of contracting infection either from other patients or from their carers. On the other hand, it is sometimes argued that the taking of precautions against infection by health care workers may be unwelcome, for example to women in labour, because it may make the experience more clinical and impersonal.

The majority of health care workers are women, including nurses, midwives, doctors, paramedical workers and ancillary workers. Their concerns about the occupational risk of infection often extend beyond themselves to their spouses and children. Women with HIV infection, however acquired, may themselves be health care workers. They will have to face possible limitations of practice because of the potential for transmission of their infection to patients, as well as risks to their own health from other infections encountered at work.

This chapter is about the risks and prevention of transmission of HIV infection in the health care setting. It reviews the data about the magnitude of the risk of occupational HIV transmission. This is followed by a discussion of the approaches to infection control for HIV infection, including the management of accidental exposures to blood. Finally, the issues concerning HIV-infected health care workers are considered.

OCCUPATIONAL TRANSMISSION OF HIV

Reports of occupational transmission

Seroconversion for HIV has been documented following injuries with needles contaminated with HIV-infected blood; the first published report was in 1984 (Anonymous 1984) and there has been a steady flow of reports since then. Table 22.1 gives a summary of reports of occupational acquisition

Table 22.1 Occupationally acquired HIV infection – documented cases to October 1992. Data from: Porter K, Heptonstall J, Gill O N 1992 Summary of published reports of occupational transmission of HIV. Internal publication of Public Health Laboratory Service, Colindale, London, October

	USA	Rest of world	Total
Seroconversion documented after specific exposure incident	31	20	51
Presumptive occupational source; no lifestyle risks identified	65	26	91
Homecare transmissions	1	3	4
Total	97	49	146

of HIV to October 1992 (Porter et al 1992). The majority of occupational seroconversions have followed needle-stick or other sharps injuries, but there have been documented seroconversions following contamination of broken skin and mucous membranes with infected blood (Centers for Disease Control 1987a, Gioannini et al 1988). It is not certain that all the presumptive cases in Table 22.1 were actually occupationally acquired; most of the health care workers concerned recalled a number of percutaneous blood exposures, some of which probably involved HIV-infected blood. A recent update from the Centers for Disease Control (1992) in the USA noted that up to September 30 1992, they had received reports of 32 documented occupational HIV infections among health care workers and a further 69 with possibly occupational infection. Of those with documented occupational infection, 84% had percutaneous exposure, 13% had mucocutaneous exposure and 3% had both. Nearly all (30) had been exposed to HIV-infected blood. Seven (22%) have subsequently developed AIDS. Of the 69 workers with possibly occupational infection, four had exposures to HIV-infected blood or laboratory material. AIDS has developed in 54 (78%) of them.

Published and officially reported cases of occupational HIV infection are very likely to be an underestimate of the true number world-wide, but nevertheless the number is small in relation to the large number of clinical contacts between health care workers and HIV-infected people.

The risk of occupational HIV transmission

Risk from a single exposure

There have been a number of large follow-up studies of health care workers who have sustained accidental exposures to HIV-infected blood. These are summarized by Porter and colleagues (1992). Among the total of 2629 in these series who sustained needle-stick injuries, there were 10 HIV infections, seven of these with documented seroconversions: a rate of 0.38% (95% confidence interval 0.18–0.70%). In these follow-up studies, no seroconversions occurred among the 538 health care workers who had 921 non-parenteral

exposures to HIV-infected blood (the upper limit of the 95% confidence interval for the transmission risk is calculated as 0.33%); the magnitude of the risk from such exposures is therefore not certain but it seems to be substantially less than after parenteral exposure.

Although there is little direct evidence, it seems likely that contact with other body fluids that are blood-stained also carries some risk of HIV transmission. And the virus is present in other body fluids to a level that implies that transmission could occur after inoculation injury or mucous membrane contact. These include: cerebrospinal, peritoneal, pericardial, pleural, synovial and amniotic fluid; and semen and vaginal secretions (Centers for Disease Control 1989, UK Health Departments 1990). There is no evidence for faeco-oral or airborne spread of HIV, nor for transmission by non-blood-stained saliva (UK Health Departments 1990). Although HIV has been found in the vapours of surgical power instruments (Johnson & Robinson 1990), the experimental model used has been criticized (Joint Working Party of the Hospital Infection Society and the Surgical Infection Study Group 1992) and there is no evidence of transmission by this route.

The risk of an individual health care worker contracting HIV infection occupationally depends not only upon the risk from a single exposure incident, but also upon the frequency of such exposures and the HIV seroprevalence in the patient population.

Frequency of needle-stick injuries and other blood exposures

Health care workers are frequently exposed to blood during their work, either directly or indirectly. Collins and Kennedy (1987) have reviewed a number of studies of the rates of needle-stick injuries among groups of health care workers, comparing the results in terms of injuries per 100 employee years. The different studies reviewed gave widely differing rates of injuries. Nurses appear to suffer the highest number of injuries, even allowing for the number of nurses employed. Other groups at risk of injury include domestic and portering staff, who risk injury from needles and other sharps not disposed of safely, and laboratory staff. Relatively few injuries in the reported studies were to doctors.

A difficulty with interpreting studies of routinely reported needle-stick injuries is the considerable under-reporting of such injuries, especially among doctors. Astbury and Baxter (1990) found a 5% reporting rate of sharps injuries among hospital staff and McGeer and associates (1990) found that less than 5% of sharps injuries were reported by medical students, interns and residents. In a recent study (Williams et al 1993) of 158 staff in an operating theatre (including doctors, nurses and operating department assistants), staff were asked how many injuries they had sustained in the last month and how many of these they had reported. Among the 119 who answered the question, a total of 26 sharps injuries had been sustained by 14 staff and a further 240 non-sharps blood exposures by 44 staff. Four of the sharps injuries had been reported (15%) and none of the other blood exposures. In this case the reporting rate did not differ between the doctors and others.

The problem of under-reporting can be overcome by questionnaire and observational studies and a number of these have been reported in recent years. Lowenfels and colleagues (1989) reported a median rate of puncture injuries among surgeons in New York, contacted by letter or telephone, of 4.2 per 1000 operating room hours, with 25% of the surgeons having injury rates of 9 or more per 1000 operating room hours. Hussain and co-workers (1988) asked 18 surgeons in Saudi Arabia to record all accidental injuries during surgery and reported that sharps injuries occurred in 5.6% of operations. Injuries were recorded by operating theatre staff in Glasgow at a rate of 1.6% per surgeon per operation, calculated to give 4.6% per operation overall (Camilleri et al 1991).

An observational study of 1307 surgical procedures at San Francisco General Hospital revealed accidental blood exposures in 6.4% of procedures and parenteral exposure to blood in 1.7%. The risk of blood exposure was highest for procedures lasting more than 3 hours, when blood loss exceeded 300 ml, and for major vascular and gynaecological procedures (Gerberding et al 1990). In a similar study of 206 procedures in Atlanta, blood exposures were observed in 30% of procedures, with percutaneous exposure in 4.9%

(Panlilio et al 1991). A prospective observational study of 1382 surgical procedures in four hospitals in the USA noted sharps injuries in 6.9% of procedures (Tokars et al 1991); the highest rate of injury was in gynaecology (10%). The high injury rate in gynaecology is probably related to the nature of the surgical procedures in this speciality, with the hands often incompletely visible in a confined space deep in the body cavity. Within specialities, there is variation between surgeons, with some sustaining far more injuries than others (Lowenfels et al 1989); this is thought to be related to individual technique.

Some studies have used glove perforations as an index of risk of skin contamination or potential sharps injury during surgery. Perforation of gloves is very common if specifically sought after a procedure. Perforation rates of between 11 and 48% have been reported among surgeons (Matta et al 1988, Brough et al 1988). A study of obstetrical and gynaecological operative procedures involving sharp instruments reported a glove perforation rate of around 30% (Doyle et al 1992).

Blood contamination of the skin or mucous membranes during surgical and emergency procedures is even more common than sharps injuries. A study in an accident and emergency department confirmed a high rate of skin and clothing contamination with blood, despite a policy of using barrier precautions for all patients (Littlechild et al 1992). A study of 226 doctors and midwives examined after undertaking or assisting at procedures in the labour suite (Kabukoba & Young 1992) identified blood or body fluid contamination of the hands, arms or face in 42%; it was also noted that 23% of the staff had broken skin and this was contaminated with blood in some cases.

Cumulative risk of occupational HIV infection

Despite the low risk of infection associated with accidental inoculation of HIV-infected blood, surgeons and others with blood and body fluid contact remain concerned about their risk of HIV infection (Shelley & Howard 1992, Gallop et al 1992). This is partly because there is a repeated risk of exposure to blood that may be infected with HIV. It is possible to calculate a figure for the cumulative risk of occupational HIV infection based on the risk from a single infected needle-stick, the seroprevalence of HIV in the patient population and the rate of needle-stick injuries. In New York, with an estimated patient HIV seroprevalence of 5%, it was estimated that the 30-year risk of HIV seroconversion among surgeons was less than 1% for 50% of the surgeons, but up to 6% for a subgroup of 10% of the surgeons with very frequent needle-stick injuries (Lowenfels et al 1989). In Amsterdam, with a lower estimated HIV seroprevalence of 0.2% among the patients, the 30-year risk of HIV seroconversion among surgeons was calculated to be 0.1% (Leentvaar-Kuijpers et al 1990). It should be remembered that these are only theoretical calculations and may be quite inaccurate. For example, the seroconversion risk after a single HIV-infected needle-stick may be lower in surgery since the seroconversions in the prospective studies were all following needle-sticks with hollow needles and most of the surgical injuries are with solid needles. It is likely that the volume of blood transferred via a solid needle injury (especially through gloves) is smaller than that transferred via a hollow needle and therefore the seroconversion risk will be lower; direct data to demonstrate this are lacking and will be difficult to accrue because the seroconversion rate is in any case so low (Royal College of Pathologists Working Group 1992).

Studies of groups of health care workers have not indicated that they have an excess risk of HIV infection. A study in a hospital in Kinshasa reported a 3% cumulative incidence over 2 years of HIV infection among the staff and concluded that this was representative of transmission in the community rather than occupational infection; this was despite poor facilities and a seroprevalence among patients of 6% in the delivery room and 39% on the female medical ward (N'Galy et al 1990). In a recent study (Centers for Disease Control 1991a), 7121 orthopaedic surgeons attending a conference in the USA were invited to be tested for HIV antibodies. Of the 3420 participants, only two were seropositive and both of these reported non-occupational risk factors. Half of the participants had operated on at least one patient known to be infected with HIV and 39% had sustained one or more needle-stick injuries during the last month. A survey of 1132 dentists

in the USA detected only one HIV-infected dentist in whom the infection might have been occupationally acquired (Klein et al 1988).

Any excess of HIV infection in an occupational group should eventually lead to an excess of people from that group with no other risk factors amongst cases of AIDS; there is no evidence of this among health care workers. Health care workers among reported cases of AIDS in the USA are not over-represented and there are not large numbers with no other apparent risk factors (Chamberland et al 1991). In France, it has been noted that there were 392 health care workers among the 14 449 AIDS cases reported up to March 1991 (Lot et al 1991). There was a non-occupational risk in 364 of the health care workers; it was thought that occupational exposure could have been the cause of infection in six of the other 26 without major risk factors. Only one had had a specific exposure with serological follow-up.

PREVENTION OF OCCUPATIONAL TRANSMISSION OF HIV

Prevention of occupational transmission of HIV depends primarily upon protecting health care workers against needle-stick injuries and other exposures to infected blood. There are two different approaches to this problem; to be effective both will require additional attention to risk reduction of procedures in the future. The question of post-exposure prophylaxis against HIV infection also needs to be considered.

General approaches to infection control for HIV infection

There are two general approaches to safe practice with regard to prevention of transmission of HIV and other blood-borne viruses: the 'traditional' infection control approach and the more recent universal precautions approach. In the traditional approach, patients or specimens known or suspected to be infected are identified and special precautions are taken in their care or processing. This approach has been advocated for reducing the risk of transmission of hepatitis B in the era before immunization became available (Hansen et al 1981) and continues to be recommended by some authorities in relation to both HIV and hepatitis B infection in laboratories (Advisory Committee on Dangerous Pathogens 1990, Health Services Advisory Committee 1991) and in operating theatres (Royal College of Surgeons of England 1990). Other official guidance in both the USA and the UK favours the universal precautions approach (Centers for Disease Control 1985, 1987b, 1988, UK Health Departments 1990). Professional bodies representing surgical specialties are moving towards recommending universal precautions, although still suggesting additional precautions for 'high risk' patients (Royal College of Obstetricians and Gynaecologists 1990, British Orthopaedic Association 1991). Recently published guidelines for staff in operating theatres (Joint Working Party of the Hospital Infection Society and the Surgical Infection Study Group 1992) take an intermediate view, recommending universal precautions in areas of high HIV seroprevalence and for certain emergency procedures but selective precautions for HIV-infected and 'high risk' patients in areas with low HIV seroprevalence.

The concept of universal precautions arose mainly as a result of the HIV epidemic and is based on the premise that patients with blood-borne infections cannot be reliably identified on the basis of their histories, so that the blood of all patients should be treated as potentially infectious; the level of precautions to be taken should depend upon a risk assessment of the procedures being undertaken rather than of the patient's infection status.

The arguments for the two approaches in relation to HIV infection have been rehearsed recently (Shanson & Cockcroft 1991). Those in favour of the selective approach argue that health care workers have a right to 'know what they are dealing with' so that they can protect themselves appropriately. It is also argued that financial constraints mean that a high level of protection can only be afforded in some cases and therefore those cases where it is necessary should be identified. A universal high standard of protection is not considered justified except in areas with a high seroprevalence of hepatitis B or HIV.

But there are difficulties with a selective approach. Identification of patients infected with HIV or hepatitis B on the basis of history is not reliable (Gordin et al 1990, Parry et al 1991). Anonymous testing of pregnant women in inner London health districts in 1990 has detected HIV infection in 0.44% (Banatvala et al 1991) and 0.32% (Chamberlain et al 1991). In both these studies most of the HIV infections were unknown to the staff caring for the women. Reliable identification of HIV-infected patients requires screening which is expensive and may divert money away from safer equipment and protective clothing. In areas of low seroprevalence of HIV and hepatitis B a screening programme would not be efficient, and in areas of high prevalence, treating all patients as infected is sensible. Awaiting test results is not feasible in emergency situations, the very situations in which exposure to blood is most likely.

Knowledge of patients' 'high risk' status does not necessarily reduce the risk of blood exposures during surgical procedures. Gerberding and associates (1990) found no difference in the rate of blood exposures overall, or in sharps injuries specifically, between known or suspected 'high risk' patients and others. In another study (Tokars et al 1991) there was a lower rate of blood exposures during surgery in identified 'high risk' patients but the numbers were small and the difference could well have occurred by chance. In the operating department at San Francisco General Hospital (Gerberding et al 1990), universal precautions were already being practised to a large extent so that it is clear that this approach is also not sufficient to prevent needle-stick injuries and other blood exposures during surgery. There is, however, evidence that practising universal (barrier) precautions reduces the frequency of non-parenteral blood exposures among trained health care workers (Fahey et al 1991); more effective barrier precautions in the labour suite have been called for (Kabukoba & Young 1992).

Several authors have reported that health care workers do not practise universal precautions even when it is official policy to do so (Baraff & Talan 1989, Kelen et al 1990). Reasons given included lack of time, a feeling that the protective clothing interfered with skilful performance of tasks and complaints that the materials were uncomfortable. In obstetrical practice, there is concern that women may object to staff wearing gowns, gloves, masks and eye protection during the natural process of childbirth. Prior discussion of these precautions and the reasons for them are clearly important. In a recent study, a majority of clinical medical students and consultants at a London hospital reported changing their clinical practice – mainly by wearing gloves and by taking care with needles – if they knew a patient was infected with HIV (Elford & Cockcroft 1991). A substantial proportion were in favour of compulsory HIV testing of patients, although this was not the practice in the hospital.

A major criticism of universal precautions is that they are expensive. However, the increased expense may not be as great as feared. The term 'universal' is misleading, suggesting the same level of precautions for every procedure. The basis of the universal precautions approach should be a risk assessment of procedures, with the level of precautions set accordingly. This can allow scarce resources to be used most effectively, with protective equipment reserved for those procedures in which it is really needed. It will avoid events such as washing down the walls of an operating theatre after a non-bloody lymph node biopsy, simply because the patient was infected with HIV.

Risk assessment and risk reduction

Whether selective or universal precautions are applied, it is necessary to consider the risks, especially of percutaneous blood exposures, in different procedures so that effective preventive action can be taken. This approach of risk assessment and risk reduction is in line with modern UK and European health and safety legislation. For example, the Control of Substances Hazardous to Health (COSHH) regulations (Health and Safety Commission 1988) require employers to assess the risk to health of employees from hazardous substances (including microbiological hazards) and to reduce the risk so far as is reasonably practicable.

Reducing the risk of sharps injuries and other blood exposures will require detailed investigation of how such incidents occur and then changes of procedures, equipment and techniques. Studies of reported incidents can help. McKinnon et al (1992) investigated a series of sharps injuries in detail and considered that pressure of work, poor

physical environment and not using correct techniques had most commonly contributed to the injuries. General guidelines for surgical practice to reduce the risk of needle-stick injuries to operators and assistants have been produced (Joint Working Party of the Hospital Infection Society and the Surgical Infection Study Group 1992). Future improvements in safe practice will require the active involvement of specialists in each field, so that feasible changes to techniques and equipment can be debated and implemented. The sorts of questions to be posed for reducing sharps injuries within a speciality include:

- Is it essential to use a sharp instrument for this procedure?
  — Can a different procedure without sharps do the job?
  — Can drugs be given by mouth etc. rather than injected?
  — Can lasers, blunt needles etc. be used?
- What evidence is there of sharps injuries in this procedure?
- Are there specific safe ways to use the sharp instrument?
  — Are they generally agreed?
  — Are juniors trained in these safe techniques?
  — Should new techniques be developed and tested?
- Is a new instrument design necessary?
- Is the user responsible for safe disposal of sharps?
- Are the sharps collection boxes suitable and conveniently placed?
- Is the system for collecting sharps containers satisfactory?
- Is the work environment satisfactory (lighting, space, noise, location of equipment, etc.)?
- What are the arrangements for investigating sharps injuries?
  — Is there encouragement to report injuries?
  — Are figures for types of injuries kept and reviewed?
  — Are injuries monitored to assess the effect of changes?

Management of blood exposure incidents

Despite all efforts to reduce the risk of needle-stick injuries and other exposures to blood at work, incidents of exposure will continue to occur. Although, as discussed above, the risk of HIV transmission from accidental blood exposures is very low, they are nevertheless a source of great anxiety to the staff involved. Psychological morbidity after blood exposures can be serious, especially if the source patient is known to be infected with HIV, and requires appropriate management from a knowledgeable and sympathetic team (Gerberding & Henderson 1992). After a significant blood exposure, it is officially recommended that the source patient should be approached and tested, with consent, for bloodborne viruses including HIV and hepatitis B (Centers for Disease Control 1989, UK Health Departments 1990). A negative result can be very reassuring for the health care worker involved. However, reviews in both the USA (Miller & Farr 1989) and the UK (Oakley et al 1992) have found that source patients are not always tested for HIV, even when it is policy to approach them. Both reviews found that logistic difficulties were the main reason for not testing source patients; it was rare for patients to refuse testing in these circumstances (Oakley et al 1992). Sometimes the clinical team responsible for the source patient may decline to approach the patient; in the UK review this was especially the case for obstetrical patients, but improved over time (Oakley K personal communication 1992).

If the source patient is HIV-positive, follow-up blood tests on the health care worker are appropriate to confirm that seroconversion has not occurred. Testing at 0, six weeks, 3 months and 6 months is a common schedule (Gerberding & Henderson 1992). The issue of postexposure prophylaxis with zidovudine arises. There is some animal evidence to suggest that zidovudine, given soon after inoculation of virus, may delay or prevent seroconversion (Ruprecht et al 1986, Tavares et al 1987) but the evidence from primates is not encouraging (Jeffries 1991). Nevertheless, it has been suggested that zidovudine should be made available to health care workers within 1 hour of an accidental inoculation of HIV-infected blood (Jeffries 1991); this has caused some consternation among occupational health specialists (Tamin et al 1991, Brown et al 1991). There are several case reports of failure of zidovudine to prevent HIV seroconversion after occupational exposure incidents (Lange et al 1990, Looke & Grove 1990, Darond et al 1991, Tait et al 1991, Jones 1991). It would require a massive study to establish whether zidovudine further reduces the low risk of seroconversion after needle-stick exposure to HIV; such a study will not be feasible. Official opinion in the USA is that zidovudine cannot 'be considered a necessary part of post exposure management' (Centers for Disease Control 1990). Similar conclusions have been reached in the UK (Consumers Association 1991, UK Health Departments 1992).

The evidence does not suggest that staff should be particularly encouraged to use zidovudine after an occupational exposure to HIV but, nevertheless, it seems reasonable to give staff the opportunity to take it if they wish. Some authors have suggested the provision of 'first dose' packs in clinical and laboratory areas (Joint Working Party of the Hospital Infection Society and the Surgical Infection Study Group 1992), but it is generally agreed that the decision to continue with prophylaxis should be taken after full discussion with a knowledgeable person, either the occupational physician or some other suitable professional. The experience in the author's hospital is that staff have decided not to take zidovudine (Oakley et al 1992); one common reason given was that they did not want to be reminded of the incident every few hours for the coming weeks. This problem was one of the reasons given for stopping zidovudine after 5 days in a recent personal account (Dobson 1992).

Management of blood exposures in relation to HIV infection is facilitated if there is a recognized protocol; this can also be explained to staff before they are involved in incidents so that they will know what to expect and can think about decisions, such as whether to take zidovudine, in advance. The protocol used in the author's hospital is shown in Figure 22.1.

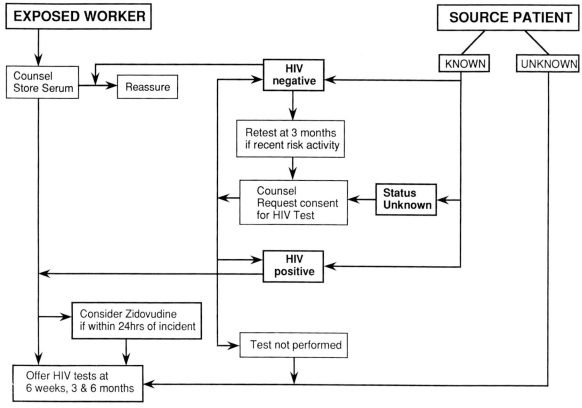

Figure 22.1   Management of accidental blood exposures in the health care setting. The procedures in relation to the risk of HIV transmission are shown; in practice, procedures for the risk of hepatitis B transmission are also applied. Source: Cockcroft A, Williams S 1993 Occupational transmission of HIV and management of accidental blood exposures. Medicine International 21: 38–40

HIV-INFECTED HEALTH CARE WORKERS

Risk of transmission to patients

It is possible for HIV infection to be transmitted from health care workers to their patients during invasive procedures, as demonstrated by the case of the Florida dentist with AIDS who was shown to have transmitted infection to five of about 1000 of his patients who were tested for HIV (Ciesielski et al 1992). The evidence suggests that the route of transmission was dentist-to-patient but the detailed means of transmission remains unclear. In contrast, there are so far no recorded cases of transmission of HIV to patients from infected health care workers in six other studies (Sacks 1985, Armstrong et al 1987, Porter et al 1990, Mishu et al 1990, Comer et al 1991, Danila et al 1991). Of the 1246 patients of these infected health care workers who were tested for HIV, one was

positive; he had other risk factors for HIV and was probably infected before the surgical procedure (Mishu et al 1990). However, it has been pointed out that this should not lead to complacency (Bird et al 1991), since all these follow-up studies were incomplete and cannot exclude the possibility of transmission to untraced patients. It is also possible that some of the few people with AIDS who have no recognized risk factors could have been infected as a result of an invasive dental or surgical procedure.

The potential for transmission of HIV from infected health care workers to patients lies in the frequency of sharps injuries during surgical and dental procedures. An observational study in the USA reported a high rate of injuries during surgical procedures and also noted that in about a third of cases the sharp instrument recontacted the patient's tissues (Tokars et al 1991). On the basis

of this, and allowing for reduction in HIV transmission because of solid needles and gloves, Bell
et al (1991) calculated that the risk of HIV transmission to a patient from an infected surgeon was
2.4–24 per million; the number of patients who
could have been infected with HIV during surgical
procedures in the USA between 1980 and 1990
was calculated as 12–129. Lowenfels and Wormser
(1991) calculated that the risk to a patient of
acquiring HIV during a 1-h procedure from an
infected surgeon was between 0.5 and 38.5 per
million. These calculated risks should be compared with the risks of anaesthetic death during
surgery (100 per million) and of acquiring HIV
infection in the USA from a transfusion of blood
screened as HIV antibody-negative (about 6.7 to
25 per million) (Ciesielski et al 1991).

In observational studies, the rate of sharps injuries to operators and the 're-entry' injury rate have
been found to be particularly high in obstetrical
and gynaecological procedures (Panlilio et al 1991,
Tokars et al 1991). Gynaecology and obstetrics are
over-represented among outbreaks of hepatitis B
infection transmitted from health care workers to
patients (Heptonstall 1991). Also by analogy with
hepatitis B transmission to patients, it is likely that
any transmission of HIV will occur in outbreaks,
with transmission rates higher than the overall calculated risks (Ciesielski et al 1991). There is
already evidence of this from the Florida dentist,
where the transmission rate seems to have been
rather high (Ciesielski et al 1992).

Prevention of HIV transmission to patients

Because there is a risk, albeit very small, of transmission of HIV from infected health care workers
to patients, official guidance in both the UK and
the USA advises that health care workers infected
with HIV should not participate in invasive procedures where there is a risk that their blood could
contact the patient's open tissues (UK Health
Departments 1991, Centers for Disease Control
1991b). The UK guidance defines invasive procedures as 'surgical entry into tissues, cavities or
organs or repair of major traumatic injuries,
cardiac catheterisation and angiography, vaginal or
caesarian deliveries or other obstetric procedures
during which bleeding may occur; the manipu-

lation, cutting or removal of any oral or perioral
tissues including tooth structure, during which
bleeding may occur'. Normal vaginal delivery itself
is not considered an invasive procedure unless a
surgical procedure is required during or after delivery. It is therefore recommended that an HIV-
infected health care worker should undertake
vaginal delivery only if other staff are available to
carry out any surgical procedure.

Screening of health care workers is not recommended in official guidance (UK Health
Departments 1991, Centers for Disease Control
1991b) and this stance has been justified by a
number of other authors (Royal College of Pathologists Working Group 1992, Joint Working Party
of the Hospital Infection Society and the Surgical
Infection Study Group 1992, Cockcroft 1992).
However, a substantial proportion of medical students and consultants (including surgeons) were
in favour of compulsory HIV testing of surgeons
in the study reported by Elford and Cockcroft
(1991). Health care workers are reminded that
they have an ethical duty to seek testing and confidential advice if they believe themselves to be at
risk of being infected with HIV and to act on that
advice (UK Health Departments 1991). It has
been pointed out that the penalties for a health
care worker in an invasive speciality of revealing
their HIV status may act as a disincentive to testing
(Cockcroft 1992); paradoxically, this could result
in a larger number of surgeons who are actually
HIV-infected continuing to operate. The effect of
the guidelines in practice needs to be monitored.
The treatment seen to be received by health care
workers who declare themselves HIV-infected, in
terms of what redeployment and protection of
income is offered, will be important in determining
whether others come forward.

The most important means of protecting
patients from HIV-infected health care workers is
the same as that for protecting health care workers
from infected patients: safe practice and particularly avoidance of sharps injuries. The specialities with high rates of injuries put both staff and
patients at risk; gynaecology and obstetrics feature
within this group. A further argument in favour of
adopting universal precautions, with a high level
of care to avoid sharps injuries for all patients, is
that this can reassure patients who are not infected

with HIV (or in a 'high risk' category) that they are being protected from possible infection in their carers.

REFERENCES

Advisory Committee on Dangerous Pathogens 1990 HIV – the causative agent of AIDS and related conditions: second revision of guidelines. HMSO, London

Anonymous 1984 Needlestick transmission of HTLV-III from a patient infected in Africa. Lancet 2: 1376–1377

Armstrong F P, Minor J C, Wolfe W H 1987 Investigation of a health care worker with symptomatic human immunodeficiency virus infection: an epidemiologic approach. Milit Med 152: 414–418

Astbury C, Baxter P J 1990 Infection risks in hospital staff from blood: hazardous injury rates and acceptance of hepatitis B immunization. J Soc Occup Med 40: 92–93

Banatvala J E, Chrystie I L, Palmer S J 1991 HIV screening in pregnancy. Lancet 337: 1218

Baraff L J, Talan D A 1989 Compliance with universal precautions in a university hospital emergency department. Ann Emerg Med 18: 654–657

Bell D M, Martone W J, Cuiver D H et al 1991 Risk of endemic HIV and hepatitis B virus (HBV) transmission to patients during invasive procedures. Proceedings of seventh International Conference on AIDS, Florence 16–21 June 1991: 37

Bird A G, Gore S M, Leigh-Brown A J et al 1991 Escape from collective denial: HIV transmission during surgery. Br Med J 303: 351–352

British Orthopaedic Association 1991 Guidelines for the prevention of cross-infection between patients and staff in orthopaedic operating theatres with special reference to HIV and the blood-borne hepatitis viruses. British Orthopaedic Association, London

Brough S J, Hunt T M, Barrie W W 1988 Surgical glove perforations. Br J Surg 75: 317

Brown E M, Caul E O, Roome A P C G et al 1991 Zidovudine after occupational exposure to HIV. Br Med J 303: 990

Camilleri A E, Murray S, Imrie C W 1991 Needlestick injuries in surgeons: what is the incidence? J Roy Coll Surg Edin 36: 317–318

Centers for Disease Control 1985 Recommendations for protection against viral hepatitis. Morbid Mortal Weekly Rep 34: 313–324, 329–335

Centers for Disease Control 1987a Update: human immunodeficiency virus infections in health care workers exposed to blood of infected patients. MMWR 36: 285–289

Centers for Disease Control 1987b Recommendations for prevention of HIV transmission in health-care settings. MMWR 36 (Suppl 2S): 1–18

Centers for Disease Control 1988 Update: universal precautions for prevention of transmission of human immunodeficiency virus, hepatitis B virus and other blood borne pathogens in health care settings. MMWR 37: 377–388

Centers for Disease Control 1989 Guidelines for prevention of transmission of human immunodeficiency virus and hepatitis B virus to health-care and public-safety workers. MMWR 38: S-6

Centers for Disease Control 1990 Public health service statement on management of occupational exposure to human immunodeficiency virus, including considerations regarding zidovudine post exposure. MMWR 39: RR-1

Centers for Disease Control 1991a Preliminary analysis: HIV serosurvey of orthopedic surgeons, 1991. MMWR 40: 309–312

Centers for Disease Control 1991b Recommendations for preventing transmission of human immunodeficiency virus and hepatitis B virus to patients during exposure-prone invasive procedures. MMWR 40: 1–9

Centers for Disease Control 1992 Surveillance for occupationally acquired HIV infection – United States, 1981–1992. MMWR 41: 823–825

Chamberlain G, Booth J, Omisakin K et al 1991 HIV screening in pregnancy. Lancet 337: 1219

Chamberland M E, Conely L J, Bush T J et al 1991 Health care workers with AIDS. JAMA 266: 3459–3462

Ciesielski C, Bell D M, Marianos D W 1991 Transmission of HIV from infected health care workers to patients. AIDS 5: S93–97

Ciesielski C, Marianos D, Ou C-Y et al 1992 Transmission of human immunodeficiency virus in a dental practice. Ann Intern Med 116: 798–805

Cockcroft A 1992 Compulsory HIV testing for surgeons? Br J Hosp Med 47: 602–604

Collins C H, Kennedy D A 1987 Microbiological hazards of occupational needlestick and 'sharps' injuries. J Appl Bacteriol 62: 385–402

Comer R W, Myers D R, Steadman C D et al 1991 Management considerations for an HIV positive dental student. J Dent Educ 55: 187–191

Consumers' Association 1991 Zidovudine in HIV infection. Drug Ther Bull 29: 81–82

Danila R N, Mackonald K L, Rhame F S et al 1991 A look-back investigation of patients of an HIV-infected physician. N Engl J Med 325: 1406–1411

Darond D E, Le-Jeunne C, Hugues F C 1991 Failure of prophylactic zidovudine after a suicidal self-inoculation of HIV infected blood. N Engl J Med 323: 1062

Dobson P 1992 Diary of a needlestick injury. Br Med J 305: 1372

Doyle P M, Alvi S, Johanson R 1992 The effectiveness of double-gloving in obstetrics and gynaecology. Br J Obstet Gynaecol 99: 83–84

Elford J, Cockcroft A 1991 Compulsory HIV antibody testing, universal precautions and the perceived risk of HIV: a survey among medical students and consultant staff at a London teaching hospital. AIDS Care 3: 151–158

Fahey B J, Koziol D E, Banks S M et al 1991 Frequency of nonparenteral occupational exposures to blood and body fluids before and after universal precautions training. Am J Med 90: 145–153

Gallop R M, Lancee W J, Taerk G et al 1992 Fear of contagion and AIDS: nurses' perception of risk. AIDS Care 4: 103–109

Gerberding J L, Littell C, Tarkington A et al 1990 Risk of exposure of surgical personnel to patients' blood during surgery at San Francisco General Hospital. N Engl J Med 322: 1788–1793

Gerberding J L, Henderson D K 1992 Management of occupational exposures to bloodborne pathogens: hepatitis B virus, hepatitis C virus and human immunodeficiency virus. Clin Infect Dis 14: 1179–1185

Gioannini P, Sinicco A, Cariti G et al 1988 HIV infection acquired by a nurse Eur J Epidemiol 4: 119–120

Gordin F M, Gibert C, Harold H P et al 1990 Prevalence of human immunodeficiency virus and hepatitis B virus in unselected hospital admissions: implications for mandatory testing and universal precautions. J Infect Dis 161: 14–17

Hansen J P, Falconer J A, Hamilton J D et al 1981 Hepatitis B in a medical center. J Occup Med 23: 338–342

Health and Safety Commission 1988 The control of substances hazardous to health regulations 1988: approved code of practice. HMSO, London

Health Services Advisory Committee 1991 Safety in health service laboratories: safe working and the prevention of infection in clinical laboratories. HMSO, London

Heptonstall J 1991 Outbreaks of hepatitis B virus infection associated with infected surgical staff. Communicable Disease Report 1: R81–85

Hussain S A, Latif A B A, Choudhary A A A A 1988 Risk to surgeons: a survey of accidental injuries during operations. Br J Surg 75: 314–316

Jeffries D J 1991 Zidovudine after occupational exposure to HIV. Br Med J 302: 1349–1351

Johnson G K, Robinson W S 1990 Human immunodeficiency virus-1 (HIV-1) in the vapors of surgical power instruments. J Med Virol 33: 47–56

Joint Working Party of the Hospital Infection Society and the Surgical Infection Study Group 1992 Risks to surgeons and patients from HIV and hepatitis: guidelines on precautions and management of exposure to blood or body fluids. Br Med J 305: 1337–1343

Jones P D 1991 HIV transmission by stabbing in spite of zidovudine prophylaxis. Lancet 338: 884

Kabukoba J, Young P 1992 Midwifery and body fluid contamination. Br Med J 305: 226

Kelen G D, DiGiovanni T A, Celentano D D et al 1990 Adherence to universal (barrier) precautions during interventions on critically ill and injured emergency department patients. J AIDS 3: 987–994

Klein R S, Phelan J A, Freeman K et al 1988 Low occupational risk of HIV infection among dental professionals. N Engl J Med 318: 86–90

Lange J M A, Boucher C A B, Hollak C E M et al 1990 Failure of zidovudine prophylaxis after accidental exposure to HIV-1. N Engl J Med 322: 1375–1377

Leentvaar-Kuijpers A, Dekker M M, Coutinho R A et al 1990 Needlestick injuries, surgeons and HIV risks. Lancet 1: 546–547

Littlechild P, Macmillan A, White M M, Steedman D 1992 Contamination of skin and clothing of accident and emergency personnel. Br Med J 305: 156–157

Looke D F M, Grove D I 1990 Failed prophylactic zidovudine after a needlestick injury. Lancet 335: 1280

Lot F, Laporte A, Bouvet E et al 1991 Differences between health care workers with AIDS and AIDS patients? Seventh International Conference on AIDS, Florence 1991: Abstr WD 4152

Lowenfels A B, Wormser G P, Jain R 1989 Frequency of puncture injuries in surgeons and estimated risk of HIV infection. Arch Surg 124: 1284–1286

Lowenfels A B, Wormser G P 1991 Risk of transmission of HIV from surgeon to patient. N Engl J Med 325: 888–889

McGeer A, Sinor A E, Low D E 1990 Epidemiology of needlestick injuries in house officers. J Infect Dis 162: 961–964

McKinnon M D, Williams S, Snashall D C et al 1992 A study of the detailed circumstances of 'sharps' injuries in health care workers. J Occup Med 34: 974–975

Matta H, Thompson A M, Rainey J B 1988 Does wearing two pairs of gloves protect operating theatre staff from skin contamination? Br Med J 297: 597–598

Miller P J, Farr B M 1989 A study of the rate of postexposure human immunodeficiency virus testing in a hospital requiring written informed consent. J Occup Med 31: 524–527

Mishu B, Schaffner W, Horan J M et al 1990 A surgeon with AIDS: lack of evidence of transmission to patients. JAMA 264: 467–470

N'Galy B, Ryder R W, Bila K et al 1990 HIV infection among employees in an African hospital. N Engl J Med 319: 1123–1127

Oakley K, Gooch C, Cockcroft A 1992 Review of incidents involving exposure to blood in a London teaching hospital, 1989–91. Br Med J 304: 949–951

Panlilio A L, Foy D R, Edwards J R et al 1991 Blood contacts during surgical procedures. JAMA 265: 1533–1537

Parry C M, Harries A D, Beeching N J et al 1991 Phlebotomy in inoculation risk patients: a questionnaire survey of knowledge and practices of hospital doctors in Liverpool. J Hosp Infect 18: 313–318

Porter J D, Cruickshank J G, Gentle P H et al 1990 Management of patients treated by a surgeon with HIV infection. Lancet 335: 113–114

Porter K, Heptonstall J, Gill O N 1992 Summary of published reports of occupational transmission of HIV to October 1992. Internal publication of Public Health Laboratory Service, Colindale, London

Royal College of Obstetricians and Gynaecologists 1990 HIV infection in maternity care and gynaecology. Royal College of Obstetricians and Gynaecologists, London

Royal College of Pathologists Working Group 1992 HIV infection: hazards of transmission to patients and health care workers during invasive procedures. Royal College of Pathologists, London

Royal College of Surgeons of England 1990 A statement by the college on AIDS and HIV infection. Royal College of Surgeons of England, London

Ruprecht R M, O'Brien L G, Rossoni L D et al 1986 Suppression of mouse viraemia and retroviral disease by 3'-azido-3'-deoxythymidine. Nature (London) 323: 467–469

Sacks J J 1985 AIDS in a surgeon. N Engl J Med 313: 1017–1018

Shanson D C, Cockcroft A 1991 Forum: testing patients for HIV antibodies is useful for infection control purposes. Rev Med Virol 1: 5–9

Shelley G A, Howard R J 1992 A national survey of surgeons' attitudes about patients with human immunodeficiency virus infections and acquired immune deficiency syndrome. Arch Surg 127: 206–212

Tait D R, Pudifin D J, Gathiram V et al 1991 Zidovudine after occupational exposure to HIV. Br Med J 303: 581

Tamin J, Menzies D, Gilbert D et al 1991 Zidovudine after occupational exposure to HIV. Br Med J 303: 581

Tavares L, Roneker C, Johnston K et al 1987 3'-azido-3'-deoxythymidine in feline leukemia virus-infected cats: a model for therapy and prophylaxis of AIDS. Cancer Res 47: 3190–3194

Tokars J, Bell D, Marcus R et al 1991 Percutaneous injuries during surgical procedures. Proceedings of the VII International Conference on AIDS, Vol 2, Florence, Italy, p 83

UK Health Departments 1990 Guidance for clinical health care workers: protection against infection with HIV and hepatitis viruses. HMSO, London

UK Health Departments 1991 AIDS – HIV infected health care workers. Recommendations of the expert advisory group on AIDS. Department of Health, London

UK Health Departments 1992 Occupational exposure to HIV and use of zidovudine. A statement from the expert advisory group on AIDS. Department of Health, London

Williams S, Gooch C, Cockcroft A 1993 Hepatitis B immunisation and blood exposure incidents among operating department staff. Br J Surg (in press)

Index